The SAGES Manual

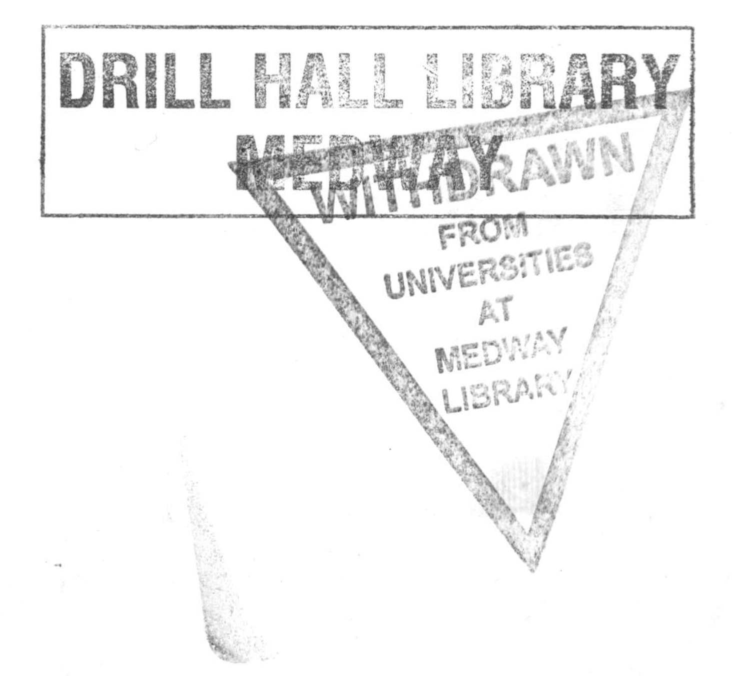

The SAGES Manual

Perioperative Care in Minimally Invasive Surgery

Richard L. Whelan, MD

Department of Surgery, Chief, Section of Colon and Rectal Surgery, New York-Presbyterian Hospital, College of Physicians and Surgeons, Columbia University, New York, New York

Editor

James W. Fleshman Jr., MD

Chief, Section of Colon and Rectal Surgery, Professor of Surgery, Division of General Surgery, Washington University School of Medicine; Co-Director, GI Center, Clinical Operations, Barnes-Jewish Hospital, St Louis, Missouri

Dennis L. Fowler, MD

New York-Presbyterian Hospital, College of Physicians and Surgeons, Columbia University, Weill Medical College of Cornell University, New York, New York

Associate Editors

With 106 Figures

Illustrations by Vaune Hatch

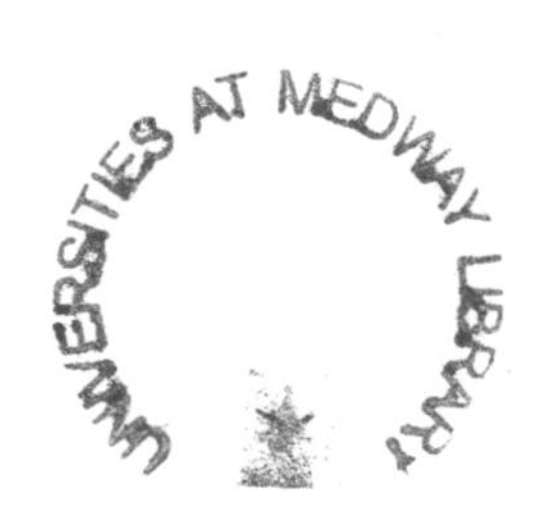

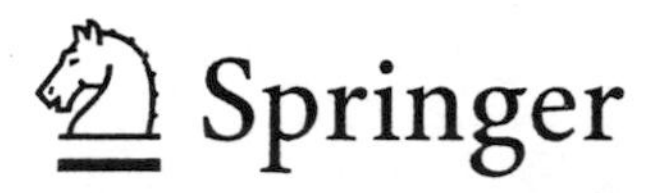

Richard L. Whelan, MD
Department of Surgery
Chief, Section of Colon and Rectal Surgery
New York-Presbyterian Hospital
College of Physicians and Surgeons
Columbia University
New York, NY 10032
USA

Dennis L. Fowler, MD
New York-Presbyterian Hospital
College of Physicians and Surgeons
Columbia University
Weill Medical College of Cornell University
New York, NY 10021
USA

James W. Fleshman Jr., MD
Chief, Section of Colon and Rectal Surgery
Professor of Surgery
Division of General Surgery
Washington University School of Medicine
and
Co-Director, GI Center
Clinical Operations
Barnes-Jewish Hospital
St Louis, MO 63110
USA

Library of Congress Control Number: 2004058965

ISBN-10: 0-387-23686-4 Printed on acid-free paper.
ISBN-13: 978-0387-23686-5

Printed in the United States of America. (BS/EB)

9 8 7 6 5 4 3 2 1 SPIN 10952139

Springer is a part of Springer Science+Business Media
springeronline.com

This manual is dedicated to the next generation of surgeons who have so enthusiastically embraced minimally invasive methods and who will further develop and refine these techniques in the years to come.

Preface

The second SAGES (Society of American Gastrointestinal Endoscopic Surgeons) manual was intended to be a companion piece for the successful first SAGES manual, edited by Carol Scott-Connor, that was published more than 4 years ago. Originally, the goal was to concentrate on tersely covered or often ignored aspects of the preoperative preparation of the patient and the operating room as well as the postoperative care of patients undergoing minimally invasive operations. It was also our intention to include a section for each procedure where several different port placement schemes would be presented and briefly discussed. Unique to this manual, the impact of the patient's body habitus (short or long, narrow or wide) on port placement is also taken into account for many of the procedures. Also unique are chapters devoted to hypothermia, port wound closure, and the management of subcutaneous emphysema and abdominal wall hemorrhage caused by trocars.

Naturally, the surgeon tends to focus on the technical aspects of the procedure, such as the operative tasks to be carried out, the order of operation, and the position of the surgeon and assistant. However, it is critical that the surgeon be aware that the CO_2 pneumoperitoneum, far more so than laparotomy, results in multiple physiologic alterations that, if not compensated for by the anesthesiologist and surgeon, may endanger the patient or prevent the laparoscopic completion of the procedure. Although most laparoscopic texts, at best, have a chapter or two on CO_2 pneumoperitoneum, a whole section of this manual has been dedicated to discussion of the physiologic ramifications of this exposure method. A well-informed surgeon is better able to work with the anesthesiologist to limit or prevent deleterious physiologic changes. It has also become clear that open and closed abdominal surgery cause immunosuppression and may have oncologic implications for the patient. The issue of port wound tumors has loomed large on the surgical landscape for more than a decade. This manual contains chapters that review the literature in these areas and will, hopefully, prove useful to readers.

The intended audience for this manual are general surgeons in training as well as already trained surgeons who are facing the often daunting task of learning how to perform advanced laparoscopic procedures. It is hoped that this manual will prove useful as a quick "lockerroom" reference for residents with limited experience heading into advanced cases in regard to setting up the operating room, positioning the patient, and selecting the port locations. On another level, we hope that this manual will also be a resource for surgeons interested in developing a thorough and well-thought-out approach to the pre- and postoperative management of minimally invasive patients or to learn more about CO_2 pneumoperitoneum and its implications.

The generation of this manual has involved hundreds of people who generously gave of their time. Although it is impossible to thank each person, I would be remiss if I did not acknowledge a number of people who were critical to the project. First, I am indebted to my co-editors, James W. Fleshman and Dennis L. Fowler, for their Herculean efforts; without them this manual could not have been completed. Their expertise both surgical and literary is greatly appreciated.

There would be no manual if not for the efforts of the expert surgeons who took the time from their busy schedules to write the chapters. Vaune Hatch, the talented artist who did all the drawings and figures for the manual, deserves a special accolade. Without complaint she made countless modifications to the figures until all were satisfied.

Finally thanks go to the SAGES Board of Governors and the Publication Committee, who entrusted this task to me. I am proud not only to have been given this responsibility but also to be part of an organization such as SAGES, which has broken much new ground over the past two decades and has consistently provided leadership and direction during a period of tremendous change in the surgical world. The SAGES family has been patient, helpful, and supportive during the entire, longer than expected, process. It has been an honor to take part in this project and to see it through to its completion.

Richard L. Whelan, MD
New York, NY
August 14, 2004

Contents

Part I: Perioperative Management and Evaluation

Part II: Intraoperative Management, Positioning, Setup, and Port Placement

Part III: Postoperative Management of the Laparoscopic Patient

Part IV: Physiologic Implications of CO_2 Pneumoperitoneum and Minimally Invasive Methods

Contributors

Arif Ahmad, MBBS, FRCS, Director of the Center for Minimally Invasive Surgery, Health Science Services, Division of General Surgery, Stonybrook University Hospital, Stony Brook, NY 11794, USA

Parswa Ansari, MD, Resident, Minimal Access Surgery Center, Department of Surgery, New York-Presbyterian Hospital, College of Physicians and Surgeons, Columbia University, New York, NY 10032, USA

Chandrakanth Are, MD, FRCS, Surgery Courtesy Staff, Bayview Medical Center, The Johns Hopkins Medical Institutions, Bayview Campus, Baltimore, MD 21224, USA

Tracey D. Arnell, MD, Assistant Professor of Surgery, Columbia University College of Physicians and Surgeons, New York-Presbyterian Hospital, New York, NY 10032, USA

Maurice E. Arregui, MD, FACS, Department of General Surgery, St. Vincent's Hospital and Healthcare Center, Indianapolis, IN 46260, USA

Robert W. Beart Jr., MD, Department of Surgery (Division of Colorectal Surgery), Keck School of Medicine, University of Southern California, Los Angeles, CA 90033, USA

James M. Becker, MD, Division of Surgery, Boston University Medical Center, Boston, MA 02118, USA

George Berci, MD, FACS, FRCS, ED (Hon), Department of Surgery, Cedars-Sinai Medical Center, Los Angeles, CA 90048, USA

Ramon Berguer, MD, Department of Surgery, University of California Davis, Martinez, CA 94553, USA

Marc Bessler, MD, Director of Laparoscopic Surgery, Assistant Attending Surgeon, New York-Presbyterian Hospital; Assistant Professor of Surgery, Columbia University College of Physicians and Surgeons, New York, NY 10032, USA

Thomas R. Biehl, MD, Department of Surgery, Virginia Mason Medical Center, Seattle, WA 98111, USA

Desmond H. Birkett, MD, Department of General Surgery, Lahey Clinic Medical Center, Burlington, MA 01805, USA

Dennis Blom, MD, Professor of Surgery, Department of Surgery, University of California, Los Angeles, CA 91024, USA

H. Jaap Bonjer, MD, University Hospital Rotterdam-Dijkzigt, Dr. Molewaterplein 40, NL-3015 GD Rotterdam, The Netherlands

Catherine Boulay, MD, Department of Surgery, Minimal Access Surgery Center, College of Physicians and Surgeons, New York-Presbyterian Hospital, Columbia University, New York, NY 10032, USA

Steven P. Bowers, MD, Department of Surgery, Emory University School of Medicine, Atlanta, GA 30322, USA

C. Braumann, MD, Department of General, Visceral, Vascular and Thoracic Surgery, Humboldt University of Berlin, Charité, D-10098 Berlin, Germany

Robert N. Cacchione, MD, Department of Surgery, University of Louisville, Louisville, KY 40292, USA

Mark P. Callery, MD, University of Massachusetts Medical Center, Worchester, MA 01655, USA

Charles Cappandona, MD, Fellow, New York Presbyterian Hospital, New York, NY 10032, USA

Joseph Carter, MD, 142 Whitman Avenue, West Gartford, CT 06107, USA

Frank H. Chae, MD, Assistant Professor of Surgery, Advanced Minimally Invasive Surgery, University of Colorado Hospital, Denver, CO 80262, USA

Jeffrey L. Cohen, MD, Department of Surgery, Connecticut Surgical Group, University of Connecticut, Hartford, CT 06106, USA

Patrick Colquhoun, MD, Department of Colorectal Surgery, Cleveland Clinic Florida, Weston, FL 33331, USA

John M. Cosgrove, MD, Chief of Surgery, Department of General Surgery, North Shore University Hospital at Forest Hills, Forest Hills, NY 11375, USA

Jorge Cueto-Garcia, MD, Cowdray Hospital and Hospital Angeles Lomas, Mexico City, Lomas Virreyes, Mexico City, DF 11000, Mexico

Karen E. Deveney, MD, Professor of Surgery, Department of Surgery, Oregon Health and Science University, Portland, OR 97239, USA

Daniel J. Deziel, MD, Senior Attending Surgeon, Professor of Surgery, Rush Medical College, Rush Presbyterian St. Luke's Medical Center, Chicago, IL 60612, USA

Michael Edye, MD, Department of Surgery, Division of Minimally Invasive Surgery, New York University School of Medicine, New York, NY 10016, USA

Daniel L. Feingold, MD, Assistant Professor of Surgery, Department of Surgery, Columbia University College of Physicians and Surgeons; New York-Presbyterian Hospital, Department of Surgery, New York, NY 10032, USA

Alessandro Fichera, MD, Assistant Professor, Biological Sciences Division, University of Chicago Medical Center; Department of Surgery, Section of General Surgery, Bernard Mitchell Hospital, Chicago, IL 60637, USA

James W. Fleshman Jr., MD, Chief, Section of Colon and Rectal Surgery, Professor of Surgery, Division of General Surgery, Washington University School of Medicine; Co-Director, GI Center, Clinical Operations, Barnes-Jewish Hospital, St Louis, MO 63110, USA

Dennis L. Fowler, MD, New York-Presbyterian Hospital, College of Physicians and Surgeons, Columbia University, Weill Medical College of Cornell University, New York, NY 10021, USA

Morris E. Franklin, MD, Clinical Professor of Surgery, University of Texas Health Science Center at San Antonio; Director, Texas Endosurgery Institute, San Antonio, TX 78222, USA

Matthew S. French, MD, Surgical Specialists of Louisiana, New Orleans, LA 70115, USA

A. Brent Fruin, MD, Division of Surgery, Boston University Medical Center, Boston, MA 02118, USA

Ali M. Ghellai, MD, Division of Surgery, Boston University Medical Center, Boston, MA 02118, USA

William Gourash, MSN, CRNP, Nurse Practitioner, Clinical and Research Associate, Department of Minimally Invasive Surgery, University of Pittsburgh Medical Center, Pittsburgh, PA 15213, USA

Frederick L. Greene, MD, Department of Surgery, Carolinas Medical Center, Charlotte, NC 28203, USA

Carsten N. Gutt, MD, Department of Surgery, University of Heidelberg, 69120 Heidelberg, Germany

Valerie J. Halpin, MD, Department of Surgery and Institue for Minimally Invasive Surgery, Washington University School of Medicine, St. Louis, MO 63110, USA

Giselle G. Hamad, MD, Assistant Professor of Surgery, University of Pittsburgh School of Medicine, Medical Director of MIS/Bariatrics, Magee-Womens Hospital of University of Pittsburgh Medical Center, Pittsburgh, PA 15213, USA

Eric J. Hazebroek, MD, University Hospital Rotterdam-Dijkzigt, Dr. Molewaterplein 40, NL-3015 D Rotterdam, The Netherlands

Christopher Heinbuch, MD, Department of General and Visceral Surgery, Ruprechts-Karls-University, Heidelberg, Germany

Stanley C. Hewlett, MD, Department of Surgery, University of Louisville School of Medicine, Louisville, KY 40202, USA

James H. Holmes IV, MD, Department of Surgery, Virginia Mason Medical Center, Seattle, WA 98111, USA

Karen D. Horvath IV, MD, Department of Surgery, University of Washington, Seattle, WA 98195, USA

John G. Hunter, MD, FACS, Department of Surgery, Emory University Hospital, Atlanta, GA 30322, USA

Sayeed Ikramuddin, MD, Department of Surgery, University of Pittsburgh Medical Center Presbyterian Hospital, Pittsburgh, PA 15213, USA

Christopher A. Jacobi, MD, PhD, Department of Surgery, Humboldt University of Berlin, Charité, D-10098 Berlin, Germany

Daniel B. Jones, MD, FACS, Chief, Minimally Invasive Surgery, Beth Israel Deaconess Medical Center, Visiting Associate Professor, Harvard Medical School, Boston, MA 02115, USA

Stephanie B. Jones, MD, Associate Professor, Department of Anesthesiology and Pain Management, University of Texas Southwestern Medical Center, Dallas, TX 75390, USA

Namir Katkhouda, MD, FACS, Department of Surgery, University of South California, Los Angeles, CA 90033, USA

Ayal M. Kaynan, MD, Fellow, Endourology and Laparoscopic Surgery, Stanford University School of Medicine, Stanford, CA 94305, USA

William E. Kelley Jr., MD, Richmond Surgical Group, Henrico Doctors' Hospital, Richmond, VA 23294, USA

Gerald M. Larson, MD, Department of Surgery, University of Louisville, Louisville, KY 40292, USA

Sang W. Lee, MD, Clinical Instructor, Department of Surgery, Section of Colon and Rectal Surgery, New York Presbyterian Hospital, Weill Medical College of Cornell University, New York, NY 10021, USA

John I. Lew, MD, Instructor in Clinical Surgery, Department of Surgery, Columbia University College of Physicians and Surgeons; New York-Presbyterian Hospital, Department of Minimal Access Surgery, New York, NY 10032, USA

Hans Lippert, MD, Otto-von-Guericke University of Medicine, 39120 Magdeburg, Germany

Kirk A. Ludwig, MD, Department of Surgery, Chief, Section of Gastrointestinal Surgery, Director, Anorectal Physiology Laboratory, Duke University Medical Center, Durham, NC 27710, USA

James D. Luketich, MD, Professor of Surgery, Department of Thoracic Surgery, University of Pittsburgh School of Medicine; Chief, Division of Thoracic and Foregut Surgery, University of Pittsburgh Medical Center Presbyterian Hospital, Pittsburgh, PA 15213, USA

Bruce V. MacFadyen Jr., MD, Professor, Department of Surgery, Medical College of Georgia, Augusta, GA 30912, USA

Sharan Manhas, MD, Department of Surgery, Minimally Invasive Surgery Program, Keck School of Medicine, University of Southern California, Los Angeles, CA 90033, USA

Peter Marcello, MD, Department of Colon and Rectal Surgery, Lahey Clinic, Burlington, MA 01805, USA

Samer G. Mattar, MD, Assistant Professor of Surgery, Mark Ravitch/Leon C. Hirsch Center for Minimally Invasive Surgery, University of Pittsburgh Medical Center Health System; Surgical Weight Loss Program, Magee-Womens Hospital of University of Pittsburgh Medical Center, Pittsburgh, PA 15213, USA

Keith P. Meslin, MD, Department of Surgery, Long Island Jewish Medical Center, New Hyde Park, NY 11040, USA

Jeffrey W. Milsom, MD, Cornell New York Presbyterian Hospital, New York, NY 10021, USA

Gamal Mostafa, MD, Department of Surgery, Carolinas Medical Center, Charlotte, NC 28203, USA

Heidi Nelson, MD, Mayo Clinic, Mayo Foundation, Division of Colon and Rectal Surgery, Rochester, MN 55905, USA

Dmitry Oleynikov, MD, Department of Surgery, University of Washington, Seattle, WA 98195, USA

James A. Olson, MD, Department of Surgery (Division of Colorectal Surgery), Keck School of Medicine, University of Southern California, Los Angeles, CA 90033, USA

Yaron Perry, MD, Division of Thoracic and Foregut Surgery, University of Pittsburgh Medical Center Presbyterian Hospital, Pittsburgh, PA 15213, USA

Joseph B. Petelin, MD, FACS, Department of Surgery, University of Kansas School of Medicine, Kansas City, KS 66160, USA

Jeffrey H. Peters, MD, Professor of Surgery, Department of Surgery, University of California, Los Angeles, CA 91024, USA

Edward H. Phillips, MD, Department of General Surgery, Cedars-Sinai Medical Center, Los Angeles, CA 90048, USA

Michael W. Potter, MD, Department of Surgery, University of Massachusetts Medical School, Worcester, MA 01655, USA

Marc A. Reymond, MD, Associate Professor of Surgery, Otto-von-Guericke University of Medicine; Department of Surgery, University Hospital, 39120 Magdeburg, Germany

Philip R. Schauer, MD, Staff Director, Bariatric Surgery Program, Department of General Surgery, Cleveland Clinic, Cleveland, OH 44195, USA

Bruce D. Schirmer, MD, Department of Surgery, University of Virginia Health System, Charlottesville, VA 22908, USA

Carol E.H. Scott-Conner, MD, Professor of Surgery, Department of Anatomy and Cell Biology, Roy J. and Lucille A. Carver College of Medicine, University of Iowa, Iowa City, IA 52242, USA

Shimul A. Shah, MD, Department of Surgery, Medical School, Harvard University, Boston, MA 02115, USA

C. Daniel Smith, MD, Chief, General and Gastrointestinal Surgery, Department of Surgery, Emory University School of Medicine, Atlanta, GA 30322, USA

Nathaniel J. Soper, MD, Department of Surgery and Institute for Minimally Invasive Surgery, Washington University School of Medicine, St. Louis, MO 63110, USA

Greg V. Stiegmann, MD, Division of Gastrointestinal Tumor and Endocrine Surgery, University of Colorado Health Sciences Center, Denver, CO 80262, USA

Arthur F. Stucchi, PhD, Division of Surgery, Boston University Medical Center, Boston, MA 02118, USA

Joseph F. Sucher, MD, Department of General Surgery/Surgical Critical Care, Clinical Fellow, University of Texas Medical School at Houston, Houston, TX 77225, USA

Lee L. Swanström, MD, Clinical Professor of Surgery, Director, Oregon Health and Science University; Department of Minimally Invasive Surgery, Legacy Health System, Portland, OR 97210, USA

Robert Talac, MD, PhD, Fellow, Division of Colon and Rectal Surgery, Mayo Clinic, Rochester, MN 55905, USA

Mark A. Talamini, MD, Associate Professor of Surgery and Director of Minimally Invasive Surgery, The Johns Hopkins University School of Medicine; Attending Surgeon, The Johns Hopkins Hospital, Baltimore, MD 21287, USA

David S. Thoman, MD, 8635 W. 3rd Street, Suite 795W, Los Angeles, CA 90048, USA

José Antonio Vazquez-Frias, MD, Departments of Surgery of The American British, Cowdray Hospital and Hospital Angeles Lomas, 01120, Mexico City, Mexico

Gary C. Vitale, MD, Department of Surgery, University of Louisville, Louisville, KY 40202, USA

David I. Watson, MB, BS, MD, FRACS, Department of Surgery, Royal Adelaide Hospital, University of Adelaide, North Terrace Adelaide, South Australia, 5000 Australia

Steven D. Wexner, MD, Chairman, Department of Colorectal Surgery, Cleveland Clinic Florida, Weston, FL 33331, USA

Richard L. Whelan, MD, Department of Surgery, Chief, Section of Colon and Rectal Surgery, New York-Presbyterian Hospital, College of Physicians and Surgeons, Columbia University, New York, NY 10032, USA

Sherry M. Wren, MD, General Surgery, VA Palo Alto Health Care System Surgical Services, Palo Alto, CA 94304, USA

Tonia M. Young-Fadok, MD, FACS, Mayo Clinic, Division of Colon and Rectal Surgery, Scottsdale, AZ 85259, USA

Part I
Perioperative Management and Evaluation

1. Preoperative Evaluation of the Healthy Laparoscopic Patient

Stephanie B. Jones, M.D.
Daniel B. Jones, M.D., F.A.C.S.

A. General Considerations

1. **The goal** of preoperative evaluation is to identify and modify risk factors that might adversely effect anesthetic care and surgical outcome.
2. **Up to 50% of patients presenting for elective surgery are regarded as "healthy."** These patients typically fall into American Society of Anesthesiologists (ASA) Physical Status I (healthy) and II (mild systemic disease). The ASA Physical Status classification (Table 1.1) is not intended to predict outcomes, nor does it incorporate risks specific to the type of surgery performed.
3. **A patient presenting without established medical diagnoses is not necessarily healthy.** He or she simply may have never previously visited a physician. Consequently, any physician visit, including preoperative evaluation, should be used as an opportunity to address routine preventive care (Table 1.2).
4. Preoperative evaluation should seek to determine absolute contraindications to laparoscopy.
   a. Inability to tolerate pneumoperitoneum
   b. Poor risk for general anesthesia
   c. Uncorrectable coagulopathy
5. The emphasis over the past decade has been a return to the use of the history and physical examination as the primary screening tools. Preoperative testing is used selectively. This approach is especially true in healthy patients.

B. History

1. **History of pulmonary disease.** Does the patient have decreased pulmonary compliance, due to obesity, scoliosis, or other restrictive lung disease? This factor may result in prohibitively high peak airway pressures after abdominal insufflation or difficulty with oxygenation. Obstructive diseases, such as asthma or chronic obstructive pulmonary

Table 1.1. American Society of Anesthesiologists Physical Status Scale.

Category	Description
I	Healthy patient
II	Mild systemic disease without functional limitation
III	Moderate to severe systemic disease with functional limitation
IV	Severe systemic disease that is a constant threat to life
V	Moribund patient unlikely to survive 24 hours with or without operation

disease, may cause inadequate gas exchange and accumulation of insufflated carbon dioxide.

2. **History of cardiac disease.** Even mild chronic hypertension can result in relative hypovolemia and possibly hypotension with pneumoperitoneum, especially at insufflation pressures greater than 15 mmHg. Carbon dioxide is a sympathetic stimulant, and may cause tachycardia or tachydysrhythmias, particularly when combined with surgical stimulation. Tachycardia may uncover otherwise asymptomatic coronary artery disease. The most significant risk to the patient is undetected aortic stenosis in the setting of potential hypotension. Any history of a murmur should be evaluated.
3. **Risk of pregnancy.** Although pregnancy may not preclude surgical treatment, port site position may need to be changed. If possible, surgery should be performed after the first trimester.
4. **History of previous abdominal operations.** An alternate port site, away from surgical scars, allows the surgeon to examine the abdominal cavity and assess the extent of adhesions.
5. **History of abnormal bleeding.** Patients should be queried regarding nosebleeds, heavy menstrual bleeding, easy bruising, or family history of bleeding disorders.

Table 1.2. Guidelines for routine preventive care.

Preventive measure	Recommended frequency
Blood pressure	Every other year in all adults
Serum cholesterol	Every 5 years for men from age 35, and women from age 45
Pap smear	At least every 3 years following onset of sexual activity
Stool for occult blood	Every year after age 40
Sigmoidoscopy	Every 3 years after age 50
Mammography ± breast exam	Every 1–2 years after age 50
Tetanus-diphtheria booster	Every 10 years
Influenza immunization	Every year after agea 65
Pneumococcal immunization	Once at age 65

6. **Difficulty with prior anesthetics.** Patients undergoing laparoscopy, especially gynecologic procedures, are at increased risk of postoperative nausea and vomiting. Aggressive antiemetic prophylaxis may be warranted, particularly for outpatients. A history of difficulty with intubation should be communicated to the anesthesiologist as well.

C. Physical Examination

1. A thorough physical examination includes assessment of the head and neck, lungs, heart, abdomen (including surgical scars), neurologic system, and vascular system. An anesthesiologist will also perform an airway evaluation.
2. Vital signs should be recorded.

D. Diagnostic Studies

1. **Diagnostic studies should be performed on a selective basis.** There are no definitive rules delineating which tests should be ordered for specific indications. The individual physician best determines this for the individual patient.
2. Test results obtained within 6 months of surgery are generally acceptable if the patient's medical history has not changed substantially. More recent tests may be required to assess a change in medical condition or therapy or to comply with the preoperative guidelines of a particular hospital or anesthesia department.
3. The impulse to routinely test every patient regardless of medical condition should be resisted. Not only is nonspecific preoperative testing expensive, it can result in morbidity when invasive testing is used to pursue false-positive results. The more tests that are ordered, the more likely a falsely abnormal result will appear.
4. Legal liability is actually greater if a test is performed but the result ignored than if it had never been done at all.
5. **Selective testing is supported by a variety of studies.**
   a. A 1985 JAMA study was one of the first to examine the question. The authors determined that 60% of the 2800 preoperative tests examined had no recognizable medical indication, and only 4 (0.2%) of the results may have been potentially significant for anesthetic or surgical management.
   b. Turnbull and Buck examined 5003 tests in 1010 otherwise healthy patients undergoing cholecystectomy. In their opinion, only 4 patients had a conceivable benefit from a preoperative screening test.
   c. Narr et al. retrospectively reviewed mostly ASA I and II patients who underwent surgery without prior laboratory studies. No

intraoperative or postoperative test was found to significantly change the surgical or medical management.

6. **Testing guidelines.** As stated previously, these are suggestions that need to be individualized for each patient.
   a. **Hemoglobin** (Hgb): Indicated if significant blood loss may be expected from the operation. Anemia may be sought in women with heavy menstrual bleeding. The lowest acceptable Hgb will vary. Otherwise healthy patients will be able to physiologically compensate for a low Hgb. This is not the case for those with limited compensatory reserve, such as patients with heart or lung disease, or the elderly.
   b. **Serum electrolytes**: Routinely check electrolytes, blood urea nitrogen (BUN), and creatinine for patients with diarrhea, renal disease, liver disease, or diabetes as well as for those receiving diuretics.
   c. **Liver function tests** are indicated for patients with known liver disease, or those undergoing planned cholecystectomy to exclude an obstructive enzyme pattern.
   d. **Coagulation profile**: While routine screening is not useful, a prothrombin time (PT) and partial thromboplastin time (PTT) should be checked in patients with a personal or family history of abnormal bleeding. These tests may also be indicated in patients with liver or renal dysfunction.
   e. **Chest X-ray** (CXR): Routine CXR is rarely helpful for abdominal laparoscopy, but should be done in patients undergoing video-assisted thoracic surgery (VATS) for baseline comparison. CXR may also be indicated in elderly patients undergoing more extensive upper abdominal surgery (e.g., laparoscopic Nissen fundoplication), or patients with recent upper respiratory infection, unstable chronic obstructive pulmonary disease (COPD), or unstable cardiac disease.
   f. **Electrocardiogram** (EKG): Coronary disease becomes more prevalent with increasing age. EKG is typically reserved for men older than 40 and women older than 50, particularly those with other risk factors such as hypertension, tobacco use, obesity, or diabetes.
   g. **Urinalysis** should be performed for urinary tract symptoms, or if a urologic procedure is planned.
   h. **Pregnancy test**: Indicated in female patients of childbearing age who have not undergone sterilization.
   i. **Human immunodeficiency virus (HIV) and hepatitis** testing is not indicated. Universal precautions should be followed in all patients.
7. The preoperative evaluation should also include **patient education.** The patient needs to know what to expect with regard to the surgery, anesthetic, and postoperative pain management. For example, patient satisfaction with same-day discharge following laparoscopic cholecystectomy has been shown to be directly related to preoperative expectations.

E. Selected References

Fleisher LA, Yee K, Lillemoe KD, et al. Is outpatient laparoscopic cholecystectomy safe and cost effective? A model to study transition of care. Anesthesiology 1999;90: 1746–1755.

Jones SB, Monk TG. Anesthesia and patient monitoring. In: Jones DB, Wu JS, Soper NJ, eds. Laparoscopic Surgery: Principles and Procedures. St. Louis: Quality Medical, 1997:28–36.

Kaplan EB, Sheiner LB, Boeckmann AJ, et al. The usefulness of preoperative laboratory screening. JAMA 1985;253:3576–3581.

Narr BJ, Warner ME, Schroeder DR, Warner MA. Outcomes of patients with no laboratory assessment before anesthesia and a surgical procedure. Mayo Clin Proc 1997; 72:505–509.

Roizen MF, Kaplan EB, Schreider BD, et al. The relative roles of the history and physical exam, and laboratory testing in preoperative evaluation for outpatient surgery: the "Starling" curve in preoperative laboratory testing. Anesth Clin N Am 1987;5:15.

Rucker L, Frye EB, Staten MA. Usefulness of screening chest roentgenograms in preoperative patients. JAMA 1983;250:3209.

Turnbull JM, Buck C. The value of preoperative screening investigations in otherwise healthy individuals. Arch Intern Med 1987;147:1101–1105.

U.S. Preventive Services Task Force. Guide to clinical preventive services: report of the U.S. Preventive Services Task Force, 2nd edition. Baltimore: Williams & Wilkins, 1996.

2. Preoperative Evaluation of Complex Laparoscopic Patients

Dmitry Oleynikov, M.D.
Karen D. Horvath IV, M.D.

Complex laparoscopic patients require careful preoperative planning for optimal outcome. These patients present unique problems that necessitate special consideration and a surgeon experienced in basic laparoscopic cases. This chapter discusses a number of such patient groups, including patients with previous abdominal surgery, significant cardiopulmonary comorbidity, obesity, and pregnancy. When evaluating any of these patients, *six questions* should be asked:

1. *Are there any contraindications to a laparoscopic procedure?*
2. *Does this patient need any additional preoperative testing? Does the surgeon need additional past medical or surgical information before surgery for planning purposes?*
3. *Does this patient need any additional preoperative medical or anesthesia planning? Will a planned postoperative ICU stay be required?*
4. *Should additional nonroutine issues be discussed with the patient as part of the informed consent?*
5. *Will the standard laparoscopic approach need to be altered in any way?*
   If the answer to the question is yes, it is recommended that the alteration be dictated into the preoperative evaluation note at the time this decision is made and not left to last-minute consideration on the day of surgery.
6. *Will this procedure require any unique equipment or staffing in the operating room that should be arranged in advance?*

A. Patient with Previous Abdominal Surgery

Few situations command as much respect as a laparoscopic procedure in a heavily scarred abdomen.

1. *Contraindications to a laparoscopic approach:*
   The only contraindication to a laparoscopic approach, in regard to patients with a history of prior abdominal operations, is a documented history of a frozen abdomen.
2. *Additional preoperative testing/and pertinent past surgical history:*
   a. Previous operative records
      1. Note the amount and type of adhesions encountered at the previous surgery.

   2. Determine the type and number of prosthetic devices used, i.e., mesh for reoperative hernia or number of stitches in a previous laparoscopic Nissen.
   b. Radiographic imaging
      1. Standard imaging before reoperative surgery, e.g., UGI for reoperative foregut surgery or CT scan for patient with diverticulitis to determine need for ureteral stenting.
      2. Ultrasound of the abdominal wall may help map adhesions preoperatively.
   c. Preoperative physical examination to appreciate the number and location of prior incisions and to look for incisional hernia(s).
3. *Additional preoperative medical/anesthesia planning:*
   Patients with a prior history of abdominal operations who are to undergo further surgery present no specific medical/anesthetic issues directly related to their past surgery. Standard evaluation should be performed as dictated by the patient's age and comorbidities.
4. *Special issues for the informed consent:*
   Regardless of type of procedure, reoperative laparoscopic surgery carries increased risks and patients should be counseled regarding them.
   a. Increased chance that conversion to an open laparotomy will be necessary.
   b. Additional ports may be required for adhesiolysis.
   c. Increased risk of enterotomy or other visceral injury.
   d. If an incisional hernia is present, patients should be consented for a simultaneous repair, if the primary laparoscopic procedure to be carried out is not classified as contaminated.
5. *Planned alterations from the standard laparoscopic approach:*
   a. Method of establishing a pneumoperitoneum in the reoperative abdomen. Options include:
      1. Veress needle entry with blind trocar insertion.
         One of the more popular methods for gaining entry into the peritoneal cavity. Caution should be used, however, especially in those with history of prior surgery, as evidence suggests a higher complication rate. If this method is to be used, the site chosen for Veress needle insertion should be well away from the prior incisions.
      2. Open/Hasson entry with blunt-tip trocar.
         Allows for a more controlled method of gaining access to the abdominal cavity and of establishing pneumoperitoneum and has been shown to have fewer complications compared with blind entry. The open/Hasson method is the preferred method in a reoperative abdomen. Also allows blunt finger dissection of local adhesions through the initial port site.
      3. Optical trocars.
         Allows visualization of the path of the trocar during insertion (Optiview, Ethicon Endosurgery, Cincinnati, OH; Visiport, USSC/Tyco Corp, Norwalk, CT). This method has not been well studied. The theoretical advantage is that by observing the trocar insertion injuries to the viscera and

vessels can be avoided. This method requires blind Veress needle insertion and insufflation before trocar insertion. This method should be carefully considered in a patient with a history of multiple prior operations or adhesions.

b. Port placement in the reoperative abdomen.
   1. Initial port placement should be well away from all abdominal wall scars, even if this port will not be of much use during the laparoscopic procedure. The right or left upper quadrant in the midclavicular line has proven to be a safe starting point.
   2. Additional ports should be placed under direct observation.

6. *Unique OR equipment or staffing:*
   a. Increased OR time.
      Laparoscopic surgery in a reoperative abdomen often requires additional OR time for establishing the pneumoperitoneum and performing adhesiolysis, similar to reoperative open surgery. If an incisional hernia is found on physical examination, extra time should also be allotted for its repair.
   b. Open instruments may be needed in case of conversion.
   c. Special tools for adhesiolysis.
      1. Additional trocars.
      2. Angled laparoscope.
      3. Ultrasonic scissors or bipolar cautery for adhesiolysis. These tools decrease the incidence of the complication known as "arcing" that can be seen with monopolar cautery, i.e., tissue damage from electrical current at a site remote from the intended area of cauterization.

B. Patients with Significant Cardiopulmonary Comorbidity

An important difference between open and laparoscopic surgery are the CO_2 pneumoperitoneum-related intraoperative physiologic effects. The CO_2 gas used for the pneumoperitoneum raises the intraabdominal pressure from 0 to 15 mmHg, resulting in hemodynamic and pulmonary function alterations. Due to the transperitoneal absorption of the insufflated CO_2 gas into the blood, a hypercarbic acidemic state results. The healthy patient is able to compensate for these changes; however, the patient with significant cardiopulmonary disease may not have the physiologic reserve to appropriately compensate. These minor physiologic stressors can have major implications in high-risk cardiopulmonary patients; thus, these patients need very close monitoring during laparoscopic surgery, even for minor procedures.

Preoperative risk stratification may be accomplished using several methods. Eagle formulated guidelines that help identify patients who are at high risk for cardiac events during noncardiac surgery (Table 2.1).

1. *Contraindications to a laparoscopic approach:*
   There are no absolute contraindications to a laparoscopic approach in a patient with significant cardiopulmonary disease.

Table 2.1. Clinical predictors of increased perioperative cardiovascular risk (myocardial infarction, congestive heart failure, death).

Major risk	Intermediate risk	Minor risk
Unstable coronary syndromes —Recent MI —Unstable or severe angina —Decompensated CHF	Mild angina pectoris (class I and II) Prior myocardial infarction by history or pathologic Q waves	Advanced age Abnormal ECG Rhythm other than sinus Low functional residual capacity
Significant arrhythmia —High-grade AV block —Symptomatic ventricular arrhythmia in the presence of underlying heart disease —SVT uncontrolled rate	Diabetes mellitus Compensated or prior CHF	History of stroke
Severe valvular disease		

MI, myocardial infarction; CHF, congestive heart failure; AV, atricoulntricular.
Source: Reprinted with permission from Eagle KA, Brundage BH, Chaitman BR, et al. Guidelines for perioperative cardiovascular evaluation for noncardiac surgery. Report of the American College of Cardiology/American Heart Association. 1996;93(6):1278–1317.

2. *Additional preoperative testing/information:*
   a. Mandatory
      1. EKG
      3. Hematocrit
      4. electrolytes
      5. Chest radiograph
   b. May be indicated (depending on the patient's history and situation)
      1. Echocardiography
      2. Stress test (standard treadmill, echo stress, thallium, etc.)
      3. Holter monitor or other arrhythmia evaluation
      4. Digoxin levels
      5. Pulmonary function testing
      6. Carotid duplex
3. *Additional preoperative medical/anesthesia planning:*
   a. Medical clearance.
      All patients in this category should be "cleared" by their primary medical doctor or cardiologist. Depending on the patient and the extent of prior cardiopulmonary evaluation, the patient may require one or more of the above-listed tests preoperatively (noted in 2b).
   b. Anesthesia considerations.
      1. Arterial line for hemodynamic and acid-base monitoring

All patients with significant cardiopulmonary disease should have an arterial line during laparoscopic surgery. This line is crucial for accurate hemodynamic monitoring in the face of increased afterload and decreased preload imposed by the pneumoperitoneum. Furthermore, the end-tidal CO_2 is **not** an accurate reflection of the arterial PCO_2 (Figure 2.1). The end-tidal CO_2 lags behind the arterial PCO_2. Patients with pulmonary disease are less able to effectively eliminate CO_2 and are thus more susceptible to acidemia with its harmful physiologic implications.

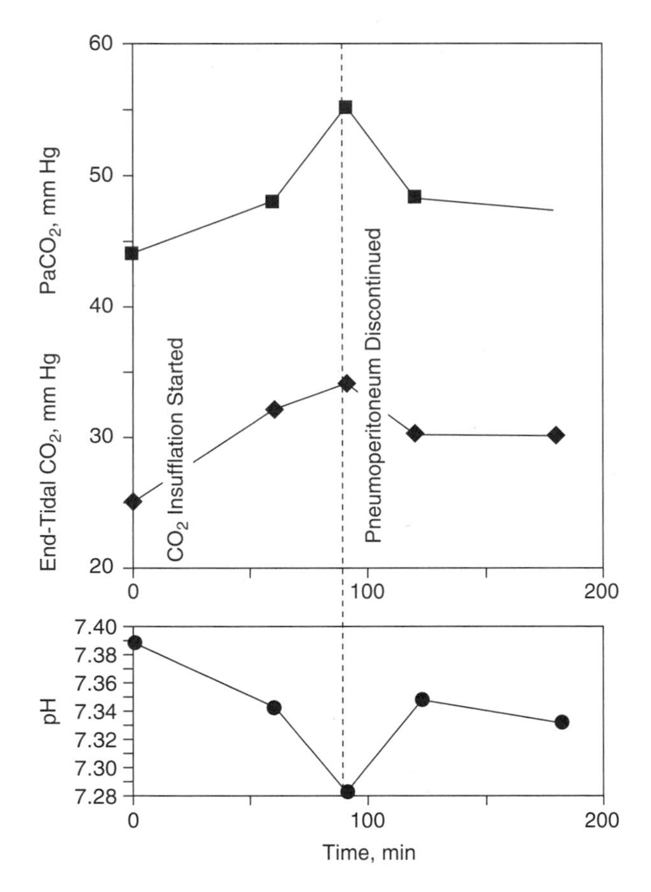

Figure 2.1. Note the nonlinear relationship between $ETCO_2$ and $PaCO_2$. A patient with an $ETCO_2$ of 35 can easily have a true $PaCO_2$ of 55 and a pH of 7.28. (*Source*: Reprinted with permission from Wittgen CM, Andrus CH, Fitzgerald SD. Analysis of the hemodynamic and ventilatory effects of laparoscopic cholecystectomy. Arch Surg 1991;126:997.)

2. Strongly consider central monitoring.
   Patients with diminished ejection fraction may benefit from central monitoring of cardiac filling by the anesthetist (Swan-Ganz catheter).

c. Pulmonary function testing and room air arterial blood gas analysis.
   1. These should be initiated in consultation with the anesthesiologist.

d. Schedule a postoperative ICU or telemetry bed.

4. *Special issues for the informed consent:*
   Regardless of the approach, surgery in this population carries increased risks of perioperative morbidity and mortality and patients should be counseled regarding these.

5. *Planned alterations from the standard laparoscopic approach:*
   a. Use lower pressures for pneumoperitoneum (10–12 mmHg).
      Human and animal experiments have demonstrated that pulmonary and hemodynamic changes are related to the pneumoperitoneum pressure. This is not a linear relationship. At *low pressures* (0–10 mmHg), relatively few changes can be detected in a normovolemic healthy adult. This relationship begins to change rapidly as intraabdominal pressure increases. At *moderate pressures* (10–22 mmHg), preload, afterload, and cardiac function are affected. Patients who are volume depleted (e.g., patients on chronic diuretic therapy) are more prone to developing significant cardiovascular alterations as a result of CO_2 pneumoperitoneum, even at low pressures. Therefore, it is important to adequately hydrate patients preoperatively, especially those patients who have undergone a bowel preparation. For patients with congestive heart failure it is crucial to avoid overresuscitation. These issues should be discussed with the anesthetist.

6. *Unique OR equipment or staffing:*
   a. Helium or nitrous oxide gas pneumoperitoneum.
      If available in your institution, use of these alternate gases for the pneumoperitoneum can minimize the effects of hypercarbia and acidemia. However, the hemodynamic alterations related to the elevated intraabdominal pressure remain the same. Further, there is a theoretical risk of gas embolism. If helium or nitrous oxide gas is to be used to establish and maintain pneumoperitoneum, then special equipment (dedicated insufflators, etc.) is usually required.
   b. Minimize OR time by soliciting the most senior assistant available.

C. Obese Patient

Obesity is defined as a body mass index (BMI) over 30 or approximately 50 lb above ideal body weight. By this definition 20% of male and 25% of female Americans are obese. Obese patients may have a number of comorbid conditions including pulmonary, cardiovascular, and metabolic disorders that need to be addressed during the preoperative evaluation. These patients also present distinct laparoscopic challenges.

1. *Contraindications to a laparoscopic approach:*
   There is no absolute contraindication to laparoscopic surgery in the obese patient.
2. *Additional preoperative testing/information:*
   a. EKG.
   b. CXR.
   c. Cessation of smoking.
   d. Attempted weight loss preoperatively, even if minimal.
   e. Cardiac and pulmonary testing as indicated in those with cardiac or pulmonary comorbidities.
3. *Additional preoperative medical/anesthesia planning:*
   a. Standard risk evaluation should be performed as dictated by the patient's age and comorbidities. Routine medical clearance is recommended.
   b. Complete muscle relaxation.
      The degree to which the abdominal wall is elevated in response to the pneumoperitoneum is maximized if the abdominal wall muscles are relaxed.
4. *Special issues for the informed consent:*
   Regardless of the specific procedure, laparoscopic surgery carries increased risks in obese patients, and the patient should be counseled regarding these.
   a. Increased chance of conversion to open laparotomy.
   b. Additional ports may be required to obtain adequate exposure.
5. *Planned alterations from the standard laparoscopic approach:*
   a. Extralong ports, trocars, and instruments may be needed.
      Body weight distribution plays an important role in gaining pneumoperitoneum and selecting appropriate ports and trocars.
      1. Female obese patients commonly have a very thick subcutaneous layer of fat with a relatively thin mesentery and omentum whereas male patients more often have a thin abdominal wall with generous mesentery and omental fat deposition.
      2. The upper abdominal wall is, most often, significantly thinner than the lower abdominal wall. Therefore, for upper gastrointestinal (GI) procedures such as Nissen fundoplication or gastric bypass extralong trocars are usually not needed; however, such trocars may be required for procedures that require lower abdominal ports.
      3. Extralong instruments may be needed for tall patients and those with a long abdominal cavity in those cases that require working in both the upper and lower abdomen. As an example, during left colectomy, splenic flexure mobilization is often necessary. The optimal port placement for the majority of the tasks that need to be accomplished during

the case is one where the most cephalad ports are at a level just above the umbilicus and the lower ports are well below the umbilicus. Standard instruments may not reach the splenic flexure from the lower port locations. The availability of extralong instruments should allow the flexure to be mobilized without having to place additional upper abdominal ports.

b. Open Hasson technique is preferable to Veress needle entry in morbidly obese patients.
The "cues" and "signs" of correct needle insertion such as initial insufflation pressures (high flow rate and a low intraabdominal pressure) and tympani over the abdomen are harder to gauge in these patients. There is greater uncertainty with blind needle insertion and blind trocar insertion techniques.

c. Place the skin incision for the initial port at the umbilicus, which is the thinnest part of the abdominal wall. Caution should be used in patients with a large pannus where the umbilicus may lie at the level of the public symphysis.

d. Angle ports toward the quadrant or area where the operation is to be carried out.
Normally, ports are placed perpendicular to the abdominal wall. In morbidly obese patients, a perpendicular trocar may result in excessive torquing of ports with gas leakage and bending of instruments.

e. Suture ports to the abdominal wall to prevent slippage.
Port slippage can lead to gas leak and subcutaneous emphysema, which further thickens the anterior abdominal wall. There are several methods for securing a port.
    1. One method is to place a skin suture near the port, tie it loosely, then wrap one end around the insufflation arm of the port and secure it to the other end of the suture with a clamp.
    2. Threaded port grips are another method of securing a port.
    3. The port can be secured via a heavy suture that is passed through the entire abdominal wall from the outside and then repassed back outside, after which one end is wrapped around the insufflation arm of the port and then secured with a clamp to the other end. This latter method, although a bit more time consuming, also prevents the abdominal wall in the area of the suture from increasing its girth as may occur when subcutaneous emphysema develops.

f. Use of increased pneumoperitoneum pressures (15–20 mmHg) to elevate a heavy anterior abdominal wall.
Elevated pressures may enlarge the operative field and improve visualization; however, the increased pressure may decrease venous return and cardiac output in patients with cardiovascular disease. For this reason, increased pneumoperitoneum pressures should only be used selectively, for brief periods. The patient must be monitored more closely when elevated pressures are utilized.

Changes in insufflation pressures must be communicated to the anesthetist. The anesthetist should be told at the start of the case to keep the surgeon informed of end-tidal CO_2 elevations, the need for high inspiratory pressures, and hypoxia. Close communication between the surgeon and the anesthetist will allow for timely adjustments of peak insufflation pressures, patient position, and the respirator settings. At times, when the end-tidal CO_2 is very high, it may be appropriate to desufflate the abdomen altogether and put the patient in reverse Trendelenburg position.

g. Deep venous thrombosis (DVT) prophylaxis.
Pneumatic compression devices + preoperative subcutaneous heparin (unless contraindicated).
Obesity is an independent risk factor for perioperative DVT formation, and therefore all patients should receive prophylaxis.

6. *Unique OR equipment or staffing:*
   a. Increased OR time.
   Laparoscopic surgery in the morbidly obese patient often requires additional OR time.
   b. Special large-size OR table.
   c. Foot boards and safety straps to avoid shifting during intraoperative positioning.
   d. Angled laparoscopes.
   e. Additional ports for exposure.
   f. Postoperative "Big Boy Bed."

D. Pregnant Patient

The pregnant patient may develop appendicitis, cholecystitis, torsion of the ovary, or a number of other problems that may require urgent or emergent surgery. When surgery is necessary in this population, minimally invasive methods can be used. Pregnancy may either lower or heighten the threshold for surgical exploration and treatment. The surgeon must determine the status of the pregnancy and inform the patient of both the routine risks and the pregnancy-related risks of surgery. The height of the gravid uterus can alter the position of the intestine and other intraabdominal organs and may necessitate a different port arrangement.

1. *Contraindications to a laparoscopic approach:*
   a) At what gestational age can laparoscopy be performed safely and effectively? Most authorities recommend avoidance of pneumoperitoneum and laparoscopy until the second trimester for indicated nonemergent operations. However, some recently published series report the safe performance of laparoscopic cholecystectomy in patients beyond the 21st week. In the second and third trimesters, because of the size of the gravid uterus, the location of the intestine and other viscera shifts in a cephalad direction. It is important to avoid manipulation of the uterus during surgery, which can induce preterm labor.

b) Although there are reports of successful laparoscopic procedures during the first 16 weeks of gestation, there are too few data to permit a recommendation for such an approach. All nonemergent surgery should be postponed until the second trimester.

2. *Additional preoperative testing/information:*
   a. Evaluation stage of pregnancy
      1. First trimester (1–14 weeks after last menstrual period). Organogenesis occurs during this time period.
         a. The viability and current location of the pregnancy should be evaluated preoperatively.
         b. Once an intrauterine pregnancy is confirmed, cardiac activity can be seen on ultrasound at the estimated gestational age of 6–7 weeks.
      2. Second trimester (14–28 weeks)
         a. Preoperative evaluation should include determination of viability and confirmation of dates.
         b. Early second trimester has traditionally been favored for elective surgical intervention because the risk of preterm labor is less than in the third trimester and because organ development is complete.
         c. Ultrasound is the best modality to document gestational age.
         d. The gestational age beyond which survival of the neonate outside of the uterus is feasible is now approaching 23 weeks in certain centers. When operating at or close to the age of viability, the opinion of an obstetric specialist should be sought. Depending on the facilities available, postoperative recovery should be carried out in the hospital obstetrics unit.
      3. Third trimester (28–42 weeks)
         a. Preoperative evaluation begins with close consultation with the treating Ob/Gyn.
         b. Due to an increased risk of preterm delivery (<37 weeks estimated gestational age), every effort should be made to postpone surgery until after delivery of the fetus, except for emergent indications.
3. *Additional preoperative medical/anesthesia planning:*
   a. An obstetrician should evaluate all pregnant patients perioperatively.
   b. Avoid fetal acidosis.
      1. Keep end-tidal CO_2 between 25 and 33 by changing minute ventilation.
      2. Consider arterial blood gas monitoring.
   c. Special anesthetic precautions should be used to avoid aspiration and hypotension.
4. *Special issues for the informed consent:*
   Large studies on the safety of laparoscopic surgery in the pregnant patient do not exist. Poor fetal outcomes and complications after laparoscopic surgical procedures are thought to be underreported. The

precise risk of premature labor and loss of pregnancy after laparoscopic surgery is unknown at this time. Despite this lack of data, patients should be informed of the following:

a. Increased chance of conversion to open laparotomy.
b. Before 14 weeks, up to 30% of known pregnancies undergo spontaneous abortion, in the absence of surgery. This is an important point that should be documented in the preoperative consent.
c. The risks relating to surgery during the first trimester include teratogenesis and a miscarriage rate of approximately 12%.
d. The risks of surgery during the second trimester include a 5%–8% risk of preterm labor.
e. The risks of surgery during the third trimester includes a risk of preterm labor and premature delivery.
f. The possibility of damaging the gravid uterus with laparoscopic instruments, ports, or trocars.

5. *Planned alterations from the standard laparoscopic approach:*
   a. Minimize operative time so that fetal acidosis is minimized. Solicit the most senior assistant available even for a "minor" case.
   b. Open/Hasson entry above the umbilicus to avoid injury to the gravid uterus.
   By the 20th week of gestation, the uterus is generally at the level of the umbilicus.
   c. Minimize pneumoperitoneum pressures to the 10–12 mmHg level.
   d. Elevation of the patient's right side during positioning to avoid inferior vena cava compression by the gravid uterus.
   e. Use angled laparoscopes to facilitate seeing around the uterus.
   f. Maternal monitoring with end-tidal CO_2 ± arterial blood gas monitioring
   Fetal acidosis is known to occur with CO_2 pneumoperitoneum, although the short- and long-term effects of this are unknown. Should the mother become acidemic, the pneumoperitoneum should be released and the patient hyperventilated to expel the CO_2 gas before continuing the procedure. It is important to note that the fetus is usually more acidemic than the mother.
   g. Routine use of pneumatic compression devises. The risk of thromboembolism is increased during pregnancy.
   h. Use a lead shield to protect the fetus during cholangiography.
   i. Fetal monitoring.
   Significant controversies in the literature exist on the merits and techniques of intraoperative fetal monitoring. At the least, pre- and postoperative fetal heart tones should be obtained and carefully documented when surgery is performed during the second and third trimesters.
6. *Unique OR equipment or staffing:*
   a. Special OR equipment is not needed for the pregnant patient.
   b. Senior assistance should be sought in the OR to minimize operative time.

E. Selected References

Curet MJ. Special problems in laparoscopic surgery. Surg Clin North Am 2000;80(4): 1093–1110.

Eagle KA, Brundage BH, Chaitman BR, et al. Guidelines for perioperative cardiovascular evaluation for noncardiac surgery. Report of the American College of Cardiology/American Heart Association Task Force on Practice Guidelines. Committee on Perioperative Cardiovascular Evaluation for Noncardiac Surgery. Circulation 1996;93(6):1278–1317.

Guidelines for laparoscopic surgery during pregnancy. Society of American Gastrointestinal Endoscopic Surgeons (SAGES). Surg Endosc 1998;12(2):189–190.

Mayol J, Garcia-Aguilar J, Ortiz-Oshiro E, De-Diego Carmona JA, Fernandez-Represa JA. Risks of the minimal access approach for laparoscopic surgery: multivariate analysis of morbidity related to umbilical trocar insertion. World J Surg 1997;21(5): 529–533.

Wittgen CM, Andrus CH, Fitzgerald SD. Analysis of the hemodynamic and ventilatory effects of laparoscopic cholecystectomy. Arch Surg 1991;126:997.

3. Preoperative Patient Instructions

Tracey D. Arnell, M.D.

A. Goals of Preoperative Patient Instructions

1. The goals of preoperative patient instructions are:
   i. Patient education. Included in this is technical information as well as information regarding appropriate expectations. Patients with realistic expectations regarding issues such as pain, recovery, length of stay, and potential complications do better.
   ii. To make patients aware of their risk factors. Involve patients in modifying risk factors that may decrease the risk of complications. (To motivate patients to alter their behavior such that they impact on their risk factors.)
   iii. To give specific instructions regarding bowel preparation, cessation of diet and fluids, management of patients' baseline medications and special surgery-related medications as well as day of surgery instructions.

B. Patient Education

1. Options. Once the decision to perform surgery is made, the surgical alternatives should be presented to the patient. In regard to surgical approach for abdominal procedures, traditional open and laparoscopic methods, including the advantages and disadvantages of each approach, are discussed.
   i. Laparoscopic resection
      1. Advantages. There are increasing data that laparoscopic methods are associated with advantages other than smaller, more **cosmetic** scars. These include a more rapid **return to normal activity**, a minor decrease in **hospital stay**, and a decrease in **wound infection** and subsequent **hernias**. Recent evidence also suggests that laparoscopic techniques are associated with significantly **better preserved immune function** as compared with open surgery.
      2. Disadvantages. Generally, **operative times** are significantly longer, although the differences decrease with increasing surgeon experience. **Cost** has traditionally been thought to be higher, although recent reports refute this. **Availability** of surgeons with adequate advanced laparoscopic training and experience is a limiting factor.

ii. General considerations
    1. Surgeon experience. Most studies support a **learning curve** regarding operative times, conversion rates, and complications.
    2. The possibility that an operation will need to be converted to an open procedure. Patients must be aware there is always a potential for conversion to an open procedure. It is not reasonable or honest to "promise" or guarantee patients that their operation will be completed laparoscopically. The conversion rate varies depending on the procedure, surgeon experience, body habitus, and pathology (Table 3.1).

2. Technical information
    i. There are many resources for general information regarding laparoscopic surgery including the **Internet**, patient **pamphlets**, and **videos**. In addition, most patients appreciate a more detailed explanation of the specific procedure to be carried out; for example, the number and location of port incisions as well as the need for an extended or additional incision in the case of hand-assisted or laparoscopic-assisted operations may be mentioned.

3. Expectations
    i. Pain. Although laparoscopic surgery is associated with decreased pain, and a decreased need for narcotics, patients should understand there will be pain and discomfort following surgery.
    ii. Diet. Depending on the procedure and the surgeon, the diet may be resumed immediately following surgery or one or several days later. In regard to intestinal surgery, most studies suggest that an oral diet is tolerated 1 to 2 days earlier after a minimally invasive procedure than after the equivalent open procedure. The extent to which the surgeon's expectations and bias impacted the postoperative management and, possibly, the short-term recovery of patients in these studies is not clear.
    iii. Hospital stay. Most published series report shorter length of stays for patients undergoing laparoscopic surgery. For intestinal surgery, the difference has not been as great as noted for procedures such as splenectomy and nephrectomy. Patients should understand that except for planned outpatient procedures (e.g., hernia) a hospital stay is generally required.

Table 3.1. Reported conversion rates.

Procedure	**Conversion rate**
Antireflux wrap	<4%
Urologic	1%–6%
Splenectomy	<3%
Roux-en-Y gastric bypass	3%–10%
Colectomy	4%–23%

iv. Resumption of normal activities. Given the limited abdominal wall trauma and more rapid "in-hospital" recovery of laparoscopic patients, it is not unreasonable to anticipate a more rapid return to normal activities. The heterogeneity of patients in regard to age and preoperative level of function as well as the lack of clear criteria defining "normal" activities for such a diverse population makes this a difficult parameter to assess. Further, the time to full recovery will vary considerably depending on the specific procedure in question.

v. Conversion. All patients must be prepared for the possibility that it may prove necessary to make a large incision and utilize traditional open methods. Therefore, only patients who are fit to undergo open surgery are candidates for laparoscopic surgery.

vi. Extended or additional incision. Depending on the particular procedure, a larger incision may be needed for specimen retrieval (i.e., colectomy, nephrectomy). Patients should understand that for these "laparoscopic-assisted" procedures this incision is mandatory. Similarly, if there is a chance that hand-assisted methods may be used then it should be made clear that a larger incision will be required.

C. Risk Factor Modification

1. Pulmonary. Patients who smoke have an increased risk of pulmonary complications such as pneumonia and prolonged intubation. This is a result of a loss of cilia with decreased clearance of airborne particles and desquamated cells. Additionally, in patients with emphysema, there is a decrease in the functional reserve capacity. Patients should be urged to stop smoking because **cessation of smoking** for at least 1 week may decrease respiratory complication rates. The preoperative use of an **incentive spirometer** is also associated with fewer pulmonary complications.
2. Bleeding. There are many prescribed and over-the-counter medications, vitamin supplements, and homeopathic medications that may alter an individual's coagulation profile. If the medications are thought to be necessary for medical reasons (i.e., aspirin in a patient with a stroke or coronary artery disease), they may be continued with an understood slightly increased risk of bleeding. Otherwise, the risk of bleeding is not warranted and they should be stopped before surgery.
3. Deep venous thrombosis (DVT). Risk factors for DVT are covered elsewhere in this manual, but there are factors that can be modified in the short term. These risk factors include **smoking**, **oral contraceptives, estrogen replacement drugs, and ambulation (the lack thereof).**

D. Specific Instructions

1. Bowel preparation. This subject is covered in Chapter 5, Part III.
2. Medications. For prescription medication, the following is a list of general recommendations.
   i. Diabetes. Usually, the patient is advised to hold the daily dose of regular insulin and administer 1/4 to 1/2 the normal daily intermediate-acting insulin dose on the morning of surgery. Patients taking a bowel preparation may need to decrease their dosage of regular insulin as determined by glucose checks. Those with poorly controlled diabetes should be admitted for management of their diabetes.
   ii. Aspirin. Unless required for medical reasons as previously described, aspirin and other platelet inactivators should be held for 7 days preoperatively.
   iii. Coumadin. The physician in charge of the patient's anticoagulation regimen should be consulted by the surgeon so that the indications for the coumadin be fully understood and so that an approach to stopping the coumadin can be agreed upon. One approach is to simply stop the coumadin 3 to 4 days before the surgery. Alternately, the patient is brought into the hospital several days preoperatively so that intravenous heparin can be given during the period when the coumadin has been held. As an alternative to in hospital I.V. heparin, subcutaneous injections of lovenox or other similar agents can be administered at home preoperatively.
   iv. Other medications. All other medications, including antihypertensives, thyroid replacement, and seizure medications, should be taken per the usual schedule.

E. Selected References

Carter JJ, Whelan RL. The immunologic consequences of laparoscopy in oncology. Surg Oncol Clin N Am 2001;10:655–677.

Lezoche E, Feliciotti F, Paganini AM, Guerrieri M, Campagnacci R, De Sanctis A. Laparoscopic colonic resections versus open surgery: a prospective non-randomized study on 310 unselected cases. Hepato-Gastroenterology 2000;47:697–708.

Lezoche E, Feliciotti F, Paganini AM, et al. Laparoscopic vs. open hemicolectomy for colon cancer. Surg Endosc 2002;16:596–602.

Lujan HJ, Plasencia G, Jacobs M, Viamonte M, Hartmann RF. Long-term survival after laparoscopic colon resection for cancer: complete five-year follow-up. Dis Colon Rectum 2002;45:491–501.

Senagore AJ, Duepree HJ, Delaney CP, Dissanaike S, Brady KM, Fazio VW. Cost structure of laparoscopic and open sigmoid colectomy for diverticular disease: similarities and differences. Dis Colon Rectum 2002;45:485–490.

Seshadri PA, Poulin EC, Schlachta CM, Cadeddu MO, Mamazza J. Does a laparoscopic approach to total abdominal colectomy and proctocolectomy offer advantages? Surg Endosc 2001;15:837–842.

Targarona EM, Gracia E, Garriga J, et al. Prospective randomized trial comparing conventional laparoscopic colectomy with hand-assisted laparoscopic colectomy: applicability, immediate clinical outcome, inflammatory response, and cost. Surg Endosc 2002;16:234–239.

4. Contraindications to Laparoscopy

Steven P. Bowers, M.D.
John G. Hunter, M.D., F.A.C.S.

A. Introduction

The applications of minimally invasive abdominal surgery continue to grow. As laparoscopic surgery becomes more advanced and more widely applied, the absolute contraindications to laparoscopy are diminishing. However, injuries to patients may occur when surgeons exceed the limitations of laparoscopic surgery and their laparoscopic skill set. This chapter discusses the present limits of laparoscopic access and the situations in which laparoscopy should be used only cautiously.

Perhaps the most difficult limitation for surgeons to recognize are the boundaries of their laparoscopic skills. Inadequate training and experience may lead to injuries. In addition, poor equipment and/or inadequate training of surgical assistants or ancillary staff should be thought of as further contraindications to advanced laparoscopic procedures. Although this chapter focuses primarily on the preoperative characteristics of the patient that make laparoscopic surgery prohibitively difficult or dangerous, it also includes a brief discussion regarding surgical judgment.

Patient limitations to laparoscopic surgery can be both anatomic and physiologic. Adverse anatomic considerations include difficult access to the abdomen, obliteration of the peritoneal space, organomegaly, intestinal distension, and the potential for dissemination or recurrence of cancer. The major physiologic obstacles to safe laparoscopy include pregnancy, increased intracranial pressure, abnormalities of cardiac output and gas exchange in the lung, and chronic liver disease and coagulopathy. While many of these conditions were formerly considered absolute contraindications to laparoscopy, they are now considered, by many surgeons, to be only relative contraindications.

B. Anatomic Limitations

1. Port access
    a. Reoperative abdomen

Especially in the reoperative abdomen, injuries can occur when placing laparoscopic ports. In several early prospective studies, there were fewer injuries when open "cut-down" access methods (Hasson technique) were employed, as compared to "blind" (Veress needle) port insertion methods [1–3]. It is now believed that the incidence of injuries is similarly small using either technique, even in the reoperative abdomen, provided the site chosen for insufflation and insertion of the first port is distant from previous abdominal incisions. If the Veress needle technique is used, failure to establish a pneumoperitoneum after two to three passes should be considered a reason to change to an open (Hasson) technique. In more than 30% of patients with a history of prior surgery, the bowel or other organs are directly adherent to the abdominal scar, rendering these areas problematic for both open and blind access methods [4–9].

The difficulty of laparoscopy in the reoperative abdomen is due to the formation of adhesions, which obliterate the peritoneal space and hinder visibility. Attempts at laparoscopy in a field previously operated upon by open technique can be very time consuming, particularly in the case of multiple previous operations or peritonitis. Many surgeons set a time limit for laparoscopic lysis of adhesions, after which conversion is carried out unless the end of the adhesiolysis is clearly in sight.

b. Intraperitoneal mesh

Because of the difficulty dissecting intestinal adhesions from prosthetic mesh, previous intraperitoneal mesh placement is considered a contraindication to laparoscopic access in that area. Conversely, it is often possible to repair recurrent ventral or inguinal hernias where mesh was used by placing trocars remote from the previous incisions and the mesh.

c. Cirrhosis and portal hypertension

In cirrhotic patients, the hazards encountered in abdominal access are often due to abdominal wall varices, and meticulous open technique is required for safe port placement [10]. In the ascites patient without portal hypertension, the Veress needle approach may be used, but it is necessary to place the patient in reverse Trendelenburg position to get the air-filled bowel away from the inferior course of the needle. In addition, it may be necessary to withdraw ascites before pneumoperitoneum can be established. Ascites becomes frothy (secondary to the albumin) when it is directly insufflated, which makes visualization difficult. Laparoscopic wounds in cirrhotic patients can be complicated by postoperative leakage of ascites. Cholecystectomy is generally considered to be prohibitively hazardous in the presence of advanced cirrhosis (Childs C) because of the abundance of large fragile collateral vessels at the liver hilum; however, laparoscopic cholecystectomy may provide an advantage over open operation in Childs A and B cirrhotic patients because of decreased wound complication rates [11,12].

2. Peritoneal space

a. Peritonitis

Early reports predicted that laparoscopic operations in the presence of bacterial peritonitis would predispose to subsequent abscess formation. However, laparoscopic appendectomy following perforation and laparoscopic closure of perforated peptic ulcers are operations that have been safely carried out with complication rates reported equivalent to the open approach [13–15].

b. Mechanical bowel obstruction

Laparoscopy in the setting of diffusely dilated small bowel loops is difficult because the working space provided by the pneumoperitoneum is reduced. Further, small bowel manipulation and retraction in this setting carries a higher risk of serosal tears or enterotomy. Although some surgeons believe laparoscopy is contraindicated for mechanical obstructions, others have reported success in selected cases and have noted wound healing benefits and early return of bowel function [16–18]. It must be accepted that the conversion rate will be high and, if complex adhesions are encountered, the surgeon should have a low threshold for laparotomy. It is helpful to decompress the bowel as much as possible preoperatively, and to start "running the bowel" at the decompressed ileocecal valve.

c. Gravid uterus

Pelvic and lower abdominal laparoscopic surgery is often not possible in the third trimester of gestation due to space considerations. Although laparoscopy has been reported, open operation is recommended. (See below for further concerns vis-à-vis laparoscopy and pregnancy.)

3. Dissemination of cancer

a. Port site recurrence

The spread of intraabdominal malignancy following laparoscopy is related to surgeon experience, tumor biology, and the completeness of resection. Laparoscopic resections for early colon cancer by skilled surgeons may be accomplished with equivalent lymphatic resection and tumor-free margins as with open operations [26]. Ongoing prospective studies suggest that laparoscopic resection of colon cancer yields equivalent long-term disease-free survival when compared to an open operation, and that port site recurrences are generally related to technical errors [19–24]. These results have been extrapolated to promote the laparoscopic resection of other intraabdominal cancers and exploratory laparoscopy has become the standard for tumor staging before resection for upper intestinal tumors [25].

b. Invasive cancers

It is generally agreed that gastrointestinal or intraabdominal malignancies that are locally invasive (into adjacent organs, the retroperitoneum, or the abdominal wall) should be resected using open techniques.

c. Tumor dissemination

Tumors with a tendency to readily disseminate in the peritoneal cavity, such as mucinous cystadenocarcinoma of the ovary and signet cell or mucinous gastrointestinal adenocarcinomas, may exhibit higher rates of implantation on peritoneal surfaces following laparoscopic resection [27–29]. This risk should be considered before laparoscopic resection of these tumors.

C. Physiologic Limitations

1. Pulmonary

a. CO_2 retention/hypoventilation

Abdominal insufflation with CO2 is associated with two potential problems. First, absorption of CO2 across the peritoneal surface may cause hypercarbia which, in turn, results in respiratory acidosisis. Second, transmission of increased intraabdominal pressure through the paralyzed diaphragm raises intrathoracic pressures by 5–15 mmHg, depending on diaphragmatic compliance. Absorption of CO2 and the ensuing hypercarbic acidosis requires intraoperative compensation by the anesthetist; increasing the minute ventilation, usually by hyperventilating the patient, lowers the PaCO2 and raises the pH. In patients with marginal pulmonary reserve, the morbidly obese, and those who require positive end expiratory pressure for adequate oxygenation, adequate compensation may not be possible and, in these cases, refractory acidosis may develop [30,31]. End-tidal CO_2 monitoring is essential in the management of the ventilation of patients undergoing laparoscopy, but may underestimate the true arterial pCO_2 by as much as 10 mmHg in the individual with chronic lung disease. Thus, arterial monitoring may be wise in these patients. In children and in patients who cannot be adequately ventilated during laparoscopic surgery, lower peak insufflation pressures should be used. If this fails, alternative measures including the use of an abdominal wall-lifting device, administration of an alternative insufflation gas such as nitrous oxide or helium, or conversion to open technique should be considered [32–34]. To date, no criteria have been developed that reliably predict intraoperative ventilatory failure during laparoscopic surgery.

2. Cardiac/circulatory

 a. Decreased venous return/metabolic acidosis

Venous return to the heart decreases in response to peritoneal gas insufflation. This effect is most prominent in hypovolemic patients, as the pneumoperitoneum will easily compress the poorly distended vena cava. In a well-hydrated patient, venous return to the heart is nearly normal. Cardiac output is decreased by impairment of venous return, and metabolic (lactic) acidosis results from decreased visceral perfusion. This may be exacerbated by the decreased capacity for respiratory compensation [35].

Laparoscopy in the elderly was once thought to be contraindicated because of the effect of pneumoperitoneum on cardiac and pulmonary physiology. With improved anesthetic techniques, these contraindications no longer exist. Several studies have confirmed the benefits of laparoscopy in the elderly, including decreased hospital stay and fewer wound and pulmonary complications when compared to traditional operative approaches [36].

 b. Hemorrhage/shock

Patients with severe cardiac disease or with profound hypovolemia may not compensate well and may manifest a dramatic fall in cardiac output with peritoneal gas insufflation. Although laparoscopy has been recommended as a diagnostic tool in some intensive care unit patients [37], laparoscopy should not be performed in patients who manifest shock, particularly from acute hemorrhage.

3. Intracranial pressure

 a. Trendelenburg position/intraabdominal pressure

Peritoneal gas insufflation can cause increased intracranial pressure during lower abdominal or gynecologic procedures that require the use of the Trendelenburg position. When accompanied by an associated acidosis, laparoscopy can cause hazardous intracranial pressure elevations in susceptible patients, especially those with acute brain injury.

 b. Ventriculoperitoneal shunt

Technical failures of ventriculoperitoneal shunts (VPS) have been reported following laparoscopic surgery. Also, a theoretical risk of intracranial insufflation exists in the case of a defective shunt valve [38,39]. Some experts recommend that in patients with VPSs requiring laparoscopic surgery, the shunt should be exteriorized before to gas insufflation and replaced following desufflation of the abdomen. In practice, the valve in the VPS is rarely incompetent, and these additional measures are believed by most neurosurgeons to be unnecessary.

4. Pregnancy
   a. Maternal/fetal effects

Peritoneal gas insufflation with CO2 has been found in laboratory studies to cause increased intrauterine pressure, decreased uterine blood flow, and maternal and fetal acidosis [40]. No long-term data are available concerning the development of the child after maternal laparoscopy, but recent clinical data suggest that adverse outcomes are rare when laparoscopy is performed in the second trimester of pregnancy [41–44].

   b. Advantages of the second trimester

Because of the possible teratogenicity of anesthetic agents, elective surgical procedures in general are contraindicated in the first trimester. In the third trimester, the risk of pre-term labor also contraindicates elective surgical procedures. The second trimester (13–26 weeks gestation) is a relatively safe period for indicated abdominal operations. Diagnostic or operative laparoscopy for appendectomy and gynecologic emergencies have been reported in all trimesters with fetal loss rates that are equivalent to open surgery [41–44]. Thus, no absolute contraindications exist, except in the late third trimester, when the gravid uterus obliterates the peritoneal space, and most indicated procedures are preceded by induction of labor or cesarean section.

5. Coagulopathy

The presence of known coagulation disorders was once considered to be a contraindication for laparoscopic surgery. This is rarely the case now, with improved surgical techniques and the development of recombinant coagulation factors. Laparoscopic splenectomy is becoming the standard approach for medically refractory immune thrombocytopenia purpura. The coagulopathy associated with congenital coagulation disorders should be corrected before operation. Uncorrected coagulopathy is a relative contraindication to both laparoscopic and open operations because of the difficulty in controlling bleeding.

D. Surgical Judgment

The laparoscopic skill set and experience of the surgeon are also important variables which must be taken into account when considering the feasibility of a particular minimally invasive operation. Also, when attempting a difficult case it is imperative that the surgical assistants be experienced. Therefore, inexperience on the part of the surgeon or assistants is a relative contraindication for advanced procedures.

Given an experienced surgeon and staff, it is also important for the surgeon to make an overall assessment early in the case as to whether it is likely or unlikely that a given case will be successfully completed using laparoscopic means. Advanced minimally invasive cases are unforgiving in that the inability to carry out just one of the many laparoscopic tasks required for the successful completion of a procedure may necessitate conversion. As an example, if, during a segmental colectomy in a patient with considerable adhesions, it becomes necessary to run the small bowel extracorpeally, to find and repair a partial-thickness enterotomy (incurred during adhesiolysis), the small bowel loops must be mobile enough to be externalized. If the small bowel is densely matted together, then, despite the fact that the anterior abdominal wall adhesions have been successfully taken down (making the laparoscopic colectomy feasible), conversion, in the end, will most likely be unavoidable. In this situation, early conversion is the logical choice. Rather than busying themselves with the parts of the operation that are feasible laparoscopically, the surgeon must be disciplined enough to make an early judgment about the steps of the operation that will be the most difficult. This process will lead to early and more timely conversions.

E. Conclusion

Contraindications to laparoscopic surgery may be anatomic or physiologic. Familiarity with and attention to the responsible factors will assure the lowest risk of adverse outcomes. The skill set and experience of the surgeons must also be taken into account when considering a minimally invasive approach. The decision to convert to an open operation must be based on the experience of the surgeon and the anatomic and physiologic constraints of the patient. Such a decision represents sound judgment and does not constitute a failure.

F. References

1. Mayol J, Garcia-Aguilar J, Ortiz-Oshiro E, et al. Risks of the minimal access approach for laparoscopic surgery: multivariate analysis of morbidity related to umbilical trocar insertion. World J Surg 1997;21(5):529–533.
2. Sigman HH, Fried GM, Garzon J, et al. Risks of blind versus open approach to celiotomy for laparoscopic surgery. Surg Laparosc Endosc 1993;3(4):296–299.
3. McKernan JB, Champion JK. Access techniques: Veress needle–initial blind trocar insertion versus open laparoscopy with the Hasson trocar. Endosc Surg Allied Technol 1995;3(1):35–38.
4. Audebert AJ, Gomel V. Role of microlaparoscopy in the diagnosis of peritoneal and visceral adhesions and in the prevention of bowel injury associated with blind trocar insertion. Fertil Steril 2000;73(3):631–635.
5. Miller K, Holbling N, Hutter J, Junger W, Moritz E, Speil T. Laparoscopic cholecystectomy for patients who have had previous abdominal surgery. Surg Endosc 1993; 7(5):400–403.
6. Gersin KS, Heniford BT, Arca MJ, Ponsky JL. Alternative site entry for laparoscopy in patients with previous abdominal surgery. J Laparoendosc Adv Surg Tech A 1998; 8(3):125–130.
7. Kumar SS. Laparoscopic cholecystectomy in the densely scarred abdomen. Am Surg 1998;64(11):1094–1096.
8. Halpern NB. The difficult laparoscopy. Surg Clin N Am 1996;76(3):603–613.

9. Halpern NB. Access problems in laparoscopic cholecystectomy: postoperative adhesions, obesity, and liver disorders. Semin Laparosc Surg 1998;5(2):92–106.
10. Abdel-Atty MY, Farges O, Jagot P, Belghiti J. Laparoscopy extends the indications for liver resection in patients with cirrhosis. Br J Surg 1999;86(11):1397–1400.
11. Yerdel MA, Koksoy C, Aras N, Orita K. Laparoscopic versus open cholecystectomy in cirrhotic patients: a prospective study. Surg Laparosc Endosc 1997;7(6):483–486.
12. Jan YY, Chen MF. Laparoscopic cholecystectomy in cirrhotic patients. Hepatogastroenterology 1997;44(18):1584–1587.
13. Khalili TM, Hiatt JR, Savar A, Lau C, Margulies DR. Perforated appendicitis is not a contraindication to laparoscopy. Am Surg 1999;65(10):965–967.
14. Navez B, Tassetti V, Scohy JJ, et al. Laparoscopic management of acute peritonitis. Br J Surg 1998;85(1):32–36.
15. Faranda C, Barrat C, Catheline JM, Champault GG. Two-stage laparoscopic management of generalized peritonitis due to perforated sigmoid diverticula: eighteen cases. Surg Laparosc Endosc Percutan Tech 2000;10(3):135–138; discussion 139–141.
16. Strickland P, Lourie DJ, Suddleson EA, Blitz JB, Stain SC. Is laparoscopy safe and effective for treatment of acute small-bowel obstruction? Surg Endosc 1999;13(7): 695–698.
17. Leon EL, Metzger A, Tsiotos GG, Schlinkert RT, Sarr MG. Laparoscopic management of small bowel obstruction: indications and outcome. J Gastrointest Surg 1998; 2(2):132–140.
18. Fazio VW, Lopez-Kostner F. Role of laparoscopic surgery for treatment of early colorectal carcinoma. World J Surg 2000;24(9):1056–1060.
19. Psaila J, Bulley SH, Ewings P, Sheffield JP, Kennedy RH. Outcome following laparoscopic resection for colorectal cancer. Br J Surg 1998;85(5):662–664.
20. Poulin EC, Mamazza J, Schlachta CM, Gregoire R, Roy N. Laparoscopic resection does not adversely affect early survival curves in patients undergoing surgery for colorectal adenocarcinoma. Ann Surg 1999;229(4):487–492.
21. Lacy AM, Delgado S, Garcia-Valdecasas JC, et al. Port site metastases and recurrence after laparoscopic colectomy. A randomized trial. Surg Endosc 1998;12(8):1039–1042.
22. Milsom JW, Bohm B, Hammerhofer KA, Fazio V, Steiger E, Elson P. A prospective, randomized trial comparing laparoscopic versus conventional techniques in colorectal cancer surgery: a preliminary report. J Am Coll Surg 1998;187(1):46–54; discussion 54–55.
23. Franklin ME Jr, Rosenthal D, Abrego-Medina D, et al. Prospective comparison of open vs. laparoscopic colon surgery for carcinoma. Five-year results. Dis Colon Rectum 1996;39(suppl 10):S35–S46.
24. The COLOR Investigators. COLOR: a randomized clinical trial comparing laparoscopic and open resection for colon cancer. Dig Surg 2000;17(6):617–622.
25. O'Brien MG, Fitzgerald EF, Lee G, Crowley M, Shanahan F, O'Sullivan GC. A prospective comparison of laparoscopy and imaging in the staging of esophagogastric cancer before surgery. Am J Gastroenterol 1995;90(12):2191–2194.
26. Moore JW, Bokey EL, Newland RC, Chapuis PH. Lymphovascular clearance in laparoscopically assisted right hemicolectomy is similar to open surgery. Aust N Z J Surg 1996;66(9):605–607.

27. Chew DK, Borromeo JR, Kimmelstiel FM. Peritoneal mucinous carcinomatosis after laparoscopic-assisted anterior resection for early rectal cancer: report of a case. Dis Colon Rectum 1999;42(3):424–426.
28. Ribeiro U Jr, Gama-Rodrigues JJ, Bitelman B, et al. Value of peritoneal lavage cytology during laparoscopic staging of patients with gastric carcinoma. Surg Laparosc Endosc 1998;8(2):132–135.
29. Gonzalez Moreno S, Shmookler BM, Sugarbaker PH. Appendiceal mucocele. Contraindication to laparoscopic appendectomy. Surg Endosc 1998;12(9):1177–1179.
30. Stuttmann R, Paul A, Kirschnik M, Jahn M, Doehn M. Preoperative morbidity and anaesthesia-related negative events in patients undergoing conventional or laparoscopic cholecystectomy. Endosc Surg Allied Technol 1995;3(4):156–161.
31. Kraut EJ, Anderson JT, Safwat A, Barbosa R, Wolfe BM. Impairment of cardiac performance by laparoscopy in patients receiving positive end-expiratory pressure. Arch Surg 1999;134(1):76–80.
32. Hunter JG, Staheli J, Oddsdottir M, Trus T. Nitrous oxide pneumoperitoneum revisited. Is there a risk of combustion? Surg Endosc 1995;9(5):501–504.
33. Fleming RY, Dougherty TB, Feig BW. The safety of helium for abdominal insufflation. Surg Endosc 1997;11(3):230–234.
34. Neuberger TJ, Andrus CH, Wittgen CM, Wade TP, Kaminski DL. Prospective comparison of helium versus carbon dioxide pneumoperitoneum. Gastrointest Endosc 1996;43(1):38–41.
35. Taura P, Lopez A, Lacy AM, et al. Prolonged pneumoperitoneum at 15 mmHg causes lactic acidosis. Surg Endosc 1998;12(3):198–201.
36. Schwandner O, Schiedeck TH, Bruch HP. Advanced age: indication or contraindication for laparoscopic colorectal surgery? Dis Colon Rectum 1999;42(3):356–362.
37. Orlando R III, Crowell KL. Laparoscopy in the critically ill. Surg Endosc 1997;11(11):1072–1074.
38. Baskin JJ, Vishteh AG, Wesche DE, Rekate HL, Carrion CA. Ventriculoperitoneal shunt failure as a complication of laparoscopic surgery. J Soc Laparoendosc Surg 1998;2(2):177–180.
39. Gaskill SJ, Cossman RM, Hickman MS, Marlin AE. Laparoscopic surgery in a patient with a ventriculoperitoneal shunt: a new technique. Pediatr Neurosurg 1998;28(2):106–107.
40. Curet MJ, Vogt DA, Schob O, Qualls C, Izquierdo LA, Zucker KA. Effects of CO_2 pneumoperitoneum in pregnant ewes. J Surg Res 1996;63(1):339–344.
41. Conron RW Jr, Abbruzzi K, Cochrane SO, Sarno AJ, Cochrane PJ. Laparoscopic procedures in pregnancy. Am Surg 1999;65(3):259–263.
42. de Perrot M, Jenny A, Morales M, Kohlik M, Morel P. Laparoscopic appendectomy during pregnancy. Surg Laparosc Endosc Percutan Tech 2000;10(6):368–371.
43. Holthausen UH, Mettler L, Troidl H. Pregnancy: A contraindication? World J Surg 1999;23(8):856–862.
44. Halpern NB. Laparoscopic cholecystectomy in pregnancy: a review of published experiences and clinical considerations. Semin Laparosc Surg 1998;5(2):129–134.

5. Perioperative Antibiotics in Laparoscopic Surgery

Tracey D. Arnell, M.D.

I. Goals

a. Prevent surgical site infections.
   i. Elimination of surgical site infections is impossible; therefore, the goal of antibiotic usage is to reduce the incidence of surgical site infections.
      1. A surgical site infection is not simply a failure of antibiotic prophylaxis.
      2. The use of laparoscopic methods may be associated with a reduction in the incidence of wound infections.
         a. Decreased postoperative immunosuppression.
         b. The role of carbon dioxide insufflation is unclear.
            i. There are conflicting results regarding laparoscopic appendectomy for appendicitis; some studies demonstrate an increase and some a decrease in surgical site infections.
            ii. Appendicitis may serve as a peritonitis model.

b. Treat existing infections, i.e., diverticulitis, appendicitis, peritonitis, etc.

c. Avoid toxicity.
   i. Allergic reactions.
   ii. Antibiotic-related infections such as *Clostridium difficile* infection.
   iii. Adverse interactions or reactions with other drugs.
   iv. Bone marrow suppression (very rare reaction to rarely used antibiotics).

d. Avoid unnecessary use.
   i. Drug resistance.
      1. Increasing incidence of resistant strains of *Staphylococcus*, enterococci (VRE), and other bacteria; this may be related to the use of broad-spectrum antibiotics as well as excessive duration of therapy.
   ii. Selection of pathogenic bacteria.
   iii. Cost considerations.
   iv. Noncompliance with antibiotic recommendations more than 50% and as high as 75%.

1. Despite multiple prospective studies and consensus statements regarding appropriate use of antibiotics, practitioners continue to deviate from recommendations.
2. Patients, at times, take antibiotics without obtaining the approval of a physician.

II. General considerations

a. Risk factors.
   i. Patient factors.
      1. Increased incidence of wound infection in the setting of:
         a. Obesity.
         b. Immunosuppression of whatever cause (diabetes, chemotherapy, steroid use, human immunodeficiency virus (HIV) infection, etc.).
         c. Advanced age.
         d. Malnutrition.
         e. Established infection in the abdomen or abdominal wall.
   ii. Technical factors.
      1. Duration of procedure in open surgery has been shown to be associated with an increased rate of infection.
         a. Although advanced laparoscopic procedures usually take more time to complete, a higher rate of surgical site infection has not been demonstrated (when compared to open results).
      2. Tissue factors.
         a. Trauma, devascularization.
         b. Inflammation.
         c. Radiation-related damage.
      3. Type of surgery: (Note: All data regarding expected rates of surgical site infection are from open surgery patients).
         a. Clean cases are associated with less than 1%–2% rate of surgical wound infection.
            i. Laparoscopic exploration, solid organ biopsy.
         b. Clean contaminated cases: less than 5% infection rate.
            i. Violation of biliary tract, uninfected urinary tract, upper intestinal surgery in the absence of stasis or achlorhydria.
         c. Contaminated cases: 10%–20% infection rate.
            i. Colorectal surgery, upper intestinal surgery with stasis or achlorhydria, cholecystitis, biliary tract stasis.

d. Infected cases: 40% infection rate.
   i. Active infection, abscess.
   ii. Examples: acute diverticulitis, gangrenous cholecystitis, appendicitis, other intestinal perforation.

b. Appropriate antibiotic choice and duration (Table 5.1).
   i. Appropriate **spectrum** for suspected source of contamination.
      1. Skin flora in clean and clean contaminated cases.
         a. Coverage may be different in hospitalized or immunosuppressed patients as well as those patients with a recent history of antibiotic usage.
      2. Intestinal flora.
         a. Gastric bacteria may include oral flora.
         b. Colonic or upper intestinal with stasis.
            i. Anaerobes and gram-negative coverage.
            ii. *Enterococcus* coverage unnecessary unless infection documented in culture of infection (i.e., abscess).
         c. Intraoperative cultures have not been found to be beneficial or necessary in guiding therapy in cases of established infection such as appendicitis. Infections in immunosuppressed patients may be an exception.
      3. Urinary tract with stasis or documented infection.
         a. Based on preoperative cultures.
         b. Expected organisms including gram-negative flora and enterococci (Table 5.1).
   ii. Maintain high tissue levels of antibiotic for the **duration** of procedure.

Table 5.1. Prophylactic antibiotic recommendations for the intestine and biliary system.

Surgery	Organism	Antibiotic	Penicillin allergic
Gastroduodenal	Gram-negative (GN) bacilli, streptococci, oropharyngeal anaerobes	First- or second-generation cephalosporin (e.g., cefazolin, cefotetan)	Fluoroquinolones and flagyl
Biliary	GN bacilli anaerobes	Cefazolin + flagyl Cefoxitin or Cefotetan	Fluoroquinolones and flagyl
Colorectal and appendix	GN bacilli anaerobes	Cefazolin + flagyl Cefoxitin or Cefotetan	Fluoroquinolones and flagyl

1. Based on the half-life of the antibiotic and duration of the procedure.
    a. Goal is to attain sufficient plasma and tissue levels before breaching the skin (within 2 hours).
    b. May require intraoperative dosing to maintain adequate levels throughout the operation depending on the half-life of the antibiotic chosen.
    c. A general recommendation is to repeat the dose of antibiotics if the surgery exceeds 4 hours.

iii. Course.
1. Prophylaxis (no established infection).
    a. No evidence to support postoperative use. A single preoperative dose is as effective.
        i. May have higher wound infection rates with increased duration of antibiotic therapy.
2. Contamination (intraoperative as well as trauma related):
    a. No evidence to support increased duration of therapy (24 hours as effective as 5 days).
3. Infection. For established infection such as perforated appendicitis or diverticulitis.
    a. Unclear if specific duration is appropriate. Traditional recommendations are being evaluated.
        i. May be based on clinical factors.
            1. Presence of temperature and leukocytosis.
            2. CT or USG (ultrasonography) evidence for collection or abscess.

III. Adjuncts to Parenteral Antibiotics

a. Bowel preparation.
    i. Common practice in cases of intestinal surgery, especially colon. Goal is to decrease the bacterial load of the colon.
        1. Mechanical "gut lavage."
            a. Many agents available.
            b. Recent data suggest it may be unnecessary and may increase infectious complication rates.
                i. Present recommendation/standard of care remains to perform bowel preparation.
        2. Oral antibiotics.
            a. Administration.
                i. Spectrum to include gram-negative and anaerobic organisms.
                ii. Given after gut lavage to prevent being washed out.

iii. Generally given as three divided doses.
b. Effectiveness.
i. Studies conflicting as to necessity when parenteral antibiotics are given. There appears to be a small advantage to administering both.
ii. High rate of intolerance and vomiting.
b. Antibiotic irrigation.
i. Intraperitoneal.
1. Very few data regarding outcomes. No evidence that there is a significant decrease in wound and intra-abdominal infections.
2. Increased rate of adhesion formation possibly.
ii. Wound.
1. Very few data.
2. May interfere with local wound inflammatory factors.

Selected References

Bailly P, Lallemand S, Thouverez M, Talon D. Multicentre study on the appropriateness of surgical antibiotic prophylaxis. J Hosp Infect 2001;49:135–138.

Balague Ponz C, Trias M. Laparoscopic surgery and surgical infection. J Chemother 2001; 13(Spec No 1):17–22.

Bozorgzadeh A, Pizzi WF, Barie PS, et al. The duration of antibiotic administration in penetrating abdominal trauma. Am J Surg 1999;177:125–131.

Colizza S, Rossi S. Antibiotic prophylaxis and treatment of surgical abdominal sepsis. J Chemother 2001;13(Spec No 1):193–201.

Esposito S. Is single-dose antibiotic prophylaxis sufficient for any surgical procedure? J Chemother 1999;11:556–564.

Farber MS, Abrams JH. Antibiotics for the acute abdomen. Surg Clin N Am 1997;77: 1395–1417.

Gilbert DN, Moellering RC, Sande MA. The Sanford Guide to Antimicrobial Therapy. Hyde Park, VT: Sanford Antimicrobial Therapy, Inc., 2002.

Gorecki P, Schein M, Rucinski JC, Wise L. Antibiotic administration in patients undergoing common surgical procedures in a community teaching hospital: the chaos continues. World J Surg 1999;23:429–432.

Lewis RT. Oral versus systemic antibiotic prophylaxis in elective colon surgery: a randomized study and meta-analysis send a message from the 1990s. Can J Surg 2002; 45:173–180.

Novelli A. Antimicrobial prophylaxis in surgery: the role of pharmacokinetics. J Chemother 1999;11:565–572.

Platell C, Hall JC. The prevention of wound infection in patients undergoing colorectal surgery. J Hosp Infect 2001;49:233–238.

Rappaport WD, Holcomb M, Valente J, Chvapil M. Antibiotic irrigation and the formation of intraabdominal adhesions. Am J Surg 1989;158:435–437.

Scher KS. Studies on the duration of antibiotic administration for surgical prophylaxis. Am Surg 1997;63:59–62.

Scott JD, Forrest A, Feuerstein S, Fitzpatrick P, Schentag JJ. Factors associated with post-operative infection. Infect Control Hosp Epidemiol 2001;22:347–351 [abstract].

Soffer D, Zait S, Klausner J, Kluger Y. Peritoneal cultures and antibiotic treatment in patients with perforated appendicitis. Eur J Surg 2001;167:214–216.

Turano A. New clinical data on the prophylaxis of infections in abdominal, gynecologic, and urologic surgery. Multicenter Study Group. Am J Surg 1992;164:16S–20S.

Part II
Intraoperative Management, Positioning, Setup, and Port Placement

Introduction to Part II: Introductory Remarks Concerning Operating Room Setup, Patient Positioning, and Port Placement Chapters

Richard L. Whelan, M.D.

A. Operating Room Setup and Patient Positioning

Not surprisingly, there is more than one way to set up the operating room and to position a patient for a given operation. It was the editor's intention to be inclusive and to present alternatives where such variety was found. It is important to realize that, in regard to operating room equipment, the available tools and resources in each hospital and, indeed, in each operating room vary. Operating rooms that are fully dedicated to minimally invasive surgery have four or five monitors that allow the surgeons to work in all four quadrants without having to move any of the monitors, booms, or towers. Furthermore, "flat screen" monitors can be easily moved without disrupting the overall operating room setup. Unfortunately, most laparoscopic surgery is not carried out in such rooms.

The majority of operating rooms have two laparoscopic monitors that are mounted on towers (on wheels) or booms. The insufflator, image processor, light source, and video recorder are usually located on one of the towers. Given these resources, when performing procedures that require working in two or more quadrants of the abdomen, it is usually necessary to move one or both towers at some point during the case. More planning is required when working under these circumstances than for a case in a room with four or more monitors. The surgeon needs to determine the order of the operation when performing a multiquadrant procedure and position the towers accordingly at the start of the case. The tower and monitor position will vary from one type of procedure to another. The operative plan should be shared with the scrub nurse, circulating nurse, and the anesthesiologist so that all can position their equipment so as to facilitate the surgery.

The purpose of the chapters that follow is to provide one or several ways to arrange the equipment and table for each specific case. The assumption has been made that each operating room has a total of two monitors. The major pieces of equipment are included in the diagrams; however, some items (suction, cautery, calf compression stocking machine) have been left out to make the drawings less cluttered and easier to understand. Although it was our goal to present several room setup alternatives, it was not possible, in some cases, to include all the possible options.

In regard to patient positioning, for a fair number of advanced procedures, the operation can be carried out with the patient in one of several positions. As examples, in the case of colectomy or antireflux surgery some surgeons place the patient in the supine position while others prefer the modified lithotomy position. The latter position allows the surgeon or assistant to stand between the legs, thereby providing an alternative vantage point from which they can dissect or retract. This decision, for colectomy or antireflux procedures, usually does not influence port positioning. There are other advanced procedures, however, such as nephrectomy or adrenalectomy, where significantly different port positioning schemes accompany each body position option. The different body positions in these instances are usually quite dissimilar, for example, supine versus lateral decubitus. Similar to operating room setup, an attempt has been made to be as inclusive as possible in regard to patient positioning.

B. Port Placement Schemes

It is important to realize that there are numerous reasonable port placement schemes for each different laparoscopic procedure. The number of ports utilized for each operation also varies from surgeon to surgeon. The factors that influence the number of ports that are required for a given advanced procedure include the patient's body habitus, the condition of the intraabdominal operative field (i.e., presence of adhesions, inflammation, atypical anatomy, etc.), the pathology, the specific operative technique utilized, and the experience of the surgeon and the assistants. Whether an assistant is to be taught how to perform the case in question is yet another important variable that influences the number of ports used in a given case; this issue is further discussed below. As a general rule most surgeons try to keep ports at least four fingerbreadths apart to prevent "sword fighting."

1. Body Habitus Considerations: The distance from the xiphoid process to the pubic symphysis varies widely, as does the width of the anterior abdominal wall, from patient to patient. In patients with a small overall abdominal wall surface area it is usually possible via a single port location to reach and work in all four quadrants. However, in a patient with a lengthy and wide abdomen, a port placed in the inferior aspect of a lower quadrant will not provide access to the more cephalad reaches of the upper quadrants. Therefore, in cases that require dissection in two or three quadrants, the port placement scheme needs to be adjusted, and/or extra ports may be needed to complete the procedure. (This occasionally is the case when taking down the splenic flexure during a sphincter-saving rectal resection.)

In depicting port placement schemes, a generic abdominal wall drawing is invariably used. Although this drawing will apply to most patients, if it is followed in patients with significantly greater abdominal wall surface area the ports will not be ideally situated. In patients with a lengthier and wider abdominal wall, the entire port placement arrangement will need to be shifted either cephalad or caudad toward the principal target quadrants. In contrast, in patients with a small abdominal wall surface area the short distance between the costal margin and the anterior superior iliac spine will leave the surgeon few choices as to where the lateral ports can go if they are to be positioned lateral to the rectus muscle and kept a reasonable distance apart. In these latter patients, regardless of a cephalad or caudad target quadrant the ports will likely be similarly positioned. In many of the ensuing chapters, a given port arrangement is depicted for three different body habitus: small, medium (average), and large anterior abdominal wall surface area patients. Figure I.1 shows a port placement scheme for a right hemicolectomy and demonstrates how the precise port positions vary based on body habitus. In this instance, the 10-mm periumbilical camera port in a small patient is best placed below the umbilicus whereas in a bigger patient with a longer and broader abdominal wall this port should be well above the umbilicus. Likewise, the proximity of the midline infraumbilical 5-mm port to the pubic symphysis also varies considerably from the petite to the large and broad abdominal wall; in the latter the port is far closer to the umbilicus than to the symphysis.

In regard to assessing a given patient relative to their body habitus, it is instructive to note the volume of gas needed to fully insufflate the abdomen after placement of the first port or Veress needle. Patients in whom only a relatively small volume of gas is required to reach the target pressure almost always have a small surface area abdomen whereas those that require a large volume of CO_2 to fully insufflate are likely to have a broad or long abdominal wall. This piece of information is useful to note and take into account when choosing port positions.

The port location arrangements for a number of advanced procedures are given in relation to the costal margin. Antireflux and morbid obesity procedures as well as nephrectomy and adrenalectomy are examples of such procedures. In these procedures, body habitus differences have less impact on the port arrangement than for an operation such as colectomy. Therefore, in the ensuing chapters, for the costal margin-based port arrangements, only a single generic body drawing is provided.

The relative position of the umbilicus in relation to the xiphoid process and the pubic symphysis varies considerably from patient to patient; the umbilicus is not always located midway between these two points. In the majority of patients the umbilicus is located within 1 to 2 cm of the midpoint between the xiphoid process and the umbilicus. However, in heavier patients the umbilicus is usually more caudally located; in some patients it may be as much as 9 cm off the midpoint (Figure II.1). Rarely, the umbilicus is located above the midpoint. When transcribing a port placement arrangement from a book or chapter there is a tendency to use the umbilicus as a main reference point. If a given port pattern is reproduced faithfully on a patient with a low-riding umbilicus for an operation where the target quadrants are in the upper abdomen, then the central periumbilical port will be poorly placed to serve as the camera port (see Figure II.2). Therefore, the surgeon must take into account the umbilical position before placing the ports. If the umbilicus is very low then the proper position for the "periumbilical" port may be 4–5 cm cephalad to the umbilicus.

It is recommended that, before choosing the port locations, the surgeon measure with a ruler the distance from the xiphoid process to the midpoint of the umbilicus as well as the distance from the pubis to the umbilicus. These measurements will provide an idea as to the overall length of the abdomen and the relative position of the umbilicus (midpoint or low- or high riding). The surgeon must also identify the target quadrant(s) and then place the ports accordingly.

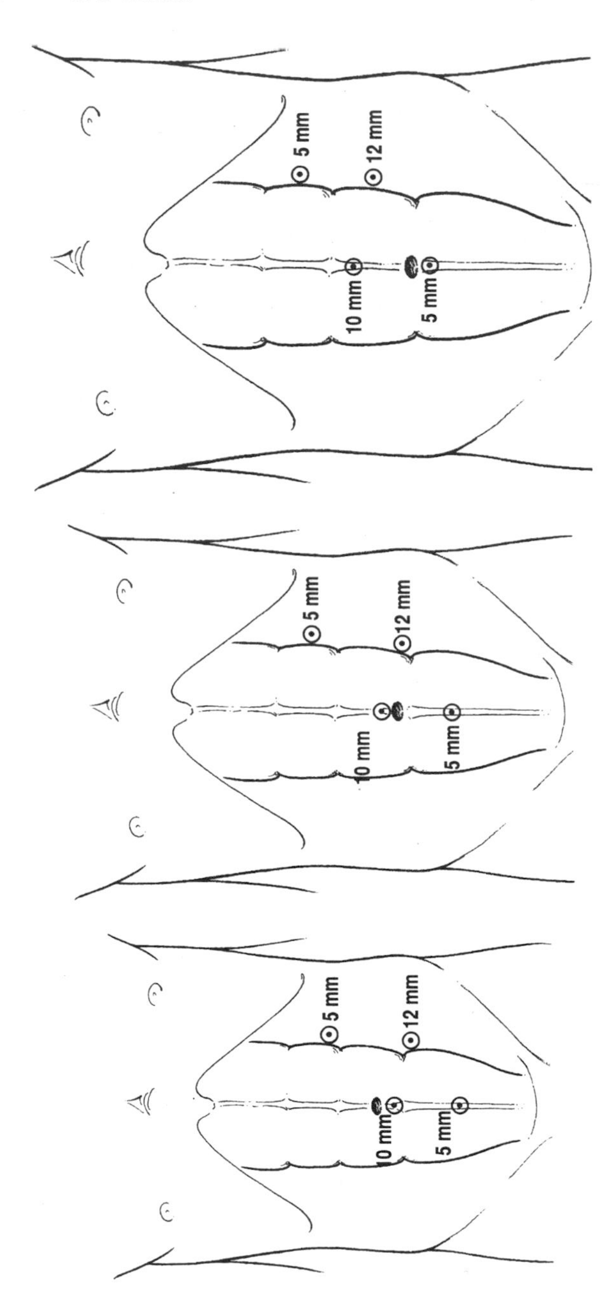

Figure II.1. Impact of body size on port placement for right hemicolectomy. The position of the ports in relation to the umbilicus and the pubic symphysis changes substantially from the small body habitus to the larger and broader abdominal wall. Note that the port locations shift cephalad, toward the target quadrant, in this case the right upper quadrant (hepatic flexure).

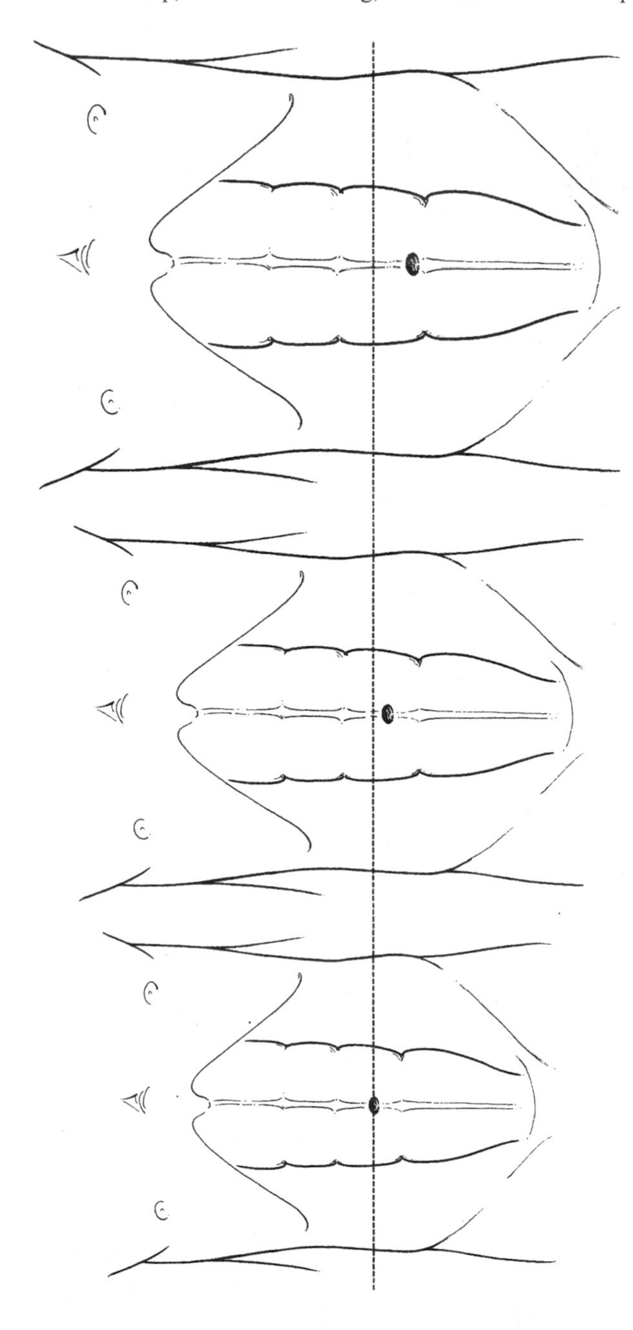

Figure II.2. These drawings demonstrate that, as stature and weight increase [and with increasing body mass index (BMI)], the position of the umbilicus, in relation to the midpoints between the xiphoid process and the pubic symphysis, shifts caudally. The umbilicus should not be used as a landmark for the midpoint between the xiphoid and the pubic symphysis.

Small bowel retraction may also be quite difficult in obese patients or in patients in whom the small bowel is distended. In patients in whom retraction of the small bowel proves difficult, it may be necessary to place an additional port so as to permit the use of an additional retractor.

2. Previous Surgery: A history of prior surgery as evidenced to by one or more abdominal scars often influences port placement. A preexisting midline scar that involves the periumbilical area prompts most surgeons to place their initial port off the midline. The finding of moderate or severe adhesions will dictate where the first few working ports are placed. As adhesiolysis is accomplished and the operative field enlarged it may be possible to revert to a more standard port placement scheme. Therefore, adhesions may mandate placement of one or more ports that would otherwise not be required.

3. Operative Team Considerations: In regard to the surgical team, if a resident or fellow is being taught advanced laparoscopic methods then it is important that they have two ports to work with so that they learn "two-handed technique." In this situation, especially if the resident is inexperienced, the teaching surgeon often also needs two ports so that she or he can guide the trainee through the procedure; therefore, a total of five ports would be needed. Consequently, for operations that can be done with four ports by an experienced team, in the teaching setting it is more likely that an extra port may be needed. Three-port methods are also feasible for some advanced procedures, provided the surgeon is sufficiently skilled and experienced. However, three-port methods do not allow for a first assistant, assuming the surgeon uses two hands, and thus are not conducive to teaching. Because the intent of this manual is to facilitate the training of surgeons, with few exceptions, three-port arrangements have not been included. By and large, four- and five-port methods are described in the chapters that follow.

4. Laparoscopic-Assisted Operations: In the case of laparoscopically assisted procedures, in which a portion of the case is done extracorporeally, there is a greater variety of port placement schemes in regard to both location of ports and the number of ports used. The extent to which a procedure is completed intracorporeally can influence the number of ports required. In general, the greater the intracorporeal component the more ports that will be required. In the case of a laparoscopically assisted colectomy, if the bowel is mobilized intracorporeally but is devascularized, resected, and reanastomosed extracorporeally, it may be feasible to do the case with three or four ports. However, if intracorporeal devascularization and bowel division is to be accomplished in the training setting, then it is more likely that five ports will be needed.

It was our goal to present the reader with a variety of port placement schemes for each operation with a brief description of how the operation can be carried out for each particular port arrangement. Unfortunately, it is impossible to include every arrangement that has been suggested or utilized.

5. Telescope Diameter: In many cases it is possible to complete an advanced laparoscopic case using a 5-mm telescope; however, the majority of surgeons utilize 10-mm telescopes. In the following chapters, unless otherwise stated, the assumption has been made that a 10-mm telescope will be utilized for all advanced cases.

6. Lateral Abdominal Ports: As a general rule, it is best to place off-midline ports beyond the lateral edge of the rectus muscle to avoid injuring the epigastric vessels. This is especially important in the lower abdominal quadrants. The majority of the port positions presented in this manual adhere to this principle; however, some do not. Specifically, the port arrangements for antireflux, gastric bypass, adrenalectomy, and nephrectomy procedures, which utilize, predominantly, the upper abdomen, include intrarectus ports. The surgeons performing these procedures do not hesitate to place ports within the rectus muscle although they do make an effort to locate and avoid the epigastric vessels by transilluminating the abdominal wall.

6. Intraoperative Management of the Laparoscopic Patient

Carol E.H. Scott-Conner, M.D.

A. Choice of Anesthesia and Monitoring of the Laparoscopic Patient

1. Because most laparoscopic surgery is done on an ambulatory or short-stay basis, these specific goals should be remembered:
   a. Prevent postoperative nausea and vomiting (PONV). Prophylactic antiemetic agents work best when administered at the appropriate time during surgery.
      1. For example, ondansetron (4 mg I.V.) is most effective when given immediately before the end of the laparoscopic procedure.
      2. Dexamethasone at a dose of 10 mg I.V. is also effective in preventing PONV.
      3. The combination of tropisetron and metoclopramide has been shown to be superior to metoclopramide alone in preventing PONV postoperatively.
   b. Rapid emergence from anesthesia.
   c. Minimal postoperative pain.
2. Laparoscopic surgery has been successfully performed under local, regional, and general anesthesia. Choice of anesthetic modality is influenced by patient and practitioner preference, the physical status of the patient, the nature of the planned surgical procedure, and the physiologic alterations associated with pneumoperitoneum. Most laparoscopic surgery is quite appropriately performed under general endotracheal anesthesia. Diagnostic laparoscopy and some brief laparoscopic procedures (e.g., laparoscopic gastrostomy) may be performed under local anesthesia. Although the use of regional anesthesia has been described, the authors of this section do not advocate it. Each modality is described here and specific considerations for laparoscopic surgery explored.
   a. **Local anesthesia.** Simple diagnostic laparoscopy and some brief laparoscopic procedures may be performed under local anesthesia. Attention must be paid to some technical points for this approach to be successful. Local anesthesia is contraindicated for the uncooperative patient, when a prolonged procedure is planned, or if the patient is allergic to local anesthetics.
      i. Raise a **skin wheal** at the initial puncture site.

ii. **Infiltrate** a cone down to the peritoneal level, including generous infiltration of the peritoneum. The pain of injection is less intense with ropivacaine than with bupivacaine.
iii. **Make the skin incision.** The Veress needle is next inserted. Ask the patient to contract their abdominal wall muscles to provide resistance to the Veress needle. Alternatively, make an open cut down and then insert a Hasson-type cannula.
iv. **Insufflate slowly** and work with thc lowcst pressure pneumoperitoneum that will permit the performance of the procedure. If possible, the insufflation pressure should be less than 10–12 mm Hg.
v. **Reflex bradycardia** may occur, necessitating desufflation or treatment with atropine.
vi. Infiltrate the second and any additional port sites required for the procedure with local anesthetic to the peritoneal level under direct vision. Raise a wheal above the peritoneum by injecting local anesthesia into the preperitoneal space.
vii. Sedative or hypnotic agents used to produce amnesia or decrease awareness may depress respiration and diminish protective airway responses. These agents potentiate the dangers of hypercapnia and aspiration inherent with pneumoperitoneum in the absence of definitive airway control. **Deep sedation** exists when the patient cannot be easily aroused but does respond purposefully following repeated or painful stimuli. In this situation, the patient's ability to independently maintain ventilatory function may be impaired and protective airway reflexes may be lost.

b. **Regional anesthesia** may be an appropriate technique for brief laparoscopic procedures that can be performed with lower insufflation pressures. However, numerous difficulties can occur with regional anesthesia in this setting. First, interventional laparoscopy requires a high level of sensory block (T4–T5). Regional anesthesia to this level also produces significant sympathetic blockade, which may result in hypotension. Breathing difficulties due to a high block may cause considerable discomfort in an awake patient whose diaphragm is already stretched and elevated because of the pneumoperitoneum. Laparoscopic procedures often require that the patient be placed in fairly steep Trendelenburg or reverse Trendelenburg position. These positions may cause cardiovascular instability in a patient whose hemodynamic compensatory mechanisms are limited because of the sympathectomy associated with regional anesthesia. Also, the Trendelenburg position further increases the pressure on the diaphragms and makes respiration more difficult. The **successful use of a regional anesthetic** (spinal or epidural anesthesia) depends on:
i. **Patient acceptance.**
ii. The **absence of contraindications**, which include:

a) Hypovolemia
b) Bleeding disorders
c) Infection close to one of the proposed port sites
d) Peripheral neurologic disease
e) Allergy to the local anesthetic agent
f) Severe pulmonary disease

iii. The **duration** of the procedure.

iv. The **skill and expertise** of the surgeon and anesthesiologist.

c. **General anesthesia with a cuffed endotracheal (ET)** tube protects the airway and also permits the anesthetist to compensate for hypercapnia by adjusting the respirator settings. Specific considerations when laparoscopy is performed under general anesthesia include:

i. **Airway protection with an ET tube** is important because high intraabdominal pressure may cause reflux of gastric contents and lead to aspiration. A face mask or laryngeal mask airway may be adequate for short diagnostic procedures (done under a low-pressure pneumoperitoneum) being carried out by surgeons with considerable experience. A history of hiatal hernia or gastroesophageal reflux is an absolute contraindication to the administration of general anesthesia unless a cuffed endotracheal tube is employed.

ii. **Hypercapnia is anticipated when a CO_2 pneumoperitoneum is utilized.** CO_2 is readily absorbed via the peritoneal surfaces. Hypercapnia causes acidosis and is associated with epinephrine release. In normal individuals, by increasing the respiratory rate, inspiratory pressure, and/or increasing the tidal volume it is almost always possible to lower the levels of CO_2 in the blood to normal levels.

iii. **Muscle relaxation** is obtained by using nondepolarizing agents in addition to establishing and maintaining an adequate depth of anesthesia. The choice of muscle relaxants depends on the length of surgery and the medical condition of the patient. Inadequate muscle relaxation will limit the exposure provided by the pneumoperitoneum. The greater the relaxation, the larger the intraabdominal working space will be.

iv. The use of **nitrous oxide** is controversial. Recent blinded studies suggest no difference in bowel distension with and without nitrous oxide. However, it is reasonable to discontinue nitrous oxide if the intraabdominal viscera are noted to be distended. Nitrous oxide levels may reach concentrations that support combustion within the bowel lumen and, therefore, under rare circumstances, has the potential to explode (Table 6.1).

3. Preoperative evaluation by a qualified anesthesia provider is required before regional or general anesthesia. This preoperative evaluation includes assessment of the ASA (American Society of

Table 6.1. Advantages and disadvantages of anesthetic modalities, with examples of laparoscopic applications.

Anesthetic modality	Advantages	Disadvantages	Examples of laparoscopic applications
Local anesthesia	• Effect limited to site of injection. • Residual analgesia if long-acting agents infiltrated. • Minimal nausea and vomiting.	• No control of airway. • Pain due to pneumoperitoneum is not blocked. • Cardiovascular reflexes are not blocked.	• Diagnostic laparoscopy. • Tubal ligation. • Laparoscopic gastrostomy.
Regional anesthesia	• Muscle relaxation. • Analgesia.	• No compensation for hypercapnia. • No control of airway. • Change in patient position may affect level of block. • Cardiovascular instability. • Recovery period. • Urinary retention. • No compensation for hypercapnia.	• Diagnostic laparoscopy. • Tubal ligation.
General anesthesia	• Control of airway. • Muscle relaxation. • Analgesia. • Loss of awareness. • Amnesia.	• Recovery period. • Postoperative nausea and vomiting. • No residual analgesic effect at site of surgery unless supplemented by local infiltration of long-acting agents.	This modality is applicable to all laparoscopic procedures, including advanced laparoscopy.

Table 6.2. The ASA Physical Status Classification System.

P1	A normal healthy patient
P2	A patient with mild systemic disease
P3	A patient with severe systemic disease
P4	A patient with severe systemic disease that is a constant threat to life
P5	A moribund patient who is not expected to survive without the operation
P6	A declared brain-dead patient whose organs are being removed for donor purposes

Source: The ASA Physical Status Classification System. http://www.asahq.org/ProfInfo/PhysicalStatus.html (Reference 1).

Anesthesiologists) physical status category (Table 6.2) as well as a more specific assessment that is outlined in Table 6.3. A discussion of the planned anesthetic modality is also included.

   a. Deep sedation (as defined above) requires the same preoperative evaluation, intraoperative monitoring, and postoperative recovery as general anesthesia.
   b. Procedures performed under local anesthesia with adjunctive use of high doses of sedating agents are, in fact, considered as risky as general anesthesia.

4. Intraoperative monitoring. Basic ASA monitors include:
   a. Breath sounds (precordial or esophageal stethoscope)
   b. Electrocardiogram (continuous)
   c. Blood pressure, pulse (continuous, noninvasive)
   d. Continuous oxygen saturation (pulse oximeter)
   e. Expired carbon dioxide (capnograph)
   f. Temperature

Table 6.3. Preoperative evaluation for laparoscopic surgery.

Systems affected by pneumoperitoneum
- Airway
- Respiratory system
- Cardiovascular system

Other relevant systems
- Central nervous system
- Endocrine system
- Gastrointestinal system

Other relevant history
- Past anesthetic experience
- Past anesthetic family history
- Allergies (particularly to local anesthetics)
- Medications

5. Other monitoring may be warranted depending on the general condition of the patient and the complexity of the procedure.
   a. Invasive monitoring may be used for patients with severe cardiopulmonary disease and those undergoing more complex procedures.
      i. Arterial catheter
      ii. Central venous line for measurement of the central venous pressure (CVP)
      iii. Swann–Ganz catheter
         a. An indwelling bladder catheter and a nasogastric tube are important for bladder and stomach decompression. Catheterization of the bladder and stomach are routinely performed in almost all laparoscopic cases. This practice deceases the chances of operative injury to the urinary bladder and stomach.
6. The anesthetist must be prepared to respond to the detrimental physiologic changes associated with pneumoperitoneum (Table 6.4).

Table 6.4. Physiologic changes associated with pneumoperitoneum and their implications for anesthesia management.

Change	Physiologic consequence	Implication for management
Elevation of diaphragm	• Decreased functional residual capacity • Increased ventilation-perfusion mismatch • Increased intrapulmonary shunting • Increased alveolar-arterial gradient	Increase mechanical ventilation and fraction of inspired oxygen
Decreased venous return with increased cardiac filling pressures	• Initial decrease in cardiac index, followed by increase due to circulating catecholamines • Cardiac axis of heart shifts, causing electrocardiographic alterations	Adequate volume load
Carbon dioxide load	• CO_2 absorbed by peritoneum must be excreted by lungs • Respiratory acidosis if CO_2 not adequately eliminated	Increase mechanical ventilation

a. **Signs of deteriorating cardiopulmonary function** include:
   i. Gradual or sudden drop in systemic blood pressure
   ii. Increasing difficulty in maintaining a normal blood pressure
   iii. Decreased pulse oximetry values
   iv. The pulse may increase, decrease, or remain the same in the face of deteriorating cardiopulmonary function
b. **Hypercapnia** is usually due to venous absorption of CO_2 from the abdominal cavity. However, the pneumoperitoneum-related complication of pneumothorax may also result in hypercapnia. Also, accidental main-stem bronchial intubation (endotracheal tube inserted too far) when combined with increased peak airway pressures may cause bronchial injury, pneumothorax, or pneumomediastinum, which can also result in hypercapnia.
c. **Hypoxia** may result from main-stem bronchus intubations, pneumothorax, atelectasis in the lung bases, venous carbon dioxide embolism, or pulmonary edema.
d. **Tachycardia and hypertension.** Hypoxia, hypercapnia, and inadequate ("light") anesthesia must be ruled out first. Tachycardia and hypertension may then be treated with increasing increments of esmolol (short-acting beta blocker) or labetalol (a mixed alpha and beta blocker).
e. Serious intraoperative problems include:
   i. **CO_2 embolism**: This serious complication is diagnosed by a sudden decrease in end-expired CO_2 partial pressure and a rapid decrease in pulse oximetry values. Despite the fact that CO_2 is highly soluble in plasma, this may be a life-threatening complication if the volume of intravascular gas is large. Precordial doppler monitoring and transesophageal echocardiography are very sensitive monitors of intravascular gas but are not routinely used during laparoscopy. Their use might be considered when it is anticipated that during the course of the surgery a large raw area will be exposed to high gas pressures or when the surgical field is vascular in a hypovolemic patient.
   ii. **Pneumothorax:** The diagnosis is made by the finding of a sudden increase in airway pressure, desaturation, and increase in end-expiratory values of CO_2 partial pressures.
   iii. **Main-stem bronchus intubations** may occur if the tip of the endotracheal tube is close to the carina. Pneumoperitoneum will shift the diaphragm and tracheobronchial tree cephalad. Thus, in the setting of a pneumothorax, the tip of the endotracheal tube, previously in the distal trachea, may be found in a main-stem bronchus.
   iv. **Other complications** include subcutaneous emphysema and facial and airway swelling (if the patient was kept in Trendelenburg position for prolonged periods of time).

References

1. The ASA Physical Status Classification System. http://www.asahq.org/ProfInfo/PhysicalStatus.html.
2. Krishnan SK, Benzon HT, Siddiqui T, Canlas B. Pain on intramuscular injection of bupivacaine, ropivacaine, with and without dexamethasone. Reg Anesth Pain Med 2000;25:615–619.
3. Liu YH, Li MJ, Wang PC, et al. Use of dexamethasone on the prophylaxis of nausea and vomiting after tympanomastoid surgery. Laryngoscope 2001;111:1271–1274.
4. Lobato EB, Glen BP, Brown MM, Bennett B, Davis JD. Pneumoperitoneum as a risk factor for endobronchial intubation during laproscopic gynecological surgery. Anesth Analg 1998;86:301–303.
5. Loughney AD, Sarma V, Ryall EA. Intraperitoneal bupivacaine for the relief of pain following day case laparoscopy. Br J Obstet Gynaecol 1994;101(5):449–451.
6. Michaloliachou C, Chung F, Sharma S. Preoperative multimodal anesthesia facilitates recovery after ambulatory laparoscopic cholecystectomy. Anesth Analg 1996;82: 44–51.
7. Micali S, Jarrett TW, Pappa P, Taccone Gallucci M, Virgili G, Vespasiani G. Efficacy of epidural anesthesia for retroperitoneoscopic renal biopsy. Urology 2000;55:590.
8. Neuman GG, Sidebotham G, Negoianu E, et al. Laparoscopy explosion hazards with nitrous oxide. Anesthesiology 1993;78(5):875–879.
9. Nishanian E, Goudsouzian NG. Carbon dioxide embolism during hip arthrography in an infant. Anesth Analg 1998;86:299–300.
10. Palter SF. Office microlaparoscopy under local anesthesia. Obstet Gynecol Clin N Am 1999;26:109–120.
11. Papadimitriou L, Livanios S, Katsaros G, et al. Prevention of postoperative nausea and vomiting after laparoscopic gynaecological surgery. Combined antiemetic treatment with tropisetron and metoclopramide versus metoclopramide alone. Eur J Anaesthesiol 2001;18:615–619.
12. Puri GD, Singh H. Ventilatory effects of laparoscopy under general anesthesia. Br J Anaesth 1992;68:211–213.
13. Tang J, Wang B, White P, Watcha MH, Qi J, Wender RH. The effect of timing of ondansetron on its efficacy, cost-effectiveness, and cost-benefit as a prophylactic antiemetic in the ambulatory setting. Anesth Analg 1998;86:274–282.
14. Tatlor E, Feinstein R, White PF, Soper N. Anesthesia for laparoscopic cholecystectomy: is nitrous oxide contraindicated? Anesthesiology 1992;76:541–543.
15. Wahba RW, Beique F, Kleiman SJ. Cardiopulmonary functions and laparoscopic cholecystectomy [Review]. Can J Anaesth 1995;42(1):51–63.
16. Wittgen CM, Andrus CH, Fizgerald SD, Baundendistel LJ, Dahms TE, Kaminski DL. Analysis of the hemodynamic and ventilatory effects of laparoscopic cholecystectomy. Arch Surg 1991;126:997–1001.

7. Summary of Intraoperative Physiologic Alterations Associated with Laparoscopic Surgery

Arif Ahmad, M.D., F.R.C.S. Eng., Edin.
Bruce D. Schirmer, M.D., F.A.C.S.

The physiologic impact of laparoscopic surgery, which is not synonymous with the physiology of pneumoperitoneum, includes the following:

1. Effect of the reduced tissue trauma by minimal access techniques, which is salutary.
2. Physiologic implications of CO_2 pneumoperitoneum, which are largely deleterious.

The laparoscopic surgeon must be aware of the physiologic consequences of laparoscopic surgery and the potential risks of pneumoperitoneum, which are traded for the benefits of minimal access techniques.

An understanding of the physiologic impact of laparoscopic surgery on the body's various systems is necessary to accurately assess and describe the risks that prospective laparoscopic surgical patients face. This knowledge becomes even more important when considering patients with significant cardiopulmonary disease or other comorbidities.

The CO_2 pneumoperitoneum exerts its physiologic effects via two different mechanisms:

1. Mechanical effects relating to increased intraperitoneal pressure.
2. Chemical effect of the gas used for insufflation, which presently in most cases is CO_2.

A. Neuroendocrine, Metabolic, and Immunologic Implications

Minimal access surgery aims to achieve correction of the disease process with a minimum of abdominal wall trauma in obtaining access to the site of the problem. Although not always synonymous with minimally invasive surgery, in most situations it is associated with a lesser magnitude of surgical injury than the equivalent traditional "open" procedure.

The metabolic response to trauma depends on the magnitude of the injury and the response of the organism to it. The neuroendocrine response and the metabolic consequences of surgery are blunted when the magnitude of injury is curtailed by minimal access techniques. The differences between open and minimal access methods are most obvious in cases in which the standard abdominal wall incision is more traumatic than the injury incurred in removing the offending organ, as in the case of cholecystectomy.

Interleukin 6 (IL-6), C-reactive protein, and leukocytosis have all been shown to be lower after laparoscopic cholecystectomy when compared to results after open cholecystectomy. This is thought to be a consequence of the limited abdominal wall injury associated with minimal access methods. Although some studies have shown lower cortisol levels after laparoscopic cholecystectomy, the majority have shown no difference in cortisol levels. Similarly, no differences in cortisol levels have been noted when patients undergoing open and laparoscopic-assisted colon resections are compared.

Immunologic implications. Systemic cell-mediated immunity is better preserved after laparoscopic procedures; this has been attributed to diminished abdominal wall trauma and to avoidance of air exposure in the peritoneal cavity. In laparoscopic cholecystectomy and colectomy patients, delayed-type hypersensitivity has been shown to be better preserved after the closed procedures than after the equivalent open procedure. Short-lived significant differences in the ratio of Th-1 and Th-2 lymphocytes have also been noted in one study of cholecystectomy patients.

Intraperitoneal cell-mediated immunity, however, appears to be impaired by pneumoperitoneum. The exact mechanism of intraperitoneal immunosuppression is unclear. Some studies have implicated CO_2 pneumoperitoneum in the impairment of intraperitoneal immunity. Macrophages incubated in CO_2 produced significantly less IL-2 and tumor necrosis factor (TNF) than those incubated in air or helium.

B. Cardiovascular Implications

Hemodynamic Changes

Both the mechanical (i.e., pressure-related) and the CO_2 absorption-related effects of CO_2 pneumoperitoneum impact the cardiovascular system.

1. **Tachycardia** is secondary to increased sympathetic discharge, hypercarbia, and impaired venous return from the abdomen and lower extremities.
2. There is an increase in the measured central venous pressure and pulmonary artery wedge pressure. These changes are artifactual and are secondary to the transmission of increased pressure from the abdomen to the mediastinum and chest. Direct measurements actually show a decrease in cardiac chamber filling and decreased venous return. Thus, there is an increase in measured preload but a decrease in actual preload. This causes a slight decrease in cardiac output. Preoperative hydration may attenuate the reduction in preload caused by pneumoperitoneum.
3. The afterload is also increased secondary to increased systemic vascular resistance (SVR) from compensatory vasoconstriction due to neurohumoral mechanisms and direct aortic compression from insufflation. Hypercarbia also possibly contributes to the vasoconstriction.

4. **Mean arterial pressure (MAP) may increase, decrease,** or remain unchanged depending on the relative effect of the pneumoperitoneum on SVR and CO. The hydration status of the patient influences the magnitude of the cardiovascular changes observed during minimally invasive procedures.

Dysrhythmias

Disturbances of the heart rhythm during minimally invasive procedures are common; they occur in 25%–47% of cases. Causes include hypercarbia, acidosis, sympathetic stimulation from decreased venous return, and vagal stimulation from stretching of the peritoneum. Moderate to severe hypercarbia can result in premature ventricular contractions (PVC), ventricular tachycardia (VT), and ventricular fibrillation. Bradyarrhythmias may occur from vagal stimulation.

Visceral Blood Flow

Blood flow to the viscera is reduced with intraabdominal pressures (IAP) of 15–20 mmHg, independent of the type of gas used for insufflation. The elevated intraabdominal pressure-related increase in SVR results in reduced visceral blood flow. The vasoconstrictive effect of CO_2 also causes reduced visceral blood flow. The clinical significance of diminished blood flow to the viscera during the procedure remains unclear.

Impact of Patient Position on Cardiopulmonary Function

Reverse Trendelenburg position:

1. Pooling of blood in the lower extremities increases hemostasis (arrest of circulation), and predisposes to deep venous thrombosis (DVT).
2. Decrease in cardiac preload occurs, due to decreased venous return secondary to the factor just mentioned. This may predispose to hypotension, especially in the setting of poor hydration or inadequate volume replacement.
3. Pulmonary function tends to improve in this position due to the caudad shift of the viscera and decreased pressure on the diaphragm. As a result, tidal volume usually increases.

Trendelenburg position:

1. Increase in preload due to increased venous return from the lower extremities and abdomen.
2. The detrimental pulmonary function changes associated with CO_2 pneumoperitoneum are accentuated when the patient is in this posi-

tion. The Trendelenburg position results in a cephalad migration of the viscera, which increases the pressure on the diaphragm and decreases the tidal volume.

Impact of Extraperitoneal Insufflation

Extraperitoneal CO_2 insufflation, which is used for inguinal hernia repair, has less of an impact on cardiopulmonary function than pneumoperitoneum. Minimal mechanical effects are noted with this mode of exposure. Thus, in patients with limited cardiopulmonary reserve there appears to be a theoretical advantage to extraperitoneal insufflation for operations such as inguinal hernia repair where an extraperitoneal approach is feasible. However, large clinical studies have not demonstrated a significant benefit of one method over the other (Table 7.1).

Table 7.1. Cardiovascular changes.

Change	Mechanism	Prevention
Tachycardia	Decreased venous return Sympathetic stimulation Hypercarbia	Pre- and intraoperative hydration Minimize stimulation Minimize hypercarbia, by increasing minute ventilation
Increased preload	Artifactual Actual chamber filling decreases	
Increased afterload	Increased systemic vascular resistance (SVR) from vasoconstriction due to: 1. Elevated intraabdominal pressure 2. Hypercarbia 3. Epinephrine release	Minimize intraabdominal pressure Gasless laparoscopy Prevent hypercarbia, by increasing minute ventilation
Dysrhythmias	Hypercarbia Sympathetic stimulation Decreased venous return	Minimize intraabdominal pressure Gasless laparoscopy Preoperative hydration
Decreased visceral blood flow	Intraabdominal pressure	Reduce intraabdominal pressure Preoperative hydration

C. Pulmonary Effects

The impact of pneumoperitoneum on pulmonary function may be divided into mechanical and chemical effects. The principal chemical effect is that the CO_2 gas is readily absorbed into the bloodstream, resulting in hypercarbia. The numerous physiologic repercussions of hypercarbia have, for the most part, been mentioned above.

The elevated intraabdominal pressure exerts important mechanical effects that impair pulmonary function. The increased pressure pushes the diaphragm upward, increases the intrathoracic pressure, and increases the work of breathing. These alterations are associated with decreased lung compliance, tidal volume, and vital capacity.

Impaired oxygenation results from reduced lung volume and atelectasis due to displacement of the diaphragm. This can be countered by increasing fractional inspiratory oxygen (FiO_2). Positive end-expiratory pressure (PEEP) will also improve oxygenation, but this may be at the cost of decreasing the preload.

The above mechanical factors will also make it more difficult to adequately ventilate the patient, especially in light of the CO_2 pneumoperitoneum-related hypercarbia. Elevating the minute ventilation by increasing tidal volume and/or the respiratory rate should improve ventilation and lower the CO_2 levels in the blood.

As mentioned earlier, the Trendelenburg position results in further embarrassment of pulmonary function by increasing the pressure on the diaphragm. Reverse Trendelenburg improves pulmonary function by decreasing the pressure on the diaphragm (Table 7.2).

D. Gastrointestinal and Hepatic Impact

As mentioned, pneumoperitoneum diminishes visceral blood flow. The risk of aspiration increases during laparoscopic procedures done under pneumoperitoneum due to the increased IAP, especially when the patient is in the Trendelenburg position or if the patient has a history of gastroesophageal reflux.

Pneumoperitoneum also decreases hepatic blood flow although the clinical significance of this temporary alteration is uncertain. Impairment or derangements in liver function have not been noted after advanced laparoscopic procedures, thus far.

E. Renal Effects

Pneumoperitoneum results in decreased renal blood flow. The clinical implications of decreased renal perfusion are likely to be most significant in patients with previously impaired renal function. In a study of patients undergoing laparoscopic cholecystectomy, renal blood flow, glomerular filtration rate, and urine output were reduced compared to open cholecystectomy. A drop in urine output is anticipated during laparoscopic cases.

Table 7.2. Pulmonary changes.

Change	Mechanism	Prevent/treat
Impaired oxygenation	Reduced lung volume, vital capacity, and atelectasis secondary to cephalad displacement of the diaphragm	Increase oxygenation With increased FiO_2 and PEEP
Impaired ventilation	As above	Increase minute ventilation on respirator
Respiratory acidosis	Hypercarbia	Avoid/rule out inadvertent preperitoneal insufflation Increase minute ventilation
Decreased tidal volume	Decreased compliance due to an increased intraabdominal pressure	Minimize intraabdominal pressure Gasless laparoscopy, reverse Trendelenburg position
Increased work of breathing	Decreased compliance	Minimize intraabdominal pressure Gasless laparoscopy Reverse Trendelenburg position

F. Body Temperature Changes

The factors responsible for intraoperative hypothermia in open cases are also applicable to laparoscopic cases. However, heat exchange from the open abdominal cavity and exposed intestines that occurs in open cases is replaced by the cooling effect of gas insufflation in laparoscopic cases.

The cooling effect of nonheated gas insufflation is significant, and laparoscopic methods have a potential of inducing greater heat loss than open cases. The carbon dioxide in the gas tank is at high pressure in the range of 3000 mmHg. When the gas enters the abdomen at a pressure of 15 mmHg, the fall in pressure is associated with significant cooling. It has been estimated that there is a drop of 0.3°C for every 50 mL CO_2 delivered. It is apparent that the cooling is more pronounced at higher flow rates and when gas leakage from the abdomen necessitates continuous insufflation of gas.

Warmed CO_2 reduces the cooling but is associated with tissue desiccation and thus requires further study.

To offset the cooling associated with pneumoperitoneum, other controllable factors should be minimized as in open surgery. Additionally, it is important to minimize gas leaks.

G. Selected References

1. Schauer P. Physiologic consequences of laparoscopic surgery. In: Eubanks S, Swanstrom L, Soper N (eds). Mastery of Endoscopic and Laparoscopic Surgery. Baltimore: Lippincott Williams & Wilkins, 2000:22–37.
2. Chekan E, Pappas T. Minimally invasive surgery. In: Townsend CM Jr, Evers KM, Beauchamp D, Mattox K (eds). Sabiston Textbook of Surgery, 16th edition. Philadelphia: Saunders, 2004. pp. 292–310.
3. Bannenberg JJ, Rademaker BM, Froeling FM. Hemodynamics during laparoscopic extra- and intraperitoneal insufflation; an experimental study. Surg Endosc 1997; 11:911–914.
4. Joris JL, Noirot DP, Legrand MJ, et al. Hemodynamic changes during laparoscopic cholecystectomy. Anesth Analg 1993;76:1067–1071.
5. Iwase K, Takenaka H, Ishizaka T, et al. Serial changes in renal function during laparoscopic cholecystectomy. Eur Surg Res 1994;25:203.
6. Safran DB, Orlando R. Physiological effects of pneumoperitoneum. Am J Surg 1994; 167:281.

8.1. Patient Positioning and Logistics in the Operating Room During Laparoscopic Biliary Surgery

George Berci, M.D., F.A.C.S., F.R.C.S, ED. (Hon.)

A. Cholecystectomy

The preoperative standard labs are routine and should be known to the operator in advance. Important information are the ultrasound findings, the status of the gallbladder (stones?), and the size and appearance of the common bile duct (CBD) (stones)?

Checklist

The surgeon must know what instruments will be needed, and make sure that the scrub nurse also knows them and that they are available in the OR. Everything should be in functioning order, including the video system. A checklist includes confirmation of the following:

1. That in case of a suspected CBD stone, the additional instruments *are in the room.*
2. These tools and the choledochoscope should be kept on a separate table.

Elective Cholecystectomy Without Preoperative Signs and Symptoms of CBD Stones

In the United States, the operator stands on the patient's left side. In Europe and other countries, the French technique was adopted with the surgeon positioned between the legs of the patient. Two TV towers are required: one for the operator (on the patient's right) and one for the assistants (on the patient's left). The nurse can follow the procedures from one of the monitors (Figure 8.1.1).

After the patient is intubated and the pneumoperitoneum is established, the trocar is successfully introduced and the telescope with the video camera is advanced, and the entire abdominal cavity is inspected. After this step, the anesthesiologist is asked to put the patient in a ***reversed Trendelenburg position***,

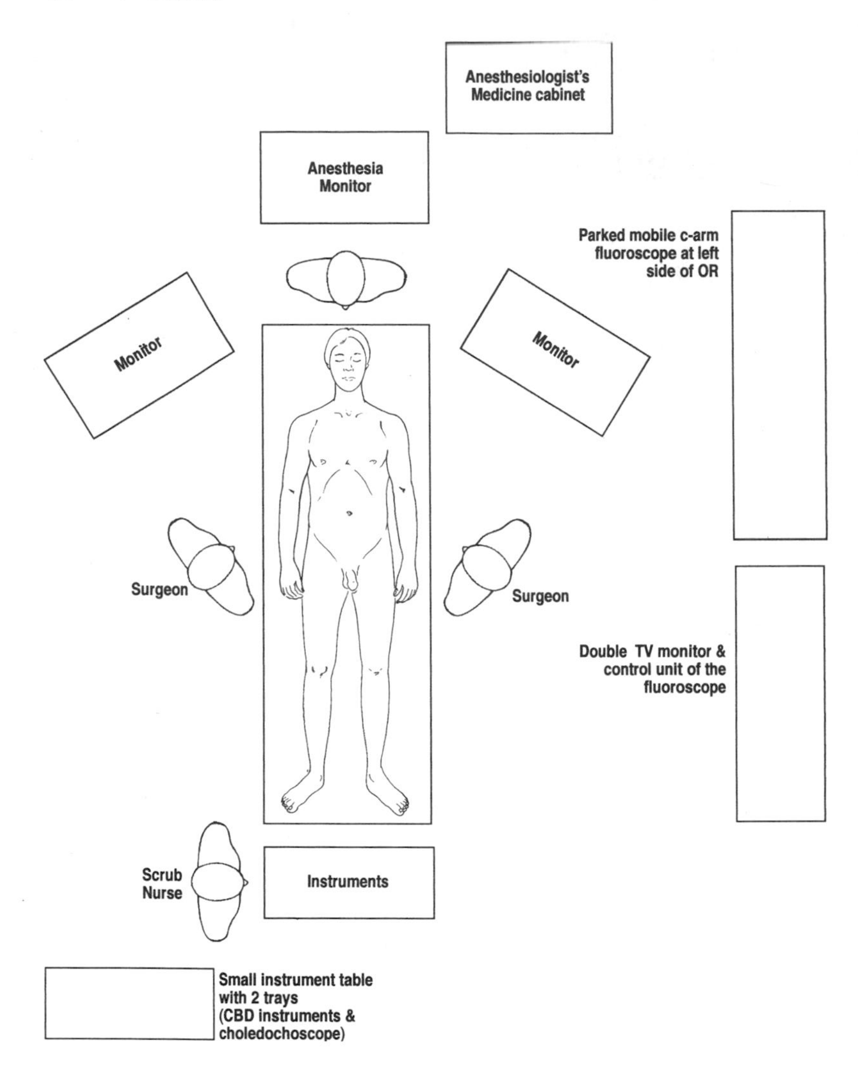

Figure 8.1.1. Schematic scaled diagram of a 20 by 16 foot operating room (OR).

which facilitates the intestinal organs and omentum to be displaced toward the pelvic area and exposes the liver with the gallbladder. Situs inversus is fortunately rare but should be considered if the gallbladder could not be located on the right side. The second, third, and fourth trocars are introduced under visual control. The anesthesiologist is asked ***at this time to rotate the table to the left***. If hemodynamic or cardiac changes are discovered and reported by the anesthesiologist, it is necessary to put the patient back into the normal horizontal position, desufflate the abdomen, and wait until normal values are obtained. The surgeon must then start over with a slower refill mode of pneumoperitoneum, not exceeding the standard intraabdominal pressure (12–14 mmHg). Make sure that the nurse prepares defogging adjuncts, such as a thermos with hot sterile water (Applied Medical Company) or the DeFogger (Novaplus Company).

Patients with a Suspicious History, Slightly Elevated Liver Function Tests, or Dilated CBD

If there exists the possibility that the surgeon will need to explore the CBD, a fluoroscope and the instrumentation for CBD exploration must be in the OR. It is highly advisable that the OR keep the necessary tools in sterile trays that are readily available. Two trays should be available (one tray: the additional accessories; the second tray: the choledochoscope.) Sometimes you can find unexpected stones (4%–5%) by routine cholangiography.

Tray 1: Two guidewires, dilating balloon catheter 5-Fr., two 3-Fr. baskets (preferably the Segura type), two 3-Fr. Fogarty balloon catheters, one stone retrieval forceps, and two 3-Fr. (blue ureteral) catheters with an end tip for cholangiography. The unused instruments can be resterilized.

Tray 2: The choledochoscope is a crucial component of transcystic or trans-CBD exploration and stone removal. It is the most accurate and successful tool for this procedure. It should be kept in a separate tray. A reducer should be included in case you insert a small choledochoscope (2.8-mm or 3.1-mm diameter) through a 5-mm trocar. A *padded grasper* should be available if you manipulate the scope with a grasper so that you do not break the fibers.

Transcystic Approach

After cholangiography documents there are stones that can be removed via the cystic duct, the cholangio catheter should be left in position. A guidewire can then be introduced under fluoroscopy through the cholangio catheter into the CBD and the cholangio catheter removed.

The next step is to introduce the dilating balloon catheter over the guidewire into the cystic duct. Inflate it to the predetermined pressure (see manufacturer instructions) and keep the cystic duct dilated for 2–3 minutes to 5.0 mm. This step will also facilitate passing the choledochoscope through any valves of Heister.

After dilation, deflate the balloon catheter, withdraw it over the guidewire, and thread the guidewire through the choledochoscope instrument channel. The guidewires are now available with soft tips on both sides (Cook Company), which make the introduction through the scope easier. If the scope is in position, you can remove the guidewire. The scope is already attached to a saline bag that is inserted into a Fenwell bag (used for emergency transfusions). The pressure applied is approximately 200 mmHg. This is required to obtain an adequate flow through this narrow channel (instrument channel diameter is only 1.2 mm). If the stone is visualized, decrease or shut off the irrigation, introduce the basket beyond the stone, open it up, and with some movements it can be easily entrapped. It is required that you have a trained assistant. Laparoscopic choledocholithotomy requires teamwork. You need a minimum of four hands and coordinated movements.

Before you start manipulations in the CBD, ask the anesthesiologist to administer 1–2 mg glucagon to relax the sphincter. If there are smaller calculi, they can be flushed through the relaxed sphincter into the duodenum using warm saline. The "push-through maneuver" with the scope is not recommended because you have to be extremely careful not to cause perforation or damage to this critical area. If stones are in the hepatic ducts or in the common hepatic duct, it is probably not possible to remove them through the transcystic duct approach because it is extremely difficult to turn around with the scope. In case of anatomic difficulties (10%), you can always inject a few milliliters of contrast material through the scope and observe the position of the scope with the fluoroscope related to the anatomy. After evacuating the duct, pull the scope back into the cystic duct, inject contrast medium through the instrument channel, and observe it on the fluoroscope to make sure that you have extracted all the stones.

Laparoscopic common bile duct exploration can successfully clear the duct in 80%–90% of cases. This eliminates additional morbidity and cost of an endoscopic retrograde cholangiopancreatography (ERCP) and papillotomy.

B. Intraoperative Fluorocholangiography (IFC)

Operative cholangiography has been debated since Mirizzi in 1933 introduced this static technique. Only a minority of surgeons accepted this important adjunct. It is also true that a static mobile unit produces only two or three films. This technique is a time-consuming process (10–20 minutes). Unfortunately, some films are not informative due to technical problems (over- or underexposure, "cutting" the anatomy due to unknown positioning, sphincter spasm, pseudocalculus sign, no contrast in the proximal ductal system). The repetition rate is 20%–30%.

The introduction of operative fluoroscopy in orthopedic surgery and the further improvement of digitized fluoroscopy in recent years made this procedure easier and faster to apply with a higher diagnostic accuracy. If the duct is cannulated it takes only a few (2–3) minutes to complete the fluorocholangiogram. The image can be immediately observed. Interesting moments can be recorded on film.

It is a prerequisite that you have a fluoroscope available on the floor. In general surgery in the majority of hospitals, orthopedic procedures are performed, and a C-arm is available in the OR. The usage has to be determined in respect to scheduling. Make sure that you get the recent model (digitized image with pulsed fluoroscopy).

Technique of Cholangiography

The patient must be repositioned in a horizontal or normal position. Dilute the contrast half and half with saline. Inject very slowly. If you inject quickly, you will immediately fill the entire ductal system and produce an overfilled or completion cholangiogram, which can result in missing stones. Go slowly, and after each 1 or 2 mL, if you see that the appearance is suspicious, expose a film.

The CBD sometimes is overlying the spine. If this is the case, the C-arm may be rotated during fluoroscopy to get the CBD into a better position. Alternatively, the patient may be rotated to the right side.

If no contrast is seen in the proximal ducts, ask the anesthesiologist to put the patient in a Trendelenburg position and repeat the cholangiogram with a slightly larger injection pressure (which should close the sphincter). If you cannot fill the proximal ductal system, then you must reevaluate why the proximal ducts have not filled. The most worrisome reason for nonfilling would be a bile duct injury. If there is extravasation of contrast material, you must reposition the catheter. However, if extravasation is significant, be aware of the possibility of ductal injury.

If contrast does not flow into the duodenum, you can administer 1 mg glucagon. The patient should be in a horizontal position for this phenomenon. In the majority of cases, the glucagon effect will open up the sphincter and contrast will flow into the duodenum. If flow into the duodenum is not accomplished, exploration (laparoscopic) is indicated.

C. Selected References

Berci G. Static cholangiography vs. digital fluoroscopy. J Surg Endosc 1995;9:1244–1248.

Berci G, Cuschieri A. Techniques of laparoscopic fluorocholangiography. In: Berci G, Cuschieri A, eds. Bile Ducts and Bile Duct Stones. Philadelphia: Saunders, 1997: 60–78.

Berci G, Hamlin GA. X-ray equipment. In: Berci G, Hamlin GA, eds. Operative Biliary Radiology. Baltimore: Williams & Wilkins, 1981:13–27.

Berci G, Morgenstern L. Laparoscopic management of common bile duct stones: a multi-institutional SAGES study. Surg Endosc 1994;8:1168–1175.

Berci G, Paz-Partlow. Laparoscopic ductal stone clearance; instrumentation. In: Berci G, Cuschieri A, eds. Bile Ducts and Bile Duct Stones. Philadelphia: Saunders, 1997: 83–97.

Carroll BJ, Friedman RL, Leiberman MA, Phillips EH. Routine cholangiography reduces the sequelae of common bile duct injuries. Surg Endosc 1996;10:1194–1197.

Hamlin GA, Berci G. The fluorocholangiogram. In: Berci G, Hamlin GA, eds. Operative Biliary Radiology. Baltimore: Williams & Wilkins, 1981:63–109.

Petelin BJ. Laparoscopic ductal stone clearance, transcystic approach. In: Berci G, Cuschieri A, eds. Bile Ducts and Bile Duct Stones. Philadelphia: Saunders, 1997: 97–109.

Traverso WL, Hauptmann E, Lynge D. Routine intraoperative cholangiography and its contribution to the selective cholangiographer. Am J Surg 1994;167:464–468.

8.2. Hepatobiliary, Cholecystectomy, and Common Bile Duct Exploration (CBDE). Includes Cholangiography and Intraoperative Choledochoscopy: Port Placement Arrangements

Dennis L. Fowler, M.D.

A. Cholecystectomy and Cholangiography

1. *Four-port cholecystectomy.* The most commonly used port placement for hepatobiliary surgery is this typical port placement for cholecystectomy (Figure 8.2.1). Cholangiography can be completed routinely or selectively through any of the typical port placements.
   a. *Port for the laparoscope.* The laparoscope is placed through a port in or near the umbilicus (port A). The size of the port will be determined by the size of laparoscope available (usually 5 mm, but sometimes 10 mm or 3 mm).
   b. *Operating port.* The primary operating port is placed just below the level of the liver and just to the right of the falciform ligament (port B). For these reasons, it is desirable to place this port after laparoscopic visualization has been established. It is not usually possible to know the exact location of the inferior margin of the liver before placing ports, and the surgery is much easier if the instruments placed through the primary operating port are aimed somewhat cephalad. This requires that the port be inferior to the inferior margin of the liver. Additionally, it is important to avoid injury of the superior epigastric artery within the right rectus sheath. Transilluminating the abdominal wall with the light of the laparoscope will often identify the location of this artery.
   c. *Assistant's ports.* The assistant's two ports are placed lateral to the rectus sheath and inferior to the inferior edge of the liver (ports C and D). It is important that the most lateral and inferior port (D) is placed sufficiently lateral that the

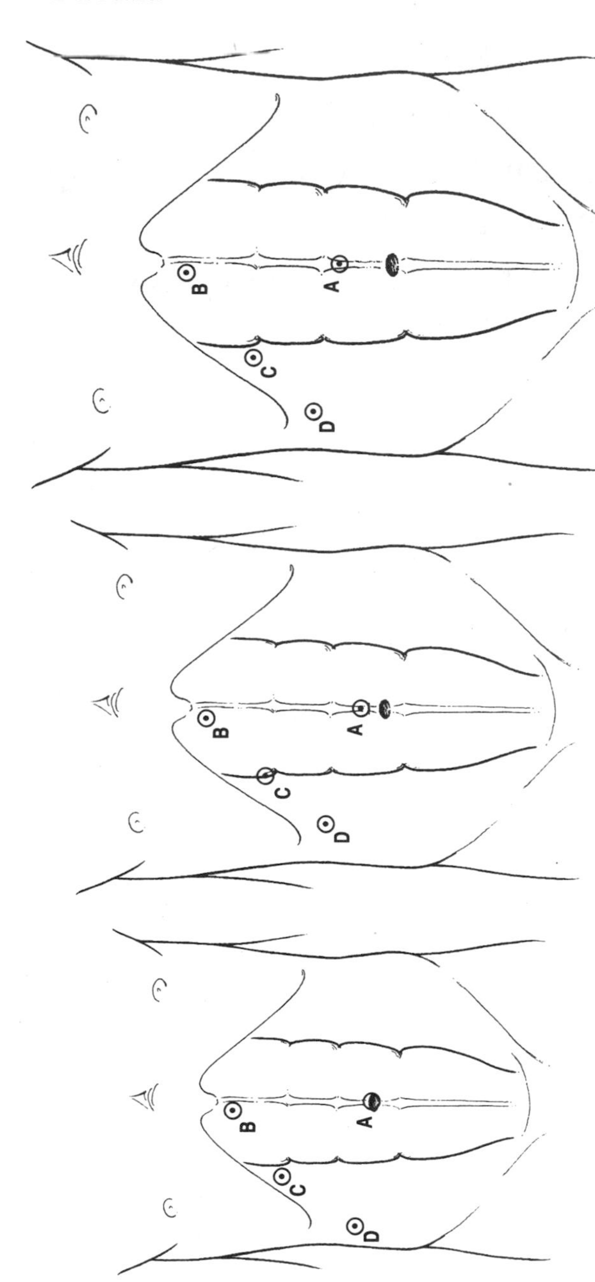

Figure 8.2.1. Four-port scheme for cholecystectomy.

instrument on the outside does not continually "bump" into the anterior superior spine of the iliac crest.

2. *Three-port cholecystectomy.* This port placement differs from the four-port technique only by eliminating one of the assistant's ports (Figure 8.2.2). The scope port (A) and operating port (B) are similarly placed. Provided a fixed arm or robot is used to manage either the retracting grasper or the laparoscope, this technique allows one surgeon to complete cholecystectomy without a human assistant. A fixed arm or a robot can be used. The single assistant's port (C) is placed lateral to the rectus sheath and inferior to the liver edge.

B. Laparoscopic Common Bile Duct Exploration (CBDE)

The typical four-port cholecystectomy setup, described above, is ideal for CBDE when cholecystectomy is also to be completed (see Figure 8.2.1).

1. *Port for the laparoscope.* The laparoscope is placed through the umbilical port as for cholecystectomy and should remain there throughout the common bile duct exploration. It is necessary to continue to visualize the bile duct and cystic duct during manipulation of instruments that are placed into the bile duct.
2. *Port for bile duct instrumentation.* Bile duct instruments (usually choledochoscope or basket) are typically placed through the upper midline port (port B). However, they can be placed through one of the assistant's ports when that provides a better angle for introduction of the instruments into the bile duct.
3. *Assistant's ports.* These ports are used for providing exposure of the common bile duct/cystic duct area. An instrument is placed on the fundus of the gallbladder to lift the liver and gallbladder anteriorly and cephalad to provide exposure. A second instrument is placed on Hartmann's pouch to provide traction on the cystic duct. Less commonly the choledochoscope might be passed through the medial assistant's port.

C. Laparoscopic Hepatic Ultrasound

If diagnostic liver/bile duct ultrasound is the only anticipated procedure, the procedure requires only two ports (Figure 8.2.3). If biopsy (other than needle biopsy) or if ablative therapy of liver lesions is anticipated, additional ports will be necessary.

1. *Port for the laparoscope.* A 10-mm port should be placed at the umbilicus (port A). Any size laparoscope can be placed through

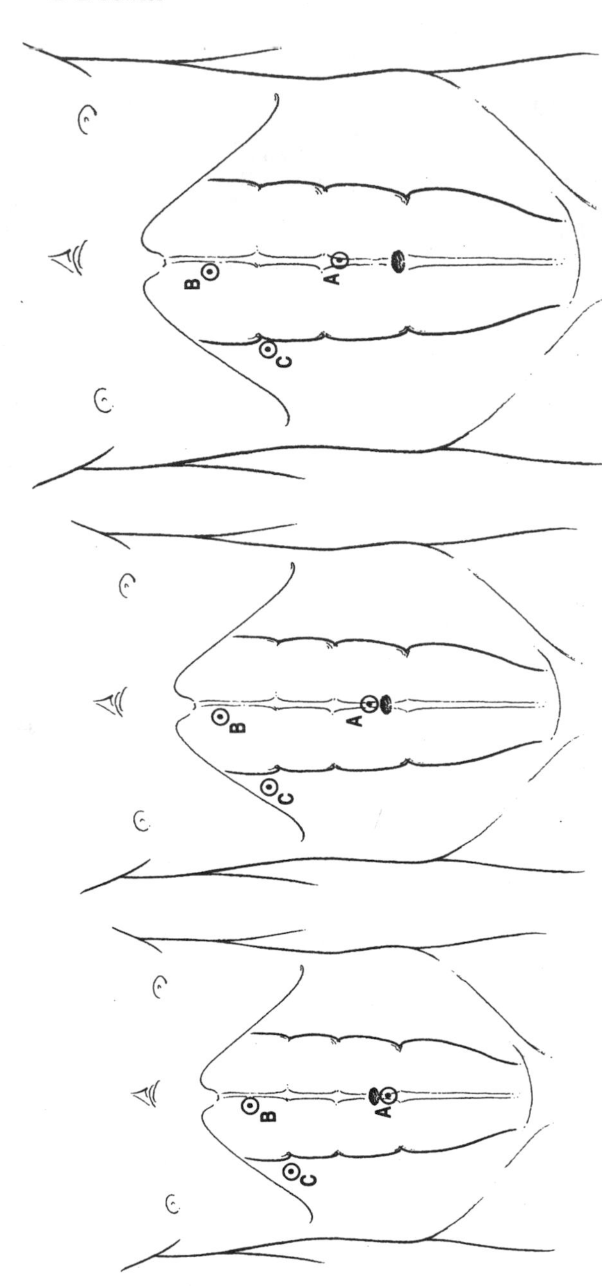

Figure 8.2.2. Three-port arrangement for cholecystectomy.

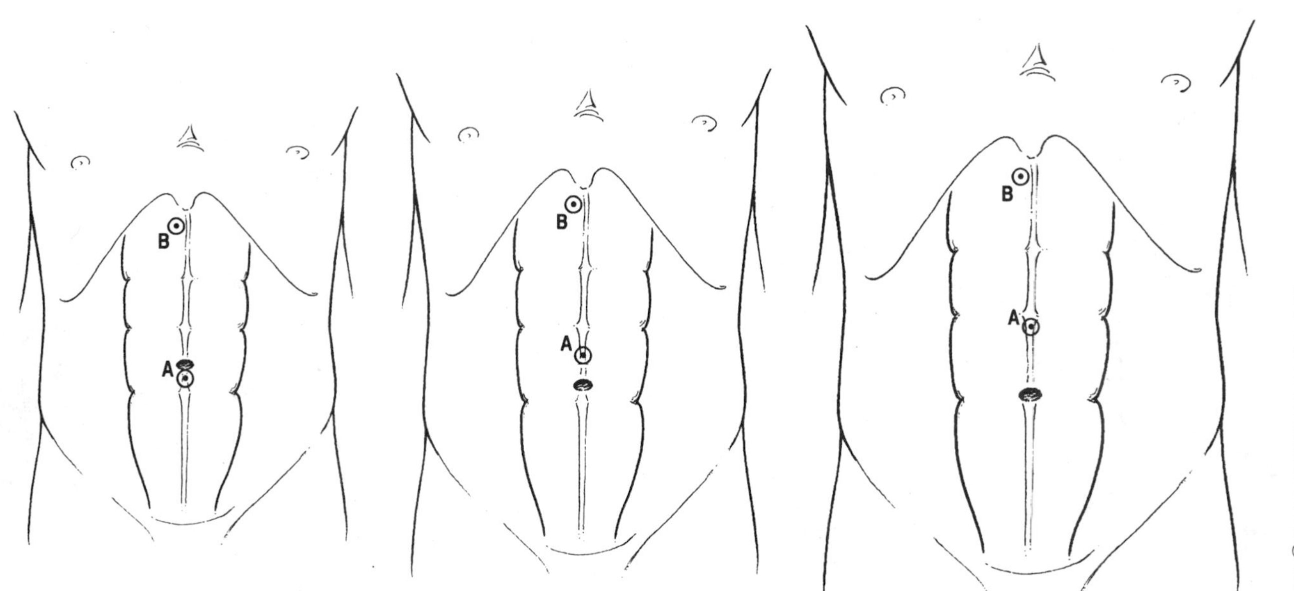

Figure 8.2.3. Two-port scheme for laparoscopic hepatic ultrasound.

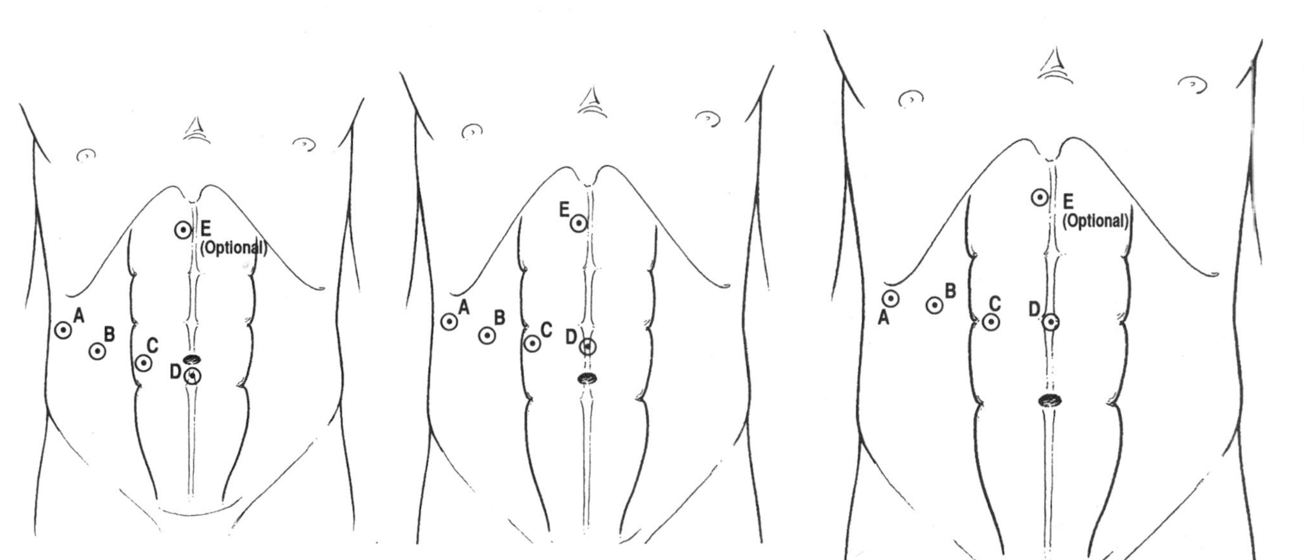

Figure 8.2.4. Five-port arrangement for common bile duct exploration and access to the duodenum.

this. However, by placing a 10-mm port, it can later be used for placement of the ultrasound probe as well.

2. *Port for the ultrasound probe.* A 10-mm port should be placed inferior to the inferior edge of the liver and just to the right of the falciform ligament (port B). Through this port, the ultrasound probe can be used to examine the liver, including identification of the vena cava and hepatic veins. The probe can then be rotated for examination of the common bile duct. Additionally, the probe can then be passed posterior to the falciform ligament for examination of the left lateral segment of the left lobe of the liver. In some situations, the laparoscope and ultrasound probe can be switched so that the ultrasound probe is introduced through the umbilicus. This facilitates a longitudinal exam of the common bile duct.

D. Alternate Port Placements for Common Bile Duct Exploration and Access to the Duodenum

If the patient has previously had a cholecystectomy, or if there is need to explore the ampulla of Vater (as for a transduodenal sphincterotomy), a more lateral set of port placements is sometimes desirable (Figure 8.2.4). This may make exposure of the common bile duct and/or Kocherization of the duodenum easier.

1. *Port for the laparoscope.* The laparoscope is placed through a port in the anterior axillary line just below the right costal margin (port A). An angled scope (30° or 45°) is usually necessary.
2. *Ports for the surgeon.* The surgeon operates through two ports in the right midabdomen (ports B and C). These ports should be placed equidistant between the scope port and the umbilicus. The surgeon can operate with either hand and assist himself/herself through the other port.
3. *Ports for the assistant.* Often, only one port at the umbilicus is necessary for the assistant to adequately expose the surgical site (port D). However, sometimes it is necessary to place a port in the upper midline through which a liver retractor can be placed (port E). In some patients this may enhance the exposure of the common bile duct and duodenum.

9.1. Operating Room Setup and Patient Positioning for Laparoscopic Gastric Bypass and Laparoscopic Gastric Banding

Philip R. Schauer, M.D., F.A.C.S.
William Gourash, C.R.N.P.
Giselle G. Hamad, M.D.
Sayeed Ikramuddin, M.D.

I. Introduction

Laparoscopic gastric bypass is one of the most technically challenging operations performed using a laparoscopic approach. It requires the completion of two intracorporeal anastomoses and advanced suturing and stapling skills. Excessive abdominal adiposity creates exposure challenges, and often instrument length may be insufficient to reach the target. To complete the operation safely and efficiently, proper patient positioning and operating setup are crucial. If these tasks are not performed optimally, the progress of the operation may be compromised and, in the worst case, patient safety jeopardized. The following recommendations regarding patient positioning and operating room setup are based on our experience of more than 1500 laparoscopic gastric bypass cases. We wish the reader to recognize that, although our approach has been proven to be safe and effective in our hands, many other approaches are suitable.

II. Operating Room Environment and Patient Positioning for Laparoscopic Gastric Bypass and Gastric Banding

A. Operating Room Equipment, Design, and Layout

An efficiently setup and organized operating room for laparoscopic bariatric surgery is critical for success. The room should be spacious enough to allow for unencumbered transfer of the morbidly obese patient to and from the operating room (OR) table. The room must be large enough to hold all the necessary equipment and to permit the unencumbered movement of the OR staff. Much of the laparoscopic visualization and insufflation equipment can be grouped together on mobile towers. Specialized operating rooms specifically for minimally invasive surgery are gaining appeal. Some of these "endosurgery suites" employ boom technology that keeps the equipment off the floor and within easy reach of the surgeon or OR staff. Efficient design of these operating rooms will likely improve overall operating efficiency and safety.

1. Voice control technology: The authors make use of voice control technology (Hermes system, Computer Motion, and Stryker Endoscopy), which serves as a centralized and simplified interface that enables the surgeon to control, via spoken commands, medical devices compatible with the voice control system. Although this type of system facilitates laparoscopic procedures, it is by no means mandatory; most advanced laparoscopic procedures are done without such technology throughout the world.
2. Robotic assistance: The authors utilize an FDA-approved surgical robot capable of holding the laparoscope and altering its position in response to a surgeon's verbal commands **(AESOP)**. The robotic device consists of two main parts: the computer controller and the articulating robotic arm. It can store in its memory several set laparoscope positions, allowing the surgeon to rapidly return or advance to optimal viewing positions. Again, whereas such a system may be helpful, it is by no means mandatory. Most surgeons do not make use of this system.

B. *The Essential Equipment*

1. Laparoscope: Laparoscopes for bariatric surgery come in various diameters (5–10 mm), lengths (32–45 cm), and angles (0°–90° orientation). An extralong laparoscope (45 cm) is sometimes necessary and very helpful in superobese patients. Angled scopes provide more flexibility in viewing internal structures and provide access to areas that would be "blind" to 0° scopes. The angled scopes require additional skills to operate and decrease light transmission slightly. For the Roux-en-Y gastric bypass, the authors typically use a 5-mm, 30° scope initially at the 5-mm entrance site to visualize the other port placements. A 10-mm-diameter, 45° angled laparoscope is used for the balance of the procedure because we have found that it provides the best viewing flexibility, especially in extremely obese patients.
2. Light source and light cable: A high-intensity light source is a requisite for a satisfactorily bright laparoscopic image. Most units employ either a xenon or metal halide bulb; these sources provide exposure that falls within the range of daylight (5500 K). Light is transmitted from the light source to the scope through a fiberoptic light cable. Any cable with more than 15% broken fibers is not suitable for a video pro-

cedure and should be replaced. Improper connection of the cable to the light source or the telescope will result in loss of significant amount of light. Light cables must be sterilized in either ethylene oxide or glutaraldehyde and should not be autoclaved.

3. Video monitor: The monitors on which the laparoscopic image is viewed should be of the highest quality. The picture should be flicker-free, with enhanced black performance for better contrast and efficient white balance circuitry that can deliver more stable color and high resolution. We use two 19-inch high-resolution color video monitors, which are placed opposite the surgeon and the assistant on towers or booms. Flat panel monitors are gaining in popularity because they are lightweight and more mobile than the standard CRT monitors; however, resolution is not on par with CRT monitors yet. The room setup shown in Figure 9.1.1 depicts the locations of two laparoscopic monitors for gastric bypass and gastric banding procedures. Advanced and dedicated minimally invasive operating rooms usually have four or more monitors, several of which are usually flat panels.
4. Insufflator: The authors recommend a high-flow insufflator capable of delivering flow rates up to 30 L/min. The rate of insufflation can be adjusted from 1 up to 20 L/min. We usually set the intraabdominal pressure at 15 mmHg but will intermittently use higher pressure (16–18 mmHg) when better exposure is needed or lower pressure when instrument length is insufficient. Gas leakage is common during laparoscopic bariatric procedures and can be very troublesome. A high-flow insufflator is recommended to accommodate for gas leakage from small air leaks at port sites, instrument exchanges, and intraabdominal suction. We usually use two insufflators set at high flow during gastric bypass procedures to provide added compensation for gas leakage. Where available, centralized delivery of CO_2 gas as opposed to the use of individual CO_2 tanks is highly preferred to eliminate interruptions for tank exchanges.
5. Laparoscopic access instruments and trocars: A Veress needle is used to establish a pneumoperitoneum in the obese patients as it is technically very difficult to perform utilizing the open cut-down (Hasson) technique due to the thick layer of subcutaneous fat. A long length Veress needle of 150 mm is used through a subcostal incision in the left upper quadrant. Correct position of the Veress needle into the abdominal cavity after it has passed through the abdominal wall can be verified by various methods, such as the water drop test. In obese patients, opening intraabdominal pressures may be high (up to 10–12 cm H_2O), and anterior traction on the abdominal wall is sometimes required to facilitate gas flow. In addition to being safe and reliable, trocars and ports for laparoscopic bariatric surgery should minimize air leaks, secure readily to the abdominal wall, allow rapid exchange of instruments of various diameters, and be of sufficient length to reach the peritoneal cavity. We use disposable ports of three sizes: 5 mm, 11 mm, and 12 mm. A spiral cannula oversheath that screws into the fascia can be inserted onto the shaft of the trocar to reduce the risk of

dislodgment. We usually secure the trocars to the skin with sutures for added security. To prevent trocar site hernias, we close all ports that are 10 mm or greater with a strong absorbable suture such as O-polysorb.

6. Laparoscopic retractors and instrument stabilizers: To expose the esophagogastric region, anterior retraction of the left lobe of the liver anteriorly is required. Many types of retraction devices are available that work sufficiently well. Most importantly, they should be strong enough to retract large, heavy livers and not traumatize the liver in the process. We use a 5-mm-diameter endoflex retractor that assumes a triangular configuration when tightened. The retractor is usually held stationary by means of an external holding device attached to the OR table (Mediflex Universal Single Flexarm System). For extremely large livers, two retractors may be necessary.
7. Laparoscopic instruments: The hand instruments are available with many different features and preferences. In general, for all our hand instruments, we prefer an in-line (as opposed to a pistol grip), ratcheted (optional) handle with finger-controlled rotation of the shaft. Many instruments are available in extralong lengths for superobese patients. Atraumatic graspers, crocodile graspers, Babcock graspers, bowel clamps, and scissors make up the essential hand instruments. A suitable clip applier, either disposable or reusable, is used to secure hemostasis; these are available in 5-mm- and 10-mm-diameter sizes.
8. Endoscopic linear stapler: An endoscopic linear stapler that generates at least two rows of staples on each side of the transected tissue is an extremely important instrument required for laparoscopic gastric bypass. It can be used to transect hollow viscera, divide highly vascular tissue (i.e., mesentery), and create an anastomosis. We use a 12-mm-diameter disposable linear stapler that applies two triple rows of staples before dividing the tissue with an advancing knife. The stapler is fired by repeated compression of the handles after disengaging the safety device/button on the shaft. The stapler can be fired multiple times (25) using disposable cartridges of various lengths (30 mm, 45 mm, 60 mm) containing staples of various heights (2.0 mm, 2.5 mm, 3.5 mm, 4.8 mm) for use with varying tissue thickness. A finger-controlled knob can rotate the shaft of the stapler. Some staplers come with cartridges that can reticulate at 45° angles.
9. Circular stapler: An endoscopic circular stapler can be used to create the gastrojejunal anastomosis (end to end or end to side). The circular staplers on the market today create a double, circular row of staples with varying diameter sizes (the most commonly used stapler diameters for bariatric surgery are between 21 and 25 mm). For the gastrojejunal anastomosis, we prefer the 21-mm-diameter size resulting in a stoma diameter of approximately 12–14 mm. The endoscopic circular staplers can be inserted directly through a dilated port site or through a large trocar. Various methods of anvil insertion into the gastric pouch have been devised, including insertion through a gastrotomy or in-

sertion through the mouth and guided into the pouch through the esophagus using a pull-wire. The later technique requires a flexible endoscope, snare, and a pull-wire.

10. Other hand instruments: Conventional endoscopic suturing technique using standard laparoscopic needle drivers and sutures are suitable for laparoscopic bariatric surgery. Alternatively suturing devices such as the Endostich (United States Surgical) may be employed to facilitate endoscopic suturing. The 10-mm-diameter, disposable Endostich utilizes a double-pointed shuttle needle with the thread mounted at the center of the needle. Double-action jaws allow the needle to be passed back and forth by squeezing the handle and maneuvering the toggle switch. We use the Endostich during the gastric bypass for approximating the bowel for the enteroenterostomy and for oversewing the gastrojejunostomy (two-layer closure). An effective and reliable suction/irrigation instrument is critical to keep the surgical field clear of pooling blood and the abdominal cavity free from smoke and vapor.
11. Energy sources for coagulation and cutting: Standard unipolar or bipolar electrocautery can be used for hemostasis and dividing tissue. For extremely vascular tissue such as mesentery, alternative energy sources such as ultrasonic coagulation may be more suitable. The Harmonic Scalpel (Ethicon Endosurgery) and the Ultrasonic Shears (United States Surgical) are ultrasonically activated instruments that provide excellent hemostasis while eliminating the problem of electrical arc injury associated with unipolar electrocautery. The instruments have a stationary jaw and a blade that vibrates at a frequency of 55,000 Hz. The mechanical action denatures collagen, forming a coagulant that instantly seals small blood vessels. Although heat is generated in the tissue through friction, the lateral spread of thermal energy is minimal (1–2 mm) as compared to electrocautery. Another reliable means of securing hemostasis and dividing mesentery and other tissue (but not bowel) is with the Ligasure Instrument (Valley Lab), which provides hemostasis via bipolar electrocoagulation and then cuts the tissue in question with a built-in knife. This device comes in both a 5-mm and a 10-mm size. During gastric bypass surgery, the authors employ an ultrasonic scissors that is used for dissection, especially along the lesser and greater curves of the stomach for gastric pouch creation. It is also used to make enterotomies in the stomach and small intestine for stapler insertion and for creating the window through the transverse mesocolon.
12. Flexible endoscope: We routinely use a flexible gastroscope at the completion of the gastric bypass procedure to examine the gastrojejunal anastomosis. After submerging the anastomosis under water, we institute intraluminal insufflation and look for air leaks. The endoscope is also useful in assessing the size and patency of the anastomosis as well as to examine for bleeding and viability of the gastric pouch. To facilitate the simultaneous use of endoscopy and laparoscopy, we prefer the use of two camera systems; one each for the laparoscope and endoscope. Both camera systems are fed through a digital mixer

so that both images are displayed on the same monitor as a "picture-in-picture" format.

C. *Patient Positioning for Gastric Bypass*

Laparoscopic gastric bypass is typically performed on patients who weigh from 250 to more than 600 pounds and may require up to 3 to 5 hours to complete. Morbidly obese patients are particularly vulnerable to position-related injury because of their size; thus, the number one rule in positioning is to provide a safe and stable platform and environment. The second rule is to use positioning to provide optimal exposure.

1. Operating table: Patient positioning for laparoscopic gastric bypass (LGBP) begins with an appropriate operating room table that can accommodate the needs of the bariatric patient. Not only must it have the capacity to support superobese patients up to 350 kg but it must also provide the steep tilt and rotation required in laparoscopy to gain adequate exposure. Table width must also be adequate to handle various body shapes. Tables with electric motors as opposed to hand cranks are highly recommended to facilitate position changes. Although it is possible to perform minimally invasive morbid obesity surgery on some standard operating tables (500-lb maximum for most), if available, it is advised that a specialized table be used for obese patients. These tables can accommodate patients who weigh 800 lb. The acquisition of such tables is logical if these cases are to be done regularly. Some table models can be controlled by the surgeon via voice activation; this feature is particularly desirable because it allows the surgeon to rapidly change table positions without relying on other operating room personnel. Important bed accessories include footboards, straps, and padding to safely secure the patient to the bed and prevent pressure injuries. Patient transfer accessories such as air transport mats can greatly aid the transfer of even the largest patients to and from the operating table.
2. Patient position: (see Figures 9.1.1, 9.1.2) Most minimally invasive bariatric experts utilize one of two patient positions for both bypass and gastric banding: either the supine position or the supine position with the legs abducted on straight leg boards (the so called "French position"). The modified lithotomy position is not recommended. The authors utilize the supine position with the legs together. Regardless of which position is chosen, it is mandatory that well-secured and padded footboards be employed. Leg straps as well as waist straps are used to secure the patient to the table. These measures will help prevent the patient from sliding down the table when placed in the reverse Trendelenburg position or when turned from side to side. The patient's weight should be evenly distributed on the table without elements of the torso or limbs "hanging over the side." A urinary catheter is then inserted, and an electrocautery grounding pad is placed, usually on the anterior thigh. Before prepping and draping, all "pressure points"

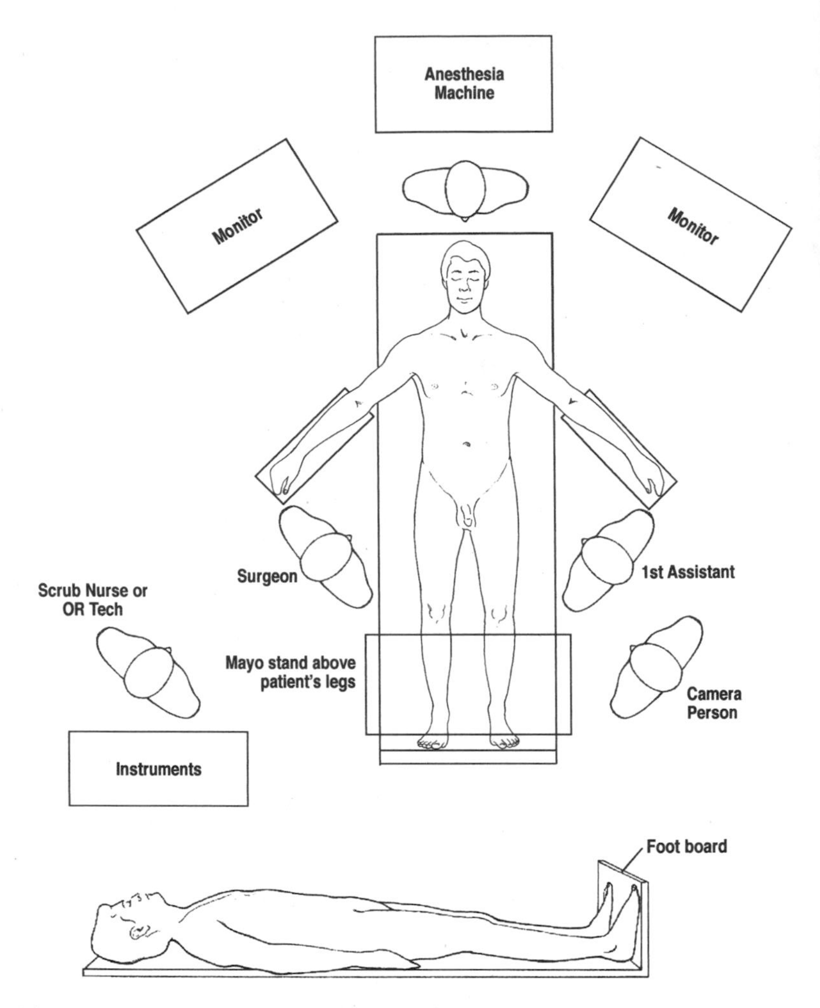

Figure 9.1.1. Operating room setup. Patient and operating room positions for laparoscopic band and laparoscopic gastric bypass. Inset shows footboard.

especially alongside the arms, hands, feet, and head should be examined and padded appropriately to avoid pressure or nerve injuries. A stationary retractor-holding device is often attached to the table and can be used to secure the liver retractor throughout the operation. It must not be in direct contact with the patient's skin to avoid pressure injury or electrocautery conduction.

a. Sequential pneumatic compression devices (SCDs) and deep vein thrombosis prophylaxis: SCDs are placed around the calves and

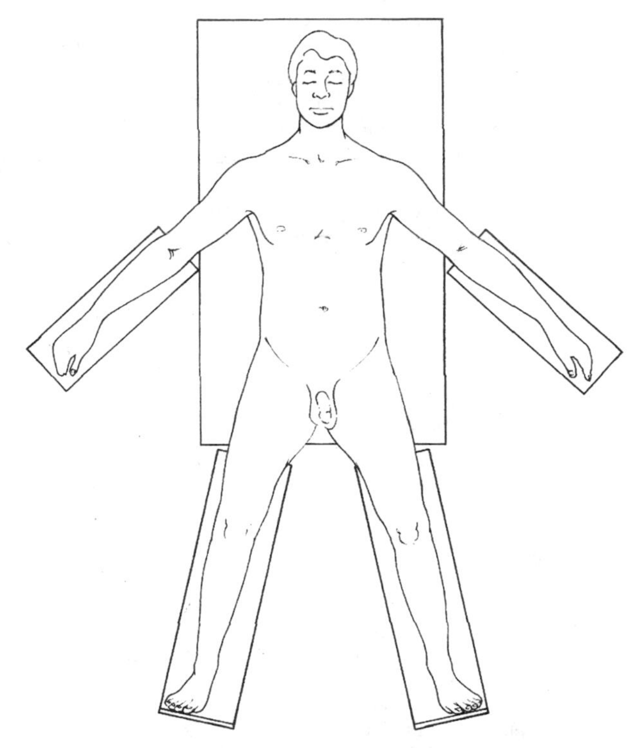

Figure 9.1.2. Alternate position of patient with legs abducted and/or flat leg boards.

thighs preoperatively. They are used throughout the anesthetic induction and the operation. SCDs, along with perioperative, low-dose heparin or low molecular weight heparin, are highly recommended to prevent venous thrombosis and pulmonary embolus, which is a rare but potentially fatal complication of morbid obesity procedures.

b. Arm positioning: The authors, most often, place the arms in the abducted position on carefully padded armboards (Figure 9.1.1). Alternatively, the right arm may be adducted or "tucked" along the patient's right side. This allows the surgeon to stand near the patient's right shoulder to perform the jejunojejunostomy in the midabdomen. A metal or plastic limb holder or "sled" may be required to secure the arm at the side.

3. Dispersement of equipment in room: Figure 9.1.1 shows the arrangement of the equipment, patient, surgeons, and staff. The anesthesia machine and equipment are in the usual position at the head of the table. One of the laparoscopic monitors is placed off the patient's left

shoulder while the second is positioned in a similar position on the right side. The table holding the surgical instruments is at the foot of the table to the patient's right side. The scrub nurse or technician stands to the right of the patient. If the supine with legs adducted position is used, then the authors suggest that the mayo stand be placed over the patient's lower legs. If the legs are abducted then the mayo stand will be off to the right side.

4. Suggested positioning of surgeons: If the supine position with legs adducted is used, the surgeon stands on the patient's right side adjacent to the operating technician while the first assistant and second assistant (camera operator) stand on the patient's left side. If the legs are placed in the abducted position then the surgeon may stand between the legs and the surgical assistants stand one on each side of the patient; the scrub nurse or technician in this scenario is also off to the side and toward the foot of the table. Patient size may be a limiting factor with the French approach as there may be limited space between the legs.

D. Conclusion

It is of paramount importance that the surgeon carefully consider both the OR setup as well as the patient's position on the operating table. Careful attention to numerous details such as the use of footboards, securing the patient to the table, and the padding of the patient is mandatory, especially in this patient population. Poor planning and positioning may necessitate time consuming and cumbersome setup and positioning adjustments during the operation.

It is also necessary that the surgeon review with the OR staff the equipment, instruments (both reusable and disposable), staplers, and tissue-cutting devices that will be or might be required during the case. Failure to do this will likely lengthen the operation and/or jeopardize the safety of the operation.

III. Selected References

1. Schauer PR, Ikramuddin S, Gourash W, Ramanathan R, Luketich J. Outcomes after laparoscopic Roux-en-Y gastric bypass for morbid obesity. Ann Surg 2000;232: 515–529.
2. Ramanathan RC, Gourash W, Ikramuddin S, Schauer PR. Equipment and instrumentation for laparoscopic bariatric surgery. In: Deitel M, Cowan GS, eds. Update: Surgery for the Morbidly Obese. Toronto: FD-Communications, 2000:277–290.
3. Schauer PR, Ikramuddin S. Laparoscopic surgery for morbid obesity. Surg Clin N Am 2001;81:1145–1179.

9.2. Minimally Invasive Procedures for Morbid Obesity: Port Placement Arrangements

Marc Bessler, M.D.
Charles Cappandona, M.D.

A. General Considerations

1. Port placement arrangements for two different procedures for morbid obesity are described in this section; laparoscopic Roux-en-Y gastric bypass and laparoscopic adjustable gastric banding.
2. Please see the preceding chapter for the details concerning the operating room setup and patient positioning options.
3. The author of this section prefers the supine position with both arms extended and with the legs placed on foot/leg boards (stirrups are not used or recommended) for both procedures. Each of these procedures can be done with either the footboards (and thus the legs) together or with the footboards apart in the abducted position. The author prefers to keep the legs together for both the gastric bypass and the banding operation. Some surgeons prefer the abducted position. Venodyne stockings are used for all cases as well.
4. The table is placed in steep reverse Trendelenburg position for both procedures.
5. Local anesthesia is injected into all wounds before incision.
6. The author places a Foley catheter for the gastric bypass procedure but not for the gastric banding operation.
7. The section author recommends the use of bladeless trocars although obviously other types of ports and trocars can be used.
8. Perioperative intravenous antibiotics and subcutaneous heparin (5000 units) are given before the start of the case.
9. The author prefers a 10-mm, 30° laparoscope for this procedure but also uses a 5-mm, 30° laparoscope early in the case.
10. The precise positions for each of the ports will be determined by the patient body habitus, the location and size of the stomach, and the liver dimensions.

B. Laparoscopic Roux-en-Y Gastric Bypass (Handsewn Gastrojejunostomy)

1. **Port arrangement A** (Figure 9.2.1)
   a. A 5-mm incision is made immediately below the left costal margin in the midclavicular line, a Veress needle is introduced into the peritoneal cavity, and the abdomen is insufflated to a pressure of 20 mmHg.
   b. A 5-mm port is placed just below the right costal margin near the midclavicular line.
   c. A 5-mm, 30° laparoscope is then inserted and proper placement of the Veress needle confirmed. The remainder of the ports are placed under direct visualization via the laparoscope.
   d. Next, the Veress needle is replaced with a blunt 5-mm port.
   e. A 10-mm port that is mainly used for the camera is placed just to the left of the midline 18 cm below the xiphoid process. At this point, the 5-mm scope is exchanged for a 10-mm, 30° laparoscope that is used for the remainder of the case.
   f. A 5-mm port is placed in the left midabdomen, just lateral to the rectus muscle.
   g. A 12-mm port is placed in the right midabdomen. It is via this port that the stomach is stapled. If a stapler with a long shaft,

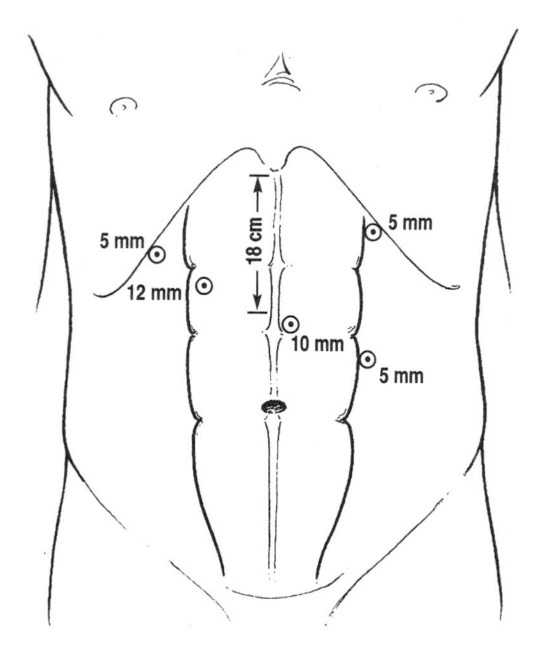

Figure 9.2.1. Laparoscopic Roux-en-Y gastric bypass (port scheme A).

which will reach further, is available then this port is placed just lateral to the rectus muscle. If a standard length stapler is to be used then this port should be placed within the rectus muscle so that the stapler will reach the proximal stomach.

h. A 5-mm subxiphoid incision is made just to the left of the falciform ligament through which the Nathanson liver retractor is placed to retract the left lobe superiorly and anteriorly (no port is placed in this location).
i. After all the ports have been placed, the insufflation pressure is lowered to 15 mmHg.
j. The surgeon and the cameraperson stands on the patient's right side while the first assistant stands on the patient's left side.

2. **Port arrangement B (Dr. William B. Inabnet's scheme)** (Figure 9.2.2)
   a. This surgeon prefers the Optiview System (Ethicon) for placement of the first port, 10 mm in size, about 15 cm below the xiphoid process, just to the right of the midline. This port is used mainly for the camera. (An alternate approach is to place a Veress needle via a transverse incision made in the left upper quadrant about 2–4 cm below the costal margin overlying the lateral portion of the left rectus muscle. Once the pneumoperitoneum has been established, the camera port, in the same location as above, is then placed in a blind fashion. The Veress needle inser-

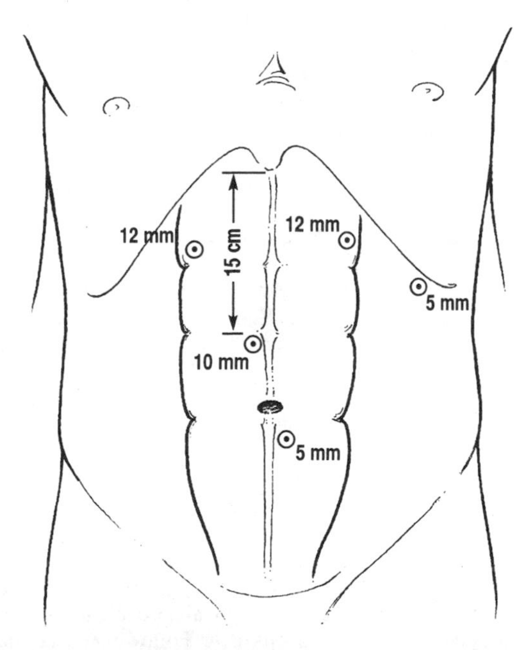

Figure 9.2.2. Alternate port scheme for gastric bypass (port scheme B).

tion site, in this case, is the site used for the left upper quadrant 12-mm port.)

b. The remainder of the ports are placed under direct visualization.

c. A 5-mm subxiphoid incision is made just to the left of the falciform ligament through which the Nathanson liver retractor is placed (no port placed in this location).

d. A 5-mm port is placed just beneath the left costal margin, usually well lateral to the rectus border (at least four fingerbreadths away from the 12-mm left upper quadrant port).

e. A 12-mm port is placed in the right upper quadrant through the rectus muscle about 2–4 cm from the costal margin.

f. A 5-mm port is placed in the left lower quadrant, just to the left of the midline, usually 1–4 cm below the umbilicus. This port is used to construct the jejunojejunostomy. In patients with very lengthy abdominal walls this port would best be positioned several centimeters above the umbilicus.

g. If the Optiview System (Ethicon) was used to place the first port, then the left upper quadrant intrarectus 12-mm port will also need to be inserted, usually 2–4 cm below the costal margin, as shown in the figure.

3. Brief description of procedure

a. Dissection is begun on the lesser curvature about 4–5 cm distal to the gastroesophageal junction and posteriorly. Several firings of a linear stapler are required to transect the stomach from this point toward the angle of His, leaving a 10- to 15-cc proximal gastric pouch.

b. The small bowel is next transected at a point 75 cm from the ligament of Treitz using a linear stapler. A stapled side-to-side enteroenterostomy is fashioned 150 cm distal from this site. The mesenteric defect is closed with a running nonabsorbable suture.

c. A window is then made in the transverse mesocolon to the left of the middle colic artery and the free stapled end of jejunum, the Roux limb, is brought up to the gastric pouch in a retrocolic, retrogastric position.

d. There are numerous ways to perform the gastrojejunostomy: a circular stapled EEA-type (End to End Anastomosis) anastomosis, a stapled side-to-side anastomosis, or a handsewn anastomosis. The author prefers a two-layer handsewn end of stomach to side of jejunum anastomosis that is performed over a 10-mm gastroscope passed transorally through the gastrotomy and the jejunostomy after the back wall of the anastomosis has been completed. After placement of a running continuous seromuscular back row with an absorbable suture, a size-matched enterotomy and gastrotomy is made. The gastrotomy is made by excising a portion of the gastric staple line. The second layer consists of full-thickness bites of the stomach and small bowel and is begun posteriorly, after which the anterior aspect is completed. An absorbable suture material is used for this running continuous layer. Following the completion of this full-thickness layer, the gastroscope is then passed from the stomach into the small bowel. Then, an anterior inverting seromuscular continuous row of absorbable sutures is placed.

e. After confirming anastomotic integrity with the saline immersion test, the transverse mesocolic window and Petersen's space are closed with interrupted and running nonabsorbable sutures, respectively. The fascial defects of all ports greater than 5 mm in size are closed. All ports and the liver retractor are removed. All skin incisions are closed in a subcuticular fashion.

C. Laparoscopic Adjustable Gastric Banding Procedure

1. **Port placement scheme A** (Figure 9.2.3)
   a. A 5-mm incision is made just below the left costal margin in the midclavicular line and a Veress needle is introduced into the peritoneal cavity, after which the abdomen is insufflated to a pressure of 20 mmHg.
   b. A 5-mm port is next placed through an incision immediately below the right costal margin in the anterior axillary line.
   c. A 5-mm, 30° laparoscope, which is used for the entire case, is then inserted and the position of the Veress needle confirmed. The Veress needle is then replaced with a 5-mm port.

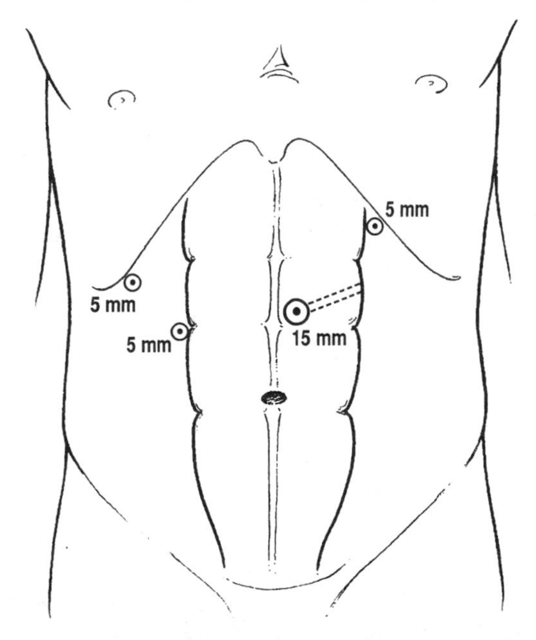

Figure 9.2.3. Port scheme A for laparoscopic adjustable gastric banding.

d. A 15-mm port is placed in the left upper quadrant within the rectus muscle well cephalad to the level of the umbilicus. This port should be at least four fingerbreadths from the left subcostal 5-mm port.
e. A 5-mm port is placed in the midright upper quadrant lateral to the rectus muscle.
f. Last, a 5-mm incision is made in the subxiphoid area just to the left of the falciform and a Nathanson liver retractor is placed to elevate the left lobe of the liver superiorly and anteriorly (no port is inserted at this location).
g. After all the ports have been placed, the insufflation pressure is lowered to 15 mmHg.
h. The surgeon stands on the patient's right side and the first assistant stands on the left side of the table.

2. **Port placement scheme B (Dr. William B. Inabnet)** (Figure 9.2.4)
   a. This surgeon prefers the Optiview System (Ethicon) for placement of the first port, 10 mm in size, about 2–4 cm above the umbilicus just to the left of the midline. This port is used mainly for the camera. (An alternate approach is to place a Veress needle via a transverse incision made in the left upper quadrant about 2–4 cm below the costal margin overlying the lateral portion of the left rectus muscle. Once the pneumoperitoneum has been

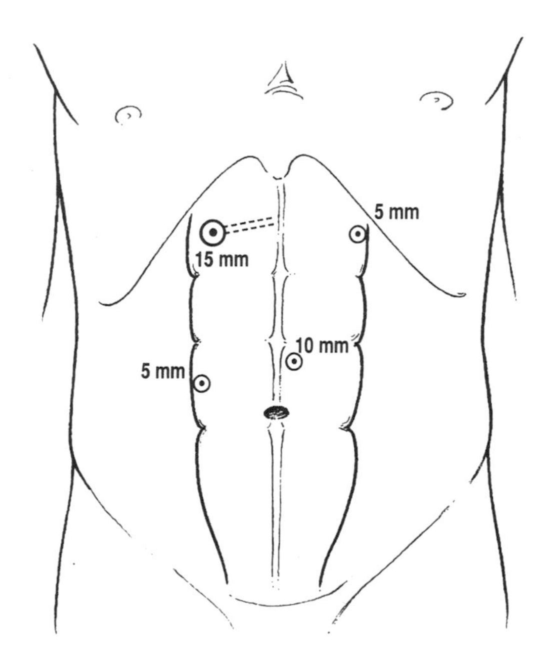

Figure 9.2.4. Port Scheme B for laparoscopic adjustable gastric banding.

established, the camera port, in the same location as above, is then placed in a blind fashion. The Veress needle insertion site, in this case, is the site used for the left upper quadrant subcostal 5-mm port.)

b. The remainder of the ports are placed under direct visualization.
c. A 5-mm subxiphoid incision is made just to the left of the falciform ligament through which the Nathanson liver retractor is placed (no port is placed in this location).
d. A 5-mm port is placed in the lower part of the right upper quadrant either through the lateral part of the rectus muscle or at the lateral margin of the rectus just above the level of the umbilicus.
e. A 15-mm port is placed in the right upper quadrant about two fingerbreadths below the costal margin. The precise location of the port is determined by the size and position of the liver and falciform ligament.

3. **Brief description of the procedure**
   a. The operation is begun by mobilizing the angle of His by dividing the attachments of the stomach to the left crus.
   b. The hepatogastric ligament is next opened in the clear space. The peritoneum overlying the most inferior aspect of the right crus is then incised and a retrogastric tunnel is bluntly dissected to the angle of His.
   c. A 10-mm Lap-Band is introduced via the 15-mm port and the tubing is grasped by an instrument placed through the retrogastric tunnel and exiting at the angle of His. The tubing and band are pulled through the tunnel until the end of the tubing can be placed through the buckle of the band, after which the buckle is closed just below the level of the gastroesophageal junction.
   d. The fundus and anterior wall of the stomach are plicated over the band with interrupted sutures, starting laterally at the angle of His and finishing medially near the lesser curvature.
   e. The 15-mm port is next removed, the fascial defect closed, and the skin incision enlarged to accommodate the reservoir for the band.
   f. For either port arrangement, a transverse tunnel through the abdominal wall is made with a 5-mm trocar that is placed via the enlarged 15-mm port skin incision and directed to the left side of the patient. The peritoneal entrance point of the 5-mm trocar should be about 4 cm to the left of the 15-mm port site.
   g. Once this tunnel has been created, the tubing from the gastric band is brought through the tunnel and out the enlarged 15-mm port skin incision. Next the tubing is secured to the reservoir (access port) for the gastric band and the excess tubing pulled back into the abdominal cavity. The access port is then positioned in a subcutaneous pocket created via the enlarged 15-mm port site. The access port is sutured to the anterior rectus fascia via four sutures.
   h. The remaining ports and liver retractor are removed and incisions are closed in the usual fashion.

10.1. Patient Positioning and Operating Room Setup for Laparoscopic Treatment of Gastroesophageal Reflux Disease

Dennis Blom, M.D.
Jeffrey H. Peters, M.D.

A. Room Setup

1. The two body positions that are utilized for minimally invasive gastroesophageal reflux disease (GERD) procedures and which are described in this chapter are the modified lithotomy and the supine position.
2. The laparoscopic equipment is set up the same way for both positions. The two video monitors are positioned at the head of the operating table on either side of the anesthesiologist (Figures 10.1.1, 10.1.2).
3. Standard laparoscopic equipment is needed. This equipment can be housed within ceiling-mounted adjustable columns in specifically designed laparoscopic operating rooms or on mobile units that can be moved between different standard operating rooms.
4. A suction/irrigation system, monopolar cautery, harmonic scalpel, or other energy source facilitate the operation.
5. Given the increased manpower needed to perform laparoscopic antireflux procedures (surgeon, first assistant, camera holder, scrub nurse/technician), there is much interest in and development of robotic assistants and adjustable table-mounted retractors and retractor holders. Several voice-controlled camera holders are now commercially available. These devices can reduce the need for extra assistance and may, in some settings, better serve the surgeon by performing repetitive, tedious tasks without fatiguing and with less motion artifact.
6. The authors **routinely use intermittent antiembolic compression devices** on both lower extremities, regardless of patient position, to improve venous return and to decrease the chances of deep vein thrombosis.
7. A urinary catheter is routinely placed after the induction of general anesthesia.
8. **Securing the patient to prevent slippage** off the table is particularly important given the 20° to 45° incline of the operating table, especially

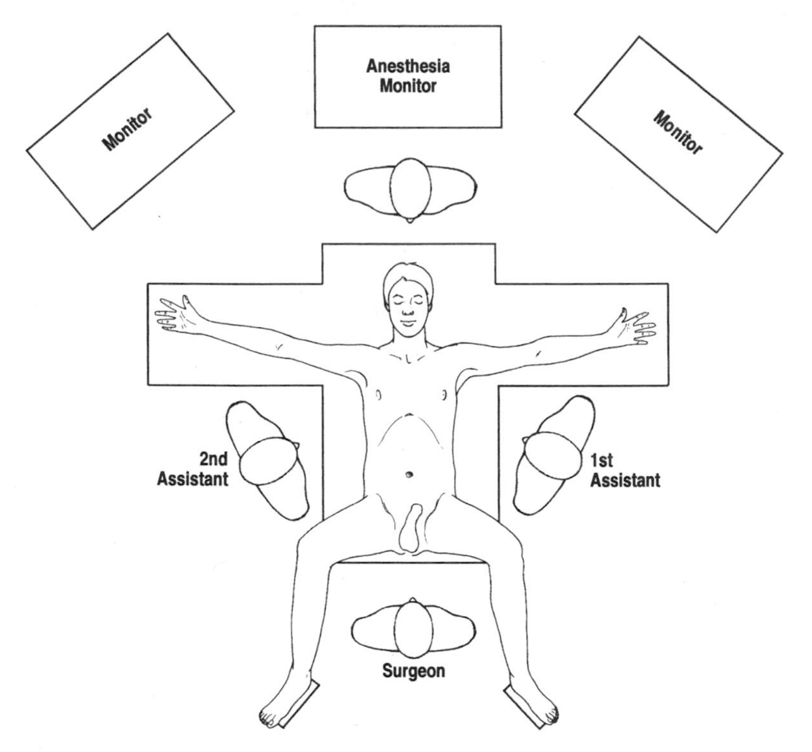

Figure 10.1.1. Operating room setup with patient in modified lithotomy position. The scrub nurse and the tables holding the operating instruments and tools would be located at the foot of the patient or just off to the side of either the left or right foot.

if the patient is obese. A number of different methods can be used to secure the patient in position.

9. A pelvic extension can be placed at the caudal end of the OR table, padded and tilted upward to act as a stop. It is far enough forward so that it does not interfere with the surgeon standing between the legs and provides excellent security against slippage.
   a. Similarly, kidney rests can be attached to the sides of the OR table, padded, and placed against the buttocks to prevent the hips from sliding downward.
   b. Another option is to use a "bean bag," which is placed under the patient; then, suction is applied to the bag. The bean bag forms a mold of the patient and helps secure the position.
   c. Alternatively, and probably least secure, is the use of a gel roll secured to the table, usually with tape, just below the patient's coccyx. Commercially available thigh straps that are designed to

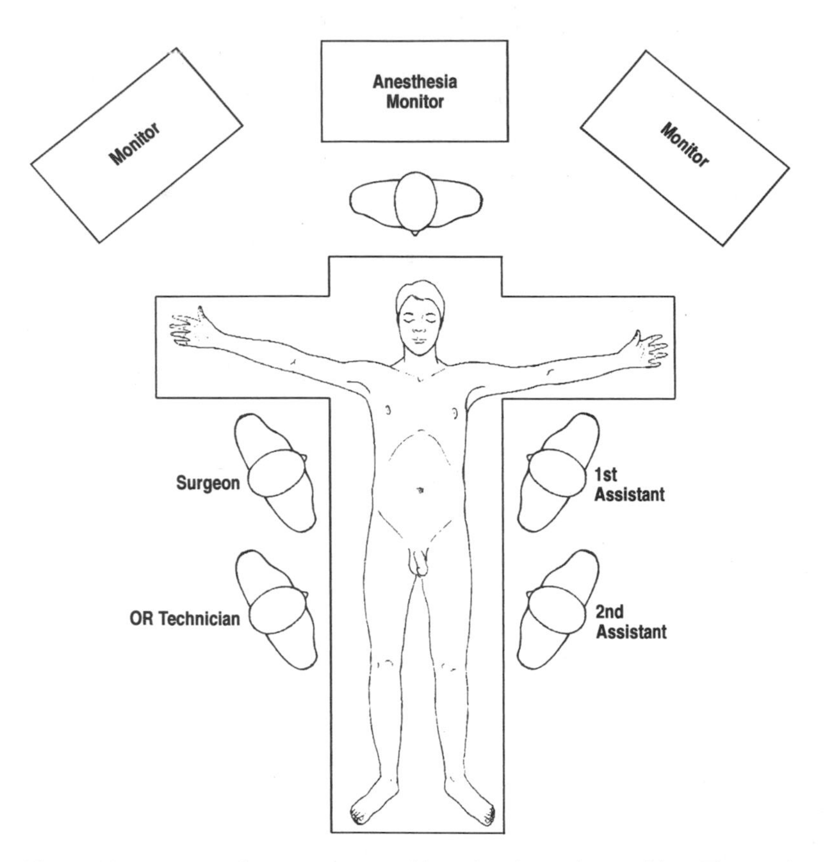

Figure 10.1.2. Operating room setup with patient in supine position. The scrub nurse and the tables holding the operating instruments and tools would be located at the foot of the patient or just off to the side of either the left or right foot.

hold the patient from sliding downward off the table may also be used.

d. In conjunction with one or several of the above measures to secure the abdominopelvic region, the chest should also be secured. Straps or tape can be placed across the padded thorax, out of the operative field, provided all potential pressure areas, such as the elbows and hands, are properly padded. An upper body convection heat device may be used to keep the patient warm throughout the procedure.

B. Patient Positioning

1. **Several options** exist for patient positioning during the performance of laparoscopic antireflux procedures.
   a. Most surgeons place the patient in a **modified lithotomy position**, with 20° to 45° of reverse Trendelenburg or with the patient's thorax elevated in a Fowler's position (Figures 10.1.1, 10.1.2). This incline allows the abdominal viscera, specifically the transverse colon and small bowel, to fall downward toward the pelvis out of the visual and operative field.
   b. The patient's arms may be padded and tucked at his sides, or abducted 90° on arm boards.
      i. The lower extremities are abducted either on a specialized fracture table or placed in stirrups with the hips and knees slightly flexed. Care must be taken not to flex the hips more than approximately 20° so that the thighs lie in the same plane as the anterior abdominal wall. Excess flexion will hinder the free movement, especially downward, of the external portions of the instruments in the lower ports (Figure 10.1.3).
      ii. When using stirrups, each of the lower extremities should be placed into the stirrups at the same time to prevent hip and back injury. Each knee should be placed in line with the contralateral shoulder. Care should be taken to avoid excessive pressure on the portion of the calf that is in contact with the stirrup. Nerve injury or pressure necrosis can result if the leg is improperly positioned. The lower legs can be secured in the stirrups in several ways:
         1. Velcro straps.
         2. Strips of broad cloth tape placed over folded towels that are placed over the anterior lower leg.
         3. Ace bandages that are wrapped around both the leg and the stirrup.
      iii. The surgeon stands between the patient's legs, allowing a coaxial approach to the operative field, with the operative field and video monitors in his line of vision. The surgeon should be free to use both hands for dissection and suturing. This position allows better triangulation of the laparoscopic instruments and is a more ergonomically comfortable and natural position.
      iv. The first assistant stands to the patient's left and the camera operator to the patient's right.
      v. The scrub nurse/technician is then free to stand to either the surgeon's right or left depending on surgeon preference and special considerations.
   c. Alternatively, the patient may be placed **supine** in a 20° to 45° reverse Trendelenburg position (see Figure 10.1.2). This position may be necessary in patients whose legs cannot be abducted and in those in whom, despite abduction of the legs, there is not

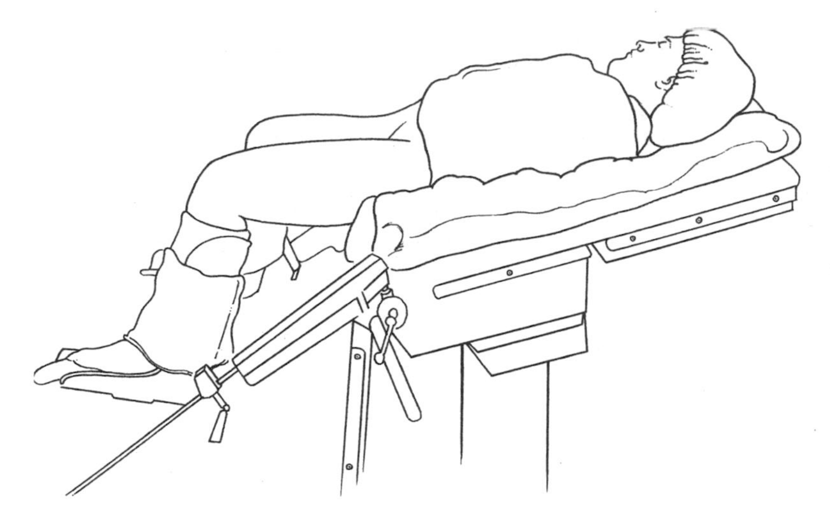

Figure 10.1.3. Side view of patient in modified lithotomy and reverse Trendelenburg position.

enough room for the surgeon to stand between the legs because of the table and/or equipment.

i. The monitors and the other equipment are positioned the same as for the modified lithotomy position.
ii. The surgeon performs the operation from the patient's right side. In this location the surgeon loses the advantages of a coaxial approach.
iii. The first assistant and the camera operator stand on the patient's left.

C. Selected References

Bowrey DJ, Peters JH. Current state, techniques and results of laparoscopic antireflux surgery. Semin Laparosc Surg 1999;6:194–212.

Peters JH, DeMeester TR, Crookes PA, et al. The treatment of gastroesophageal reflux with laparoscopic fundoplication: prospective evaluation of 100 consecutive patients with typical symptoms. Ann Surg 1998;228:40–50.

Soper NJ. Laparoscopic management of hiatal hernia and gastroesophageal reflux. Curr Probl Surg 1999;36:765–840.

Underwood RA, Dunnegan DL, Soper NJ. Prospective randomized trial of bipolar electrosurgery vs. ultrasonic coagulation for division of the short gastric vessels during laparoscopic Nissen fundoplication. Surg Endsoc 1999; 3:763–768.

10.2. Port Placement Arrangements for Gastroesophageal Reflux Disease Surgery

Jorge Cueto-Garcia, M.D.
José Antonio Vazquez-Frias, M.D.

A. Introduction

1. A total of four different port arrangements for gastroesophageal reflux disease (GERD) procedures are presented and briefly described in this chapter.
2. **Positioning**: As mentioned in the previous chapter, either the supine or the modified lithotomy position can be used for minimally invasive GERD procedures. The authors of this chapter recommend the modified lithotomy position. The so-called European position allows the surgeon to stand between the legs and provides excellent frontal vision for antireflux procedures. This position can also be used for cardiomyothomy, vagotomies, placement of the adjustable gastric band, reoperations in the esophageal hiatus, etc.
3. **OR table**: As for other advanced laparoscopic procedures, it is important that the operating table permit the patient to be placed in steep Fowler's position (reverse Trendelenburg) as well as to allow sharp lateral angulation ("airplaning") to provide adequate exposure.
4. **Establishment of pneumoperitoneum**: Regardless of which specific port arrangement is used, the pneumoperitoneum can be established through one of the epigastric port sites with a Veress needle unless there has been previous open abdominal surgery, in which case the initial puncture is done in the left upper quadrant. The authors recommend infiltration of the trocar sites with 2% lidocaine with epinephrine (2–3 mL) to decrease postoperative pain as well as to limit the metabolic response to trauma [1].
5. Although most other advanced laparoscopic procedures make use of a periumbilical port, this position is not often used in GERD operations because of the long distance between this site and the esophageal hiatus. Most instruments cannot reach the latter easily through a port at the umbilicus. One exception to this is in the pediatric patient in whom the periumbilical area is usually used to insert a 5- or 10-mm trocar.
6. **Intrarectus ports**: Most of the port arrangements presented in this chapter call for the placement of one or several ports through the rectus muscle. For GERD procedures it is usually necessary to make use

of such ports. It is important to avoid placing these ports too lateral within the rectus muscle in order to prevent an injury to the epigastric vessels.

B. Port Placement 1

1. It is advised that the patient be placed in the modified lithotomy position (see Figure 10.1.1) and that the surgeon stand between the patient's legs.
2. The initial trocar (5 or 10 mm) is placed 4–5 cm above the umbilicus and 3–4 cm to the right of the midline (intra-rectus) in a patient with average build (middle body drawing of Figure 10.2.1). Subsequently, this port is used for instruments held in the left hand of the surgeon.
3. A 5- or 10-mm laparoscope (a 30° is recommended) is introduced and a complete examination of the abdominal cavity is carried out. The remaining trocars are then placed under direct visualization.
4. A 5- or 10-mm port is next inserted just below the costal margin, in the midline or 2–3 cm to the left of the midline. This port will be used mainly for the laparoscope.
5. In the right upper quadrant just a few centimeters below the costal margin in the midclavicular line, a 5- or a 10-mm trocar is inserted that will be used for the liver retractor.
6. In the left upper quadrant, a few centimeters below the costal margin, in the midclavicular line, a 5-mm port is placed. A retractor is placed through this port and used to provide exposure of the gastroesophageal area.
7. The last port, 5 or 10 mm in size, is inserted through the left rectus muscle in the left upper quadrant at the level of the initial trocar and will be used for the right hand of the surgeon.
8. This arrangement provides for a comfortable, ergonomic position for both hands of the surgeon, and has advantages not only for the dissection, but also very importantly for suturing the plication [2, 3].

C. Port Placement 2

The following is a description of an alternative port arrangement that has been shown to be successful [4] (Figure 10.2.2).

1. This port placement puts the laparoscope lower in the abdomen, just cephalad and to the left of the umbilicus.
2. The surgeon's hands work through ports placed higher on the abdomen. The left hand controls an instrument through a 5-mm subcostal (or subhepatic, depending on size of the liver) port just to the right of the midline, and the right hand controls an instrument through a 5-mm subcostal port in the left upper quadrant lateral to the rectus muscle.

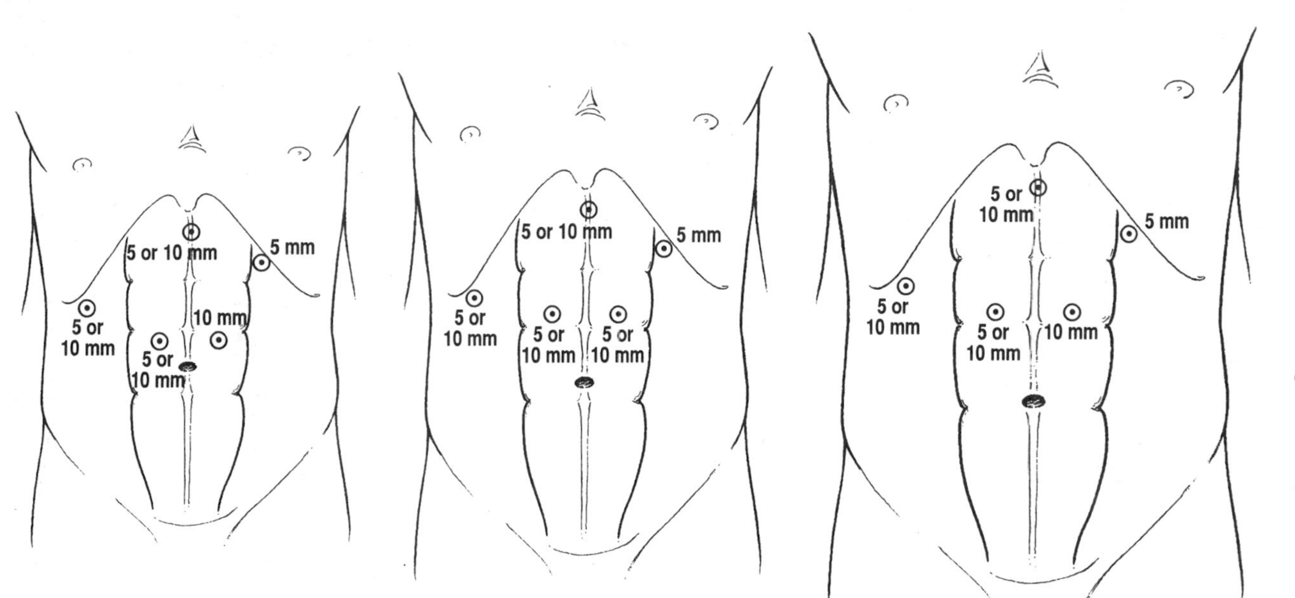

Figure 10.2.1. Port arrangement 1 for antireflux surgery. Depending on the body habitus of the patient, the surgeon's preference, and the available equipment, either 5- or 10-mm trocars can be used.

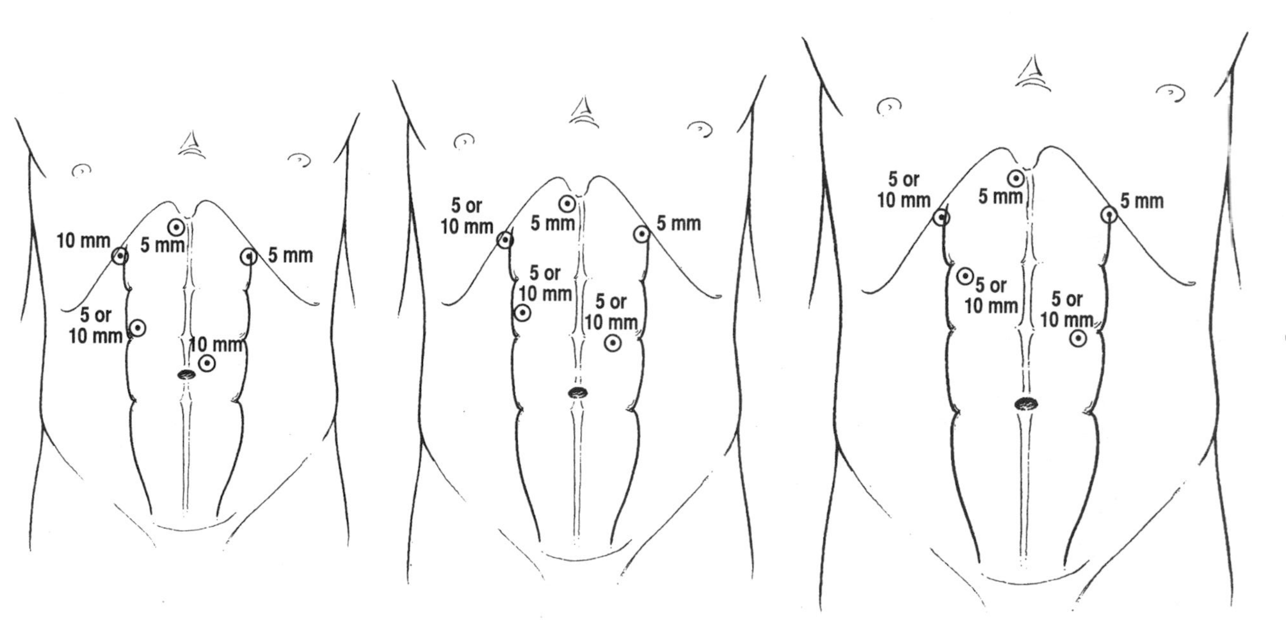

Figure 10.2.2. Port arrangement 2 for gastroesophageal reflux disease (GERD) procedures. (Suggested by A.E. Cuschieri [4].)

3. The liver retracting and assisting ports for the assistant are in the right upper quadrant.

D. Port Placement 3

In pediatric patients, because there is less distance between the umbilicus and the esophageal hiatus, a port at the umbilicus is usually appropriate. Otherwise, pediatric port arrangements are similar to the arrangements used in adults. Depending on the size of the patient, 3-mm instruments may be used for all ports except for the port through which suturing is completed. For suturing, a 5- or 10-mm port may be necessary (Figure 10.2.3).

1. The laparoscope is placed through a port at the umbilicus.
2. The surgeon's left hand utilizes the ports near the xiphoid process while the right hand controls instruments inserted via the left subcostal ports.
3. Liver retraction is accomplished through a port in the right upper quadrant; the other assistant works through a port in the lower left upper quadrant at the lateral edge of the rectus muscle.

E. Port Placement 4

With this placement, the laparoscope and the instruments in the surgeon's hands are in the same location as port placement 2.

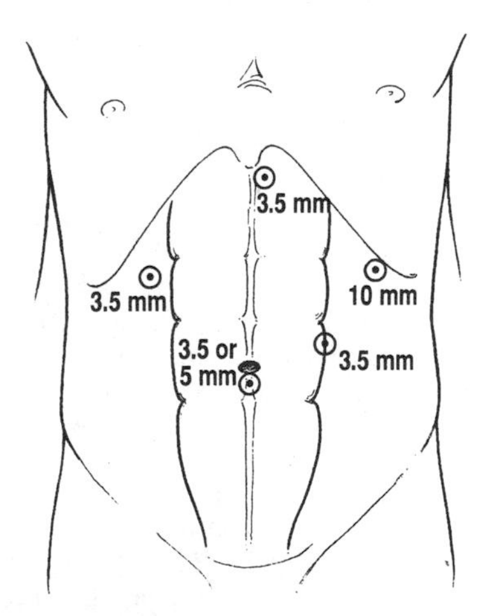

Figure 10.2.3. Port arrangement 3 (for pediatric, very young, and/or short patients; five-port scheme). The umbilicus is used for one of the trocar sites. The trocars used can be 3, 5, or 10 mm in diameter.

1. The laparoscope is placed through a port placed well superior to and just to the left of the umbilicus (Figure 10.2.4).
2. The surgeon's hands control instruments through ports in the upper abdomen. The surgeon's left hand controls an instrument through a port placed below the costal margin just a bit to the right of the upper midline. Some patients have a large lateral segment of the left lobe of the liver, requiring that this port be placed somewhat more caudally. The surgeon's right hand controls an instrument place through a port just below the left costal margin in the left upper quadrant.
3. The liver retractor is placed through a port in the right upper quadrant.
4. The assistant manipulates a retractor/grasper placed through the port in the left midabdomen at the lateral border of the rectus muscle.

F. Placement of Additional Trocars

In very complicated situations such as those of intense periesophagitis [2, 3], obesity, paraesophageal hernia, etc., or when otherwise needed, an additional trocar may be placed. The purpose of this port is usually to provide better exposure.

The location for this additional port will be determined by the nature of the condition requiring the additional port. It should be placed away from the other ports, yet provide access for retraction of omentum, liver, stomach, or whatever is limiting exposure. There is no specific prescribed location for this additional port. Making use of an added port has proved to be invaluable in many patients. When an additional procedure is planned, such as a cholecystectomy (8% in our series [2, 3]), the right upper quadrant port is placed more laterally and an extra 3- or 5-mm trocar is placed in the right anterior axillary line to provide traction of the fundus of the gallbladder. Vagotomy usually can be done with the arrangement already described.

G. Reoperations in the Esophageal Hiatus

Reoperations of the esophageal hiatus are being performed more frequently. If the previous procedure was laparoscopic, the initial puncture can be tried with the Veress needle in the umbilicus. Otherwise, it is best to insufflate via a left upper quadrant insertion site. After a careful inspection of the abdomen the extent and severity of the adhesions is evaluated. With careful and diligent blunt and sharp dissection using the bipolar electrocautery or the harmonic scissors, the areas selected for the placement of the trocars are carefully cleared of adhesions. Special care must be taken to avoid injury to the transverse colon. Among 23 reoperations for failed GERD procedures, there have been no conversions to laparotomy.

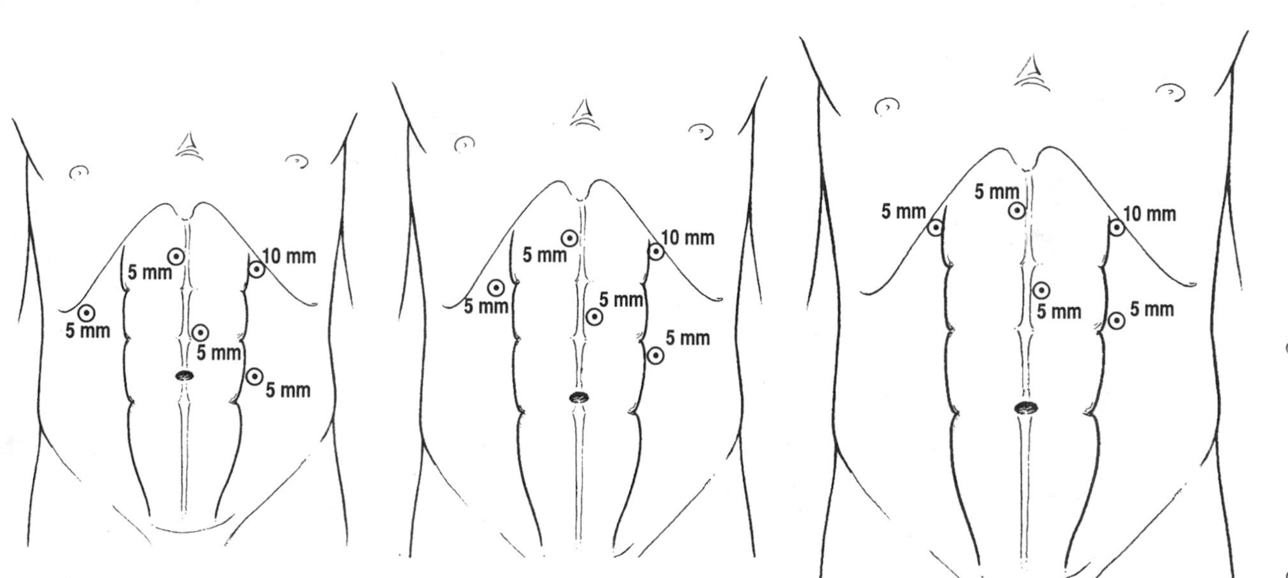

Figure 10.2.4. Port arrangement 4. This alternative plan for port placement uses four 5-mm ports and one 10-mm port.

H. References

1. Pasqualucci A, Contardo R, Da Broi U, Colo F. The effects of intraperitoneal local anesthetic on analgesic requirements and endocrine response after laparoscopic cholecystectomy: a randomized double-blind controlled study. J Laparoendosc Surg 1994;4:405–412.
2. Cueto J, Weber A. Procedimientos antirreflujo. In: Cirugía Laparoscópica. México: McGraw Hill Interamericana, 1997:68–79.
3. Cueto J, Swanstrom L. Antireflux procedures. In: Cueto J, Gagner M, Jacobs M, eds. Laparoscopic Surgery. New York: McGraw-Hill (in press).
4. Cuschieri AE. Hiatal hernia and reflux esophagitis. In: Hunter JG, Sackier JM, eds. Minimally Invasive Surgery. New York: McGraw-Hill, 1993:87–111.

I. Selected References

Bowrey DJ, Blom D, Crookes D, et al. Risk factors and the prevalence of trocar site herniation after laparoscopic fundoplication. Presentation No. S-79. SAGES Scientific Session 2000, Atlanta, GA, March 29–April 1, 2000.

Cueto J, Melgoza C, Weber A. A simple and safe technique for closure of trocar wounds using a new instrument. Surg Laparosc Endosc 1996;6(5):392–393.

Cueto J, Vázquez JA, Nevarez R, Poggi L, Zundel N. Laparoscopic repair of traumatic diaphragmatic hernia. Surg Laparosc Endosc Percutaneous Tech 2001;11(3): 209–212.

Mealy K, Hylan J. Small bowel obstruction following laparoscopic cholecystectomy. Eur J Surg 1991;157:675–676.

Weber A, Muñoz J, Garteiz D, Cueto J. Use of subdiaphragmatic bupivacaine instillation to control postoperative pain after laparoscopic surgery. Surg Laparosc Endosc 1997; 7(1):6–8.

11.1. Minimally Invasive Esophageal Resection: Patient Position and Room Setup

James D. Luketich, M.D.
Yaron Perry, M.D.

A. Patient Position and Room Setup

1. Laparoscopic transhiatal esophagectomy
   a. Position the patient supine on the operating table (Figure 11.1.1).
   b. The surgeon stands on the patient's right side and the assistant stands on the left.
   c. Another option is to position the patient in the modified lithotomy position with the legs extended in stirrups, the hips minimally flexed, and the thighs parallel to the abdomen. The surgeon can stand between the abducted legs.
   d. Whether in supine or modified lithotomy position, the table is placed in reverse Trendelenburg (20°–30° head up).
   e. A video monitor is placed at the head of the table on each side of the patient.
   f. The scrub nurse and the instrument table can be positioned at the foot of the table or off the left or right foot of the table.
2. Thoracoscopic and laparoscopic esophagectomy
   a. Thoracoscopic stage:
      1. The patient is intubated with a double-lumen endotracheal tube for single lung ventilation and positioned in the left lateral decubitus position (Figure 11.1.2). The patient is held on the bed using a bean bag and cloth tape. The right arm is placed on pillows or supported with a bar and an axillary roll is placed under the left axilla. The position is similar to that used for a right posterolateral thoracotomy.
      2. The surgeon stands on the patient's right side and the assistant stands on the left.
      3. Video monitors are placed on both sides of the head of the operating table.
      4. The middle and upper portions of the esophagus are mobilized with thoracoscopic access through the right chest.
   b. Laparoscopic stage:
      1. After the thoracoscopic stage has been completed, the patient is placed in the supine position as for a totally laparo-

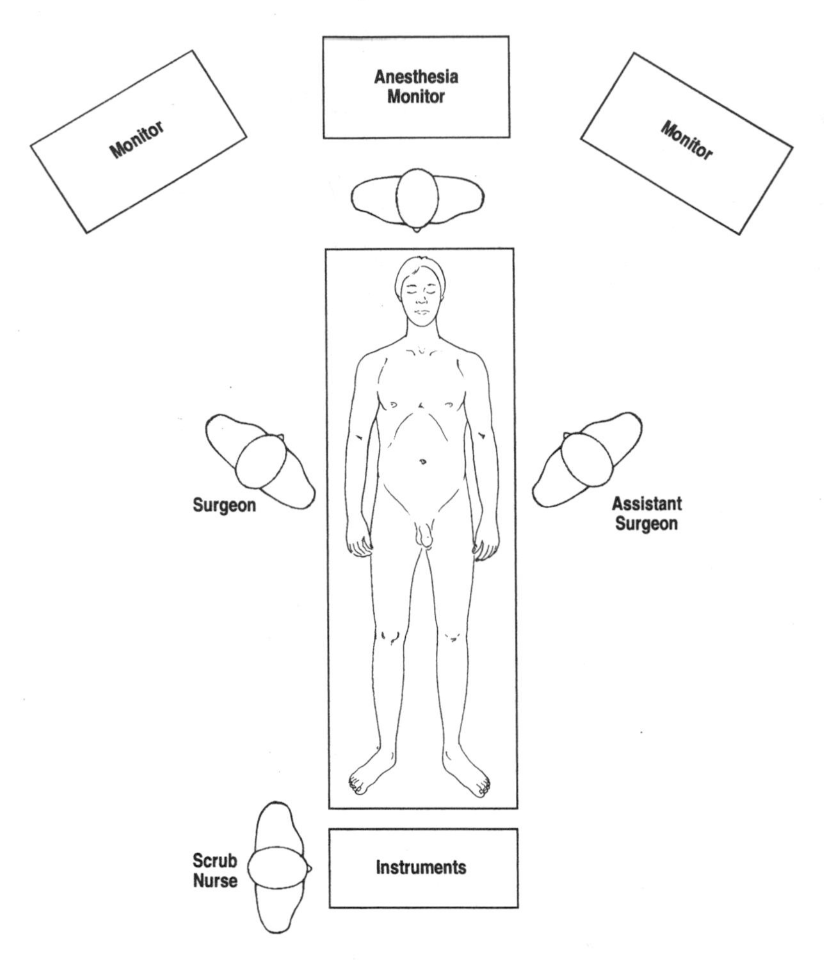

Figure 11.1.1. Patient position and operating room setup for laparoscopic transhiatal esophagectomy.

scopic esophagectomy (Figure 11.1.1), to permit the laparoscopic portion of the operation.

2. The surgeon stands on the patient's right side and the assistant stands on the left. The modified lithotomy position is also an option as described in Section A.3 (above). In this case, the surgeon may stand between the patient's legs.
3. The surgical technique is the same as for the totally laparoscopic technique except that only the lower esophagus is mobilized with access through the hiatus because the middle and upper parts of the esophagus are mobilized using thoracoscopy as described above.

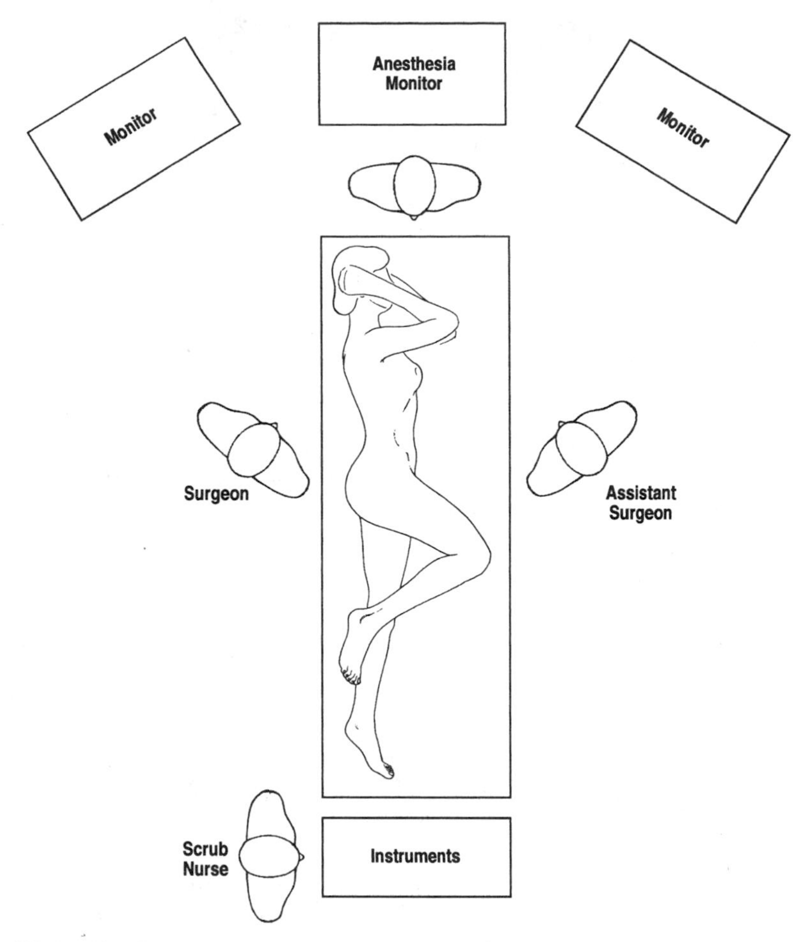

Figure 11.1.2. Operating room setup for thoracoscopic stage of thoracoscopic/laparoscopic esophagectomy.

B. Equipment

a. A double lumen endotracheal tube is essential for the thoracoscopic portion of the procedure.
b. A liver retractor is necessary for the abdominal portion of the procedure.
c. Standard laparoscopic/thoracoscopic instruments (including staplers, clip appliers, and energy sources) are routinely used for this procedure.

11.2. Port Placement for Minimally Invasive Esophagectomy

James D. Luketich, M.D.
Yaron Perry, M.D.

A. Introduction

Two different minimally invasive approaches to esophagectomy are presented in this chapter; in both methods the intraabdominal portion of the case is carried out laparoscopically. The first method, the transhiatal approach, avoids entry into the chest; in this case the operation is completed via a neck incision. In contrast, the second method calls for part of the case to be completed via thoracoscopic means. Regardless, a single port arrangement suffices for the transabdominal portion of both the transhiatal and the thoracoscopic/laparoscopic esophagectomy.

B. Port Placement 1: Laparoscopic Transhiatal Esophagectomy

1. Port placement arrangement
   a. Five abdominal ports should be placed (Figure 11.2.1).
   b. The initial port (5 or 10 mm) is placed cephalad and to the left of the umbilicus after the abdomen has been insufflated with a Veress needle at this site. This port is used for the laparoscope.
   c. An assistant's port (5 or 10 mm) is introduced at the costal margin lateral to the rectus abdominus muscle on the left.
   d. A 5-mm port is placed on the right side in the anterior axillary line just below the costal margin. This port is used for a 5-mm liver retractor to hold the lateral segment of the left lobe of the liver anteriorly and cephalad. This step will provide exposure to the esophageal hiatus.
   e. Another 5-mm port is placed at the lateral edge of the right rectus abdominus muscle just caudal to the costal margin. This port is used by the surgeon's left hand.
   f. A 12-mm port is placed superior and to the right of the umbilicus. This port is used by the surgeon (right hand) and must be 12 mm to accommodate the linear stapler.

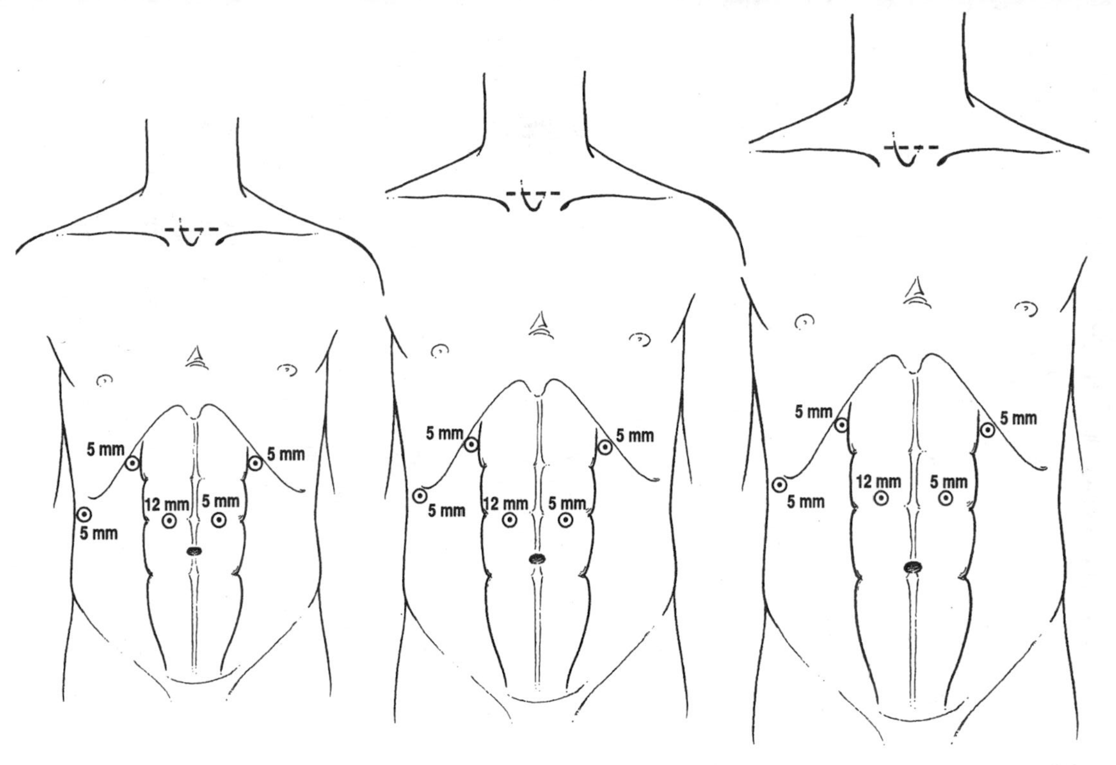

Figure 11.2.1. Port arrangement for abdominal portion of both laparoscopic transhiatal esophagectomy and for thoracoscopic/laparoscopic esophagectomy (five ports).

2. Brief description of procedure: The procedure includes the following parts:
   a. Mobilize the stomach by dividing the short gastric arteries, the left gastric artery, and the greater and lesser omentum.
   b. Kocherize the duodenum.
   c. Mobilize the esophagus through the hiatus.
   d. Make a neck incision to remove the esophagus, pull the stomach through the mediastinum, and create an anastomosis between the pharynx or proximal esophagus and the fundus of the stomach.

B. Port Placement 2: Combined Thoracoscopic and Laparoscopic Esophagectomy

1. Port placement
   a. Thoracoscopic portion (Figure 11.2.2)
      i. Four thoracic trocars are introduced. The camera port (5 or 10 mm) is placed at the seventh intercostal space at the midaxillary line.
      ii. A 5-mm port for the ultrasonic shears is placed at the eighth or ninth intercostal space, 2 cm behind the posterior axillary line.
      iii. One 5-mm port is placed behind the tip of the scapula.
      iv. An additional 5-mm port, for a retractor, is placed in the fourth intercostal space at the anterior axillary line.
      v. Next, a single retracting suture, 0-surgitek (US Surgical), is placed in the central tendon of the diaphragm and brought out of the inferior, anterior chest wall through a 1-mm skin nick using a suitable port closure device (suture passer).
   b. Laparoscopic Portion
      i. After the thoracoscopic portion of the case has been completed, the patient is repositioned into the supine position.
      ii. Next, five abdominal ports are placed on the anterior abdominal in the same locations as described for transhiatal esophagectomy (see Figure 11.2.1).

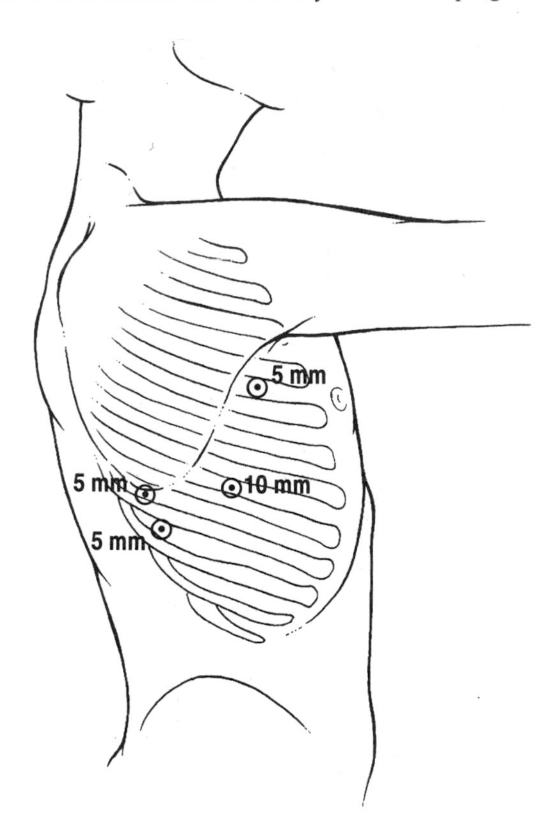

Figure 11.2.2. Port arrangement for the thoracoscopic portion of the combined thoracoscopic/laparoscopic esophagectomy. Ports are placed through the chest wall as described in text. None are placed below costal margin.

C. Selected References

Gerhart CD. Hand-assisted laparoscopic transhiatal esophagectomy using the dexterity pneumo sleeve. J Soc Laparoendosc Surg 1998;2(3):295–298.

Gossot D, Toledo L, Cortes A. Minimal access esophagectomy: where are we up to? Semin Laparosc Surg 2000;7(1):2–8.

Lerut T. Esophageal surgery at the end of the millennium. J Thorac Cardiovasc Surg 1998; 116(1):1–20.

Luketich JD, Nguyen NT, Schauer PR. Laparoscopic transhiatal esophagectomy for Barrett's esophagus with high grade dysplasia. J Soc Laparoendosc Surg 1998; 2(1):75–77.

Luketich JD, Nguyen NT, Weigel T, Ferson P, Keenan R, Schauer P. Minimally invasive approach to esophagectomy. J Soc Laparoendosc Surg 1998;2(3):243–247.

Luketich JD, Schauer PR, Christie NA, et al. Minimally invasive esophagectomy. Ann Thorac Surg 2000;70(3):906–912.

Nguyen NT, Schauer PR, Luketich JD. Combined laparoscopic and thoracoscopic approach to esophagectomy. J Am Coll Surg 1999;188(3):328–332.

Nguyen NT, Schauer P, Luketich JD. Minimally invasive esophagectomy for Barrett's esophagus with high-grade dysplasia. Surgery 2000;127(3):284–290.

Nguyen NT, Follette DM, Wolfe BM, Schneider PD, Roberts P, Goodnight JE Jr. Comparison of minimally invasive esophagectomy with transthoracic and transhiatal esophagectomy. Arch Surg 2000;35(8):920–925.

Sammartino P, Chirletti P, Calcaterra D, et al. Video-assisted transhiatal esophagectomy for cancer. Int Surg 1997;82(4):406–410.

Swanstrom LL, Hansen P. Laparoscopic total esophagectomy. Arch Surg 1997;132(9): 943–949.

Urschel JD. Ischemic conditioning of the stomach may reduce the incidence of esophagogastric anastomotic leaks complicating esophagectomy: a hypothesis. Dis Esophagus 1997;10(3):217–219.

Urschel JD. Esophagogastric anastomotic leaks: the importance of gastric ischemia and therapeutic applications of gastric conditioning. J Invest Surg 1998;11(4):245–250.

Watson DI, Davies N, Jamieson GG. Totally endoscopic Ivor Lewis esophagectomy. Surg Endosc 1999;13(3):293–297.

Watson DI, Jamieson GG, Devitt PG. Endoscopic cervico-thoraco-abdominal esophagectomy. J Am Coll Surg 2000;190(3):372–378.

Willson P, Montgomery P, Mochloulis G, Tolley NS, Rosin RD. Laparoscopically-assisted total pharyngolaryngo-oesophagectomy. Br J Surg 1997;84(6):870–871.

Yahata H, Sugino K, Takiguchi T, et al. Laparoscopic transhiatal esophagectomy for advanced thoracic esophageal cancer. Surg Laparosc Endosc Percutan Tech 1997; 7(1):13–16.

12.1. Hernia Repair: Patient Positioning and Operating Room Setup

David S. Thoman, M.D.
Edward H. Phillips, M.D.

A. Room and Equipment Setup

1. Inguinal hernia repair
   a. An adjustable operating table capable of Trendelenburg positioning is required.
   b. A movable cart with the following equipment is placed at the patient's feet:
      i. Large color monitor
      ii. Proccssing unit for camera
      iii. Light source
      iv. Insufflator
      v. Video cassette recorder (optional)
      vi. Color printer (optional)
   c. The monitor should be at a comfortable height facing the patient.
   d. The camera cord, light cord, and insufflation tubing are fastened to the drapes at the patient's knees and run directly to the instrument cart.
   e. The electrocautery unit and suction are best placed near the head and brought off either side. This allows the surgeon and assistant to change sides without negotiating cords and tubing.
   f. A mayo stand with instruments is placed over the patient's lower legs and appropriately adjusted for Trendelenburg positioning.
   g. Basic instruments:
      i. 30° 10-mm or 5-mm laparoscope
      ii. Veress needle, Hasson cannula, or an optical nonbladed trocar
      iii. Dissecting balloon (totally extraperitoneal approach only)
      iv. Fine laparoscopic grasping forceps with electrocautery potential
      v. Blunt locking atraumatic graspers
      vi. Laparoscopic scissors
      vii. Long laparoscopic needle for local anesthetic injection
      viii. Hernia mesh stapler

ix. One or two sheets of permanent mesh
x. Three working ports (diameter based on technique)

2. Incisional hernia repair
   a. Monitor position will vary based on hernia location and size. Likely to require repositioning during case because mesh must be anchored or sutured circumferentially.
   b. The position of the surgeon, first assistant, and cameraperson (if utilized) about the table will also vary during the case.
   c. Supine position again is utilized.
   d. Foley catheter is selectively used.
   e. As explained in next chapter, the number of ports required will vary.

B. Patient Preparation and Positioning

1. All patients should have had nothing to eat or drink for at least 6 hours before induction of anesthesia.
2. Bowel preparation may be considered for patients with multiple prior abdominal procedures but is generally not necessary.
3. Venous thromboembolism prophylaxis is not routinely used, although some surgeons routinely use pneumatic compression boots or subcutaneous heparin. There is little available information; however, the risk seems to be minimized with the short operative time and the liberal use of Trendelenburg. Patients at high risk may benefit from prophylaxis.
4. The patient voids before surgery, making routine **bladder catheterization** unnecessary unless there are bilateral hernias.
5. **Nasogastric drainage** is unnecessary, unless peritonoscopy is performed and gastric dilatation is present.
6. A first-generation cephalosporin, or equivalent, is given 30 minutes before incision.
7. The **supine position** is uniformly utilized for inguinal and incisional hernia repair. It is important to pad all bony prominences.
8. The arms should be padded and tucked at the sides if possible.
9. A retaining strap is placed at the midthigh level.
10. The abdomen is shaved from umbilicus to pubis.
11. An electrocautery grounding pad is placed on the patient away from the field.
12. **Antiseptic skin preparation** of the entire abdomen, genital region, and upper thighs is performed, in case scrotal manipulation is necessary.
13. **Draping** is done to limit the amount of lower abdominal skin exposed. This helps prevent inadvertent contact of the mesh with skin before implantation.
14. For unilateral inguinal hernias, the operating surgeon stands on the contralateral side. For bilateral hernias, the surgeon may remain on the left side or can switch sides (Figure 12.1.1).

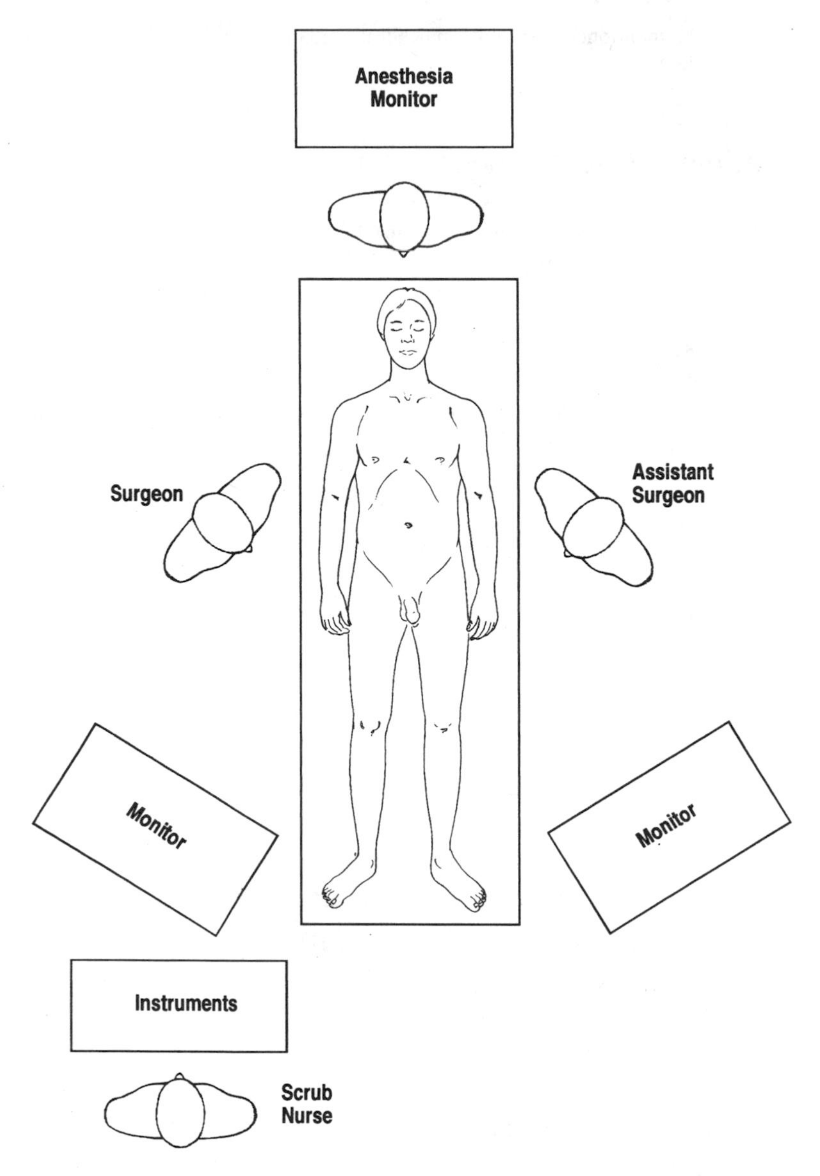

Figure 12.1.1. Typical operating room setup for laparoscopic inguinal hernia repair (surgeon positioned for a left inguinal hernia repair).

15. As mentioned, for incisional hernia repair the staff positions around the table will vary.

C. Selected References

Airan MC. Equipment setup and troubleshooting. In: Scott-Conner CEH, ed. The SAGES Manual. New York: Springer-Verlag, 1999:1–11.

Crawford DL, Phillips EH. Totally extraperitoneal laparoscopic herniorrhaphy. In: Zucker KA, ed. Surgical Laparoscopy. Philadelphia: Lippincott Williams & Wilkins, 2001: 571–584.

Fallas MJ, Phillips EH. Laparoscopic near-total preperitoneal hernia repair. In: Phillips EH, Rosenthal RJ, eds. Operative Strategies in Laparoscopic Surgery. New York: Springer-Verlag, 1995:88–94.

12.2. Hernia: Port Placement Arrangements

David S. Thoman, M.D.
Edward H. Phillips, M.D.

A. Transabdominal Preperitoneal (TAPP) Repair

1. The optical port (5–10 mm) is placed just below the umbilicus in the midline.
2. Place two additional 10-mm working ports lateral to the rectus sheath on either side at the level of the umbilicus. (Figure 12.2.1). These may be used to pass the mesh into the abdomen and to accommodate the hernia stapler.
3. Alternatively, a 5-mm helical tacker may be used, allowing for 5-mm lateral ports. The mesh can then be passed blindly through the 10-mm optical port. There are also data to support not fixing the mesh, although migration has been observed.

B. Near-Total Preperitoneal Repair

1. Pneumoperitoneum is established with the Veress needle technique, and an optical port (5–10 mm) is placed at the umbilicus.
2. A 10-mm incision is made just superior to McBurney's point on the right side of the abdomen. This point corresponds to the site of a preperitoneal fat pad commonly located in this position (Figure 12.2.2).
3. A Kelly clamp is then used to dissect through the oblique muscles until the peritoneum is reached.
4. A large mayo clamp is then used to develop this preperitoneal space, creating a pathway for a blunt-tipped 10-mm trocar.
5. A blunt grasper and CO_2 are used to develop the preperitoneal space toward the internal ring.
6. The procedure is duplicated on the left side at the mirror-image location.
7. The optical port is then repositioned into the preperitoneal space under direct vision, while the pneumoperitoneum is released.

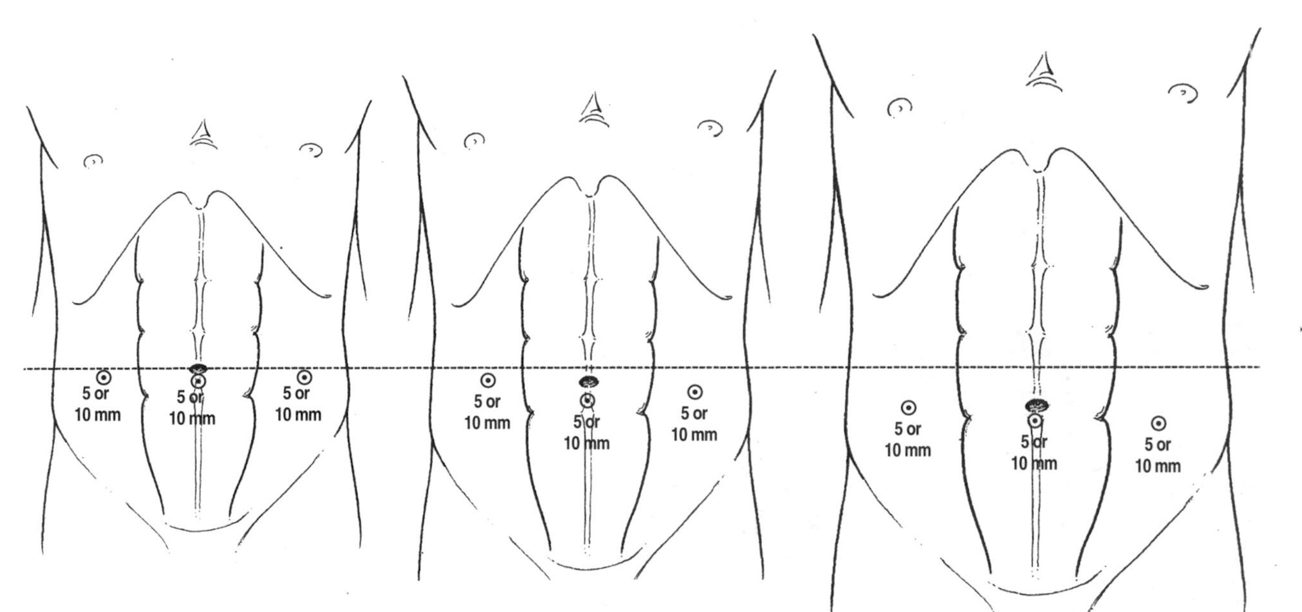

Figure 12.2.1. Port arrangement for transabdominal preperitoneal repair (TAPP).

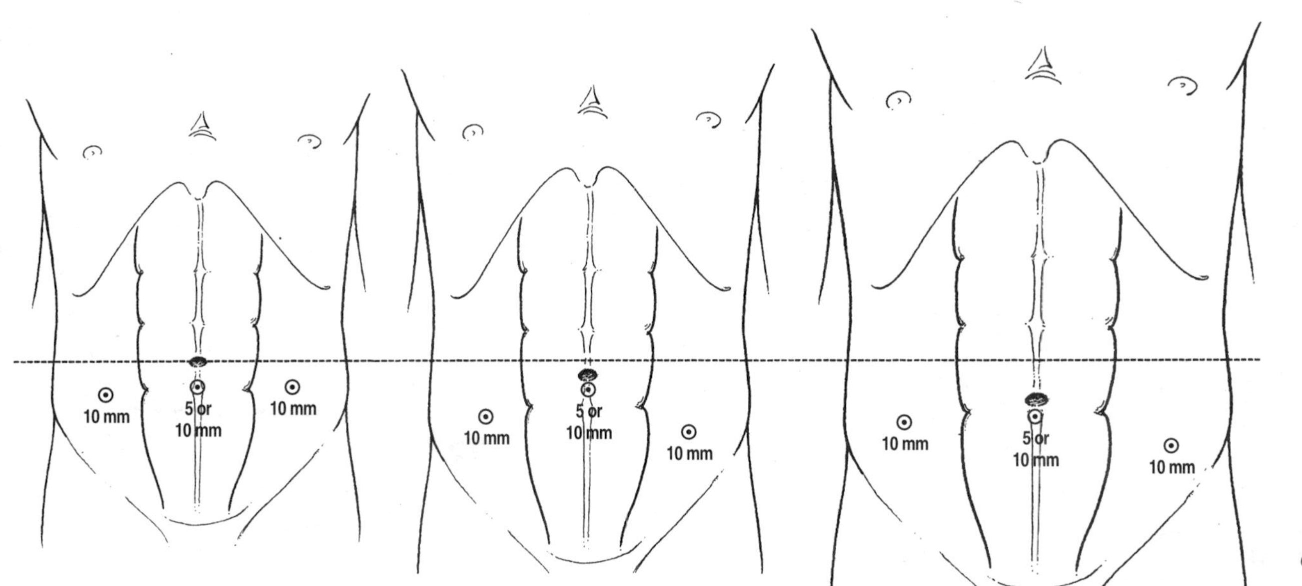

Figure 12.2.2. Port placement scheme for near-total preperitoneal repair (note that lateral ports are more caudally located than in the scheme depicted in Figure 12.2.1).

C. Totally Extraperitoneal Repair

1. The initial incision is made infraumbilically to accommodate a 10-mm port. The anterior rectus sheath is opened on the ipsilateral side and the muscle is retracted laterally to expose the posterior sheath. Stay sutures may be placed in the anterior fascia to secure the port and limit CO_2 leakage.
2. Dissection is carried toward the symphysis pubis, opening the space between the peritoneum and the transversalis fascia. This may be done with a dissecting balloon or manually.
3. Once the preperitoneal space is insufflated, two additional working ports are placed under direct vision in one of the following arrangements.
   i. A 5-mm port is placed one fingerbreadth above the symphysis pubis in the midline and a 5- or 10-mm working port is inserted midway between the 5-mm port and the umbilicus *(depending on the size of the fixating stapler or tacker to be used)*.
   ii. A 5- or 10-mm working port is placed midway between the symphysis pubis and the umbilicus (Figure 12.2.3A) *(depending on the size of the fixating stapler or tacker to be used)*, and a 5-mm port placed lateral to the rectus on the ipsilateral side (Figure 12.2.3B).
4. As mentioned, a 5-mm helical tacker may be used, or the mesh simply not anchored or fixed, reducing the minimum number of 10-mm ports to one.

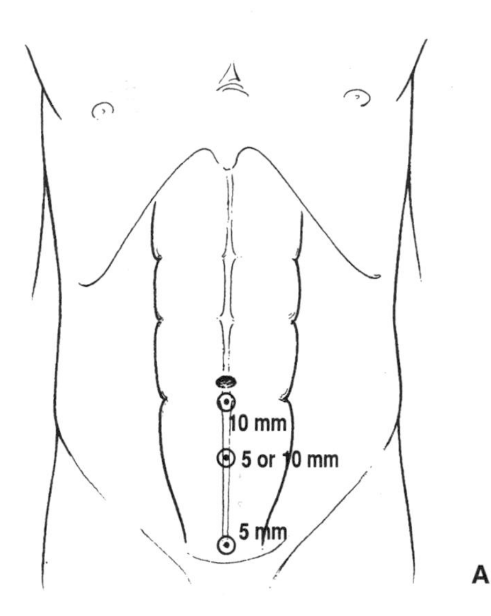

Figure 12.2.3A. Port placement scheme for total extraperitoneal repair.

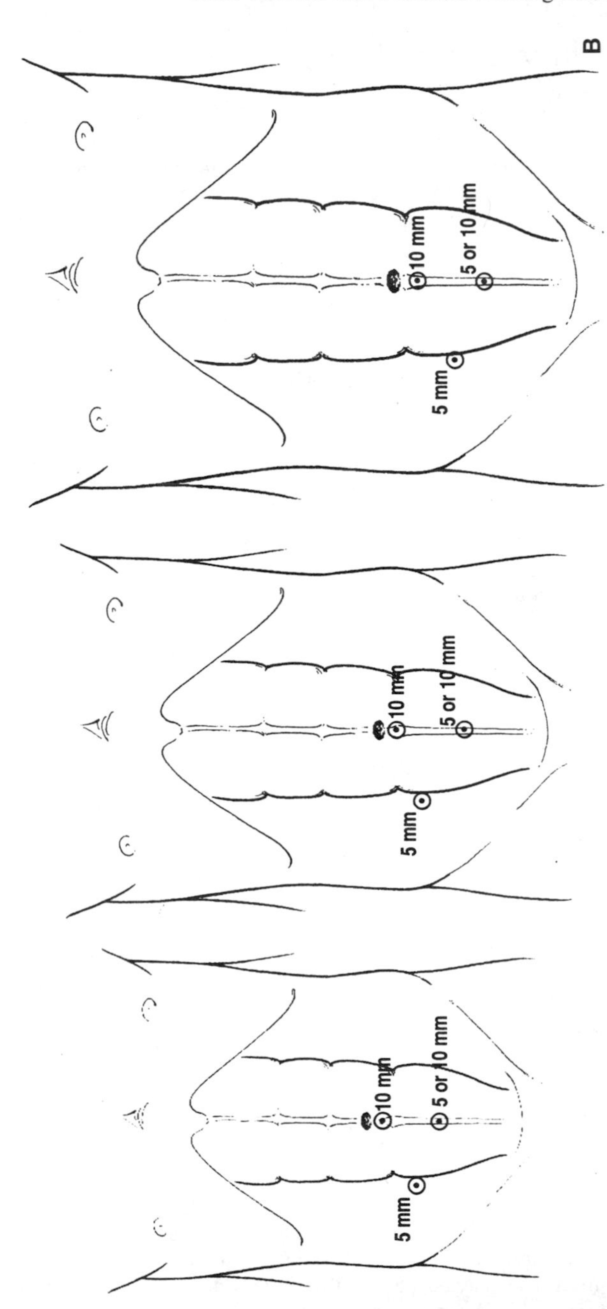

Figure 12.2.3B. *Continued*

Brief Operative Description of Inguinal Hernia Repair

Regardless of the approach, laparoscopic repair includes the following steps.

1. After access to the preperitoneal space, the preperitoneal space is developed to a large enough area to accommodate a sizeable piece of mesh.
2. The preperitoneal dissection includes reduction of the space (direct, indirect, or femoral).
3. The dissection must include exposure of midline between the rectus abdominus muscles, Cooper's ligament, the direct space, the internal inguinal ring, the gonadal vessels, and either the vas deferens or the round ligament, and enough space lateral, superior, and inferior to the internal ring to place mesh.
4. The peritoneum must be dissected away from the gonadal vessels sufficiently proximal for the mesh to fit posterior and inferior to the peritoneum.
5. The mesh is introduced into the preperitoneal space through one of the 10-mm ports.
6. The mesh is often, but not always, fixed with tacks or staples, depending on surgeon preference.
7. The peritoneum is either closed or allowed to roll up onto the mesh as desufflation occurs.

D. Ventral Hernia Repair

Port Placement 1

1. The site farthest from the edge of the hernia defect is found on the right or left lateral abdominal wall. The open Hasson technique is used to place a lateral 10-mm port midway between costal margin and the iliac crest. (Figure 12.2.4).
2. On the same side, under direct visualization, two 5-mm ports are placed, one as far superior and lateral as possible and one inferior and lateral.
3. Rarely, a fourth 5-mm port is required on the contralateral side.

Port Placement 2

1. A site for entry is chosen as far lateral and superior as possible (Figure 12.2.5). Either the Veress needle technique or Hasson technique may be used. This may be a 5- or 10-mm port, depending on the size of the laparoscope to be used.

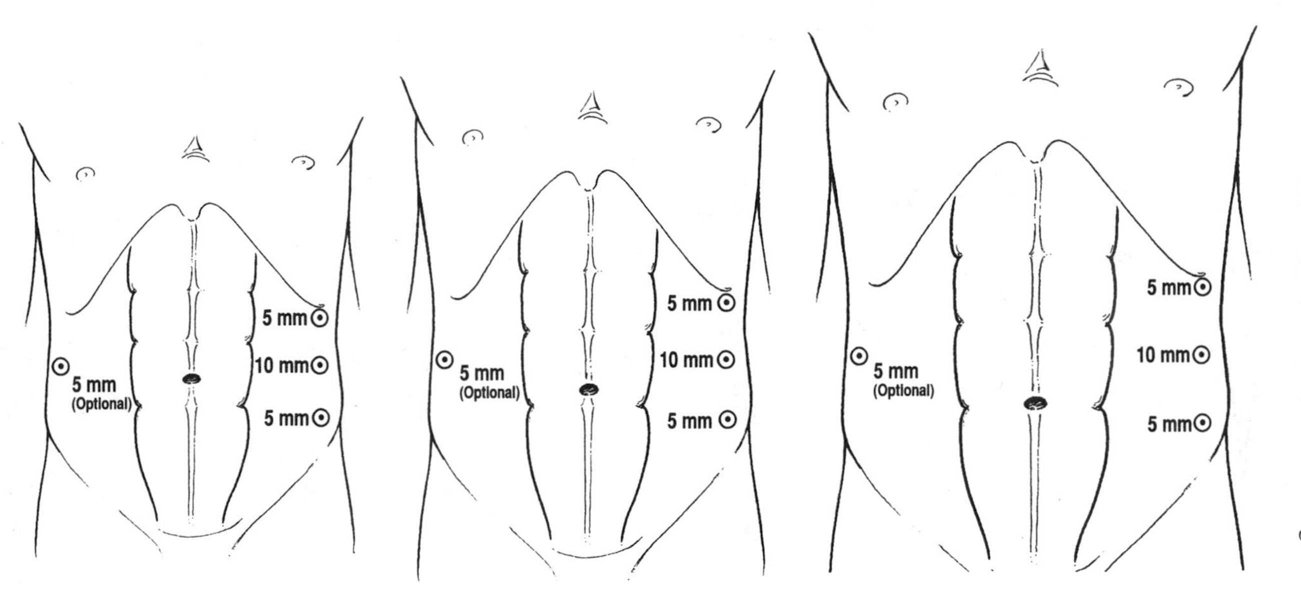

Figure 12.2.4. Port placement scheme for ventral hernia repair.

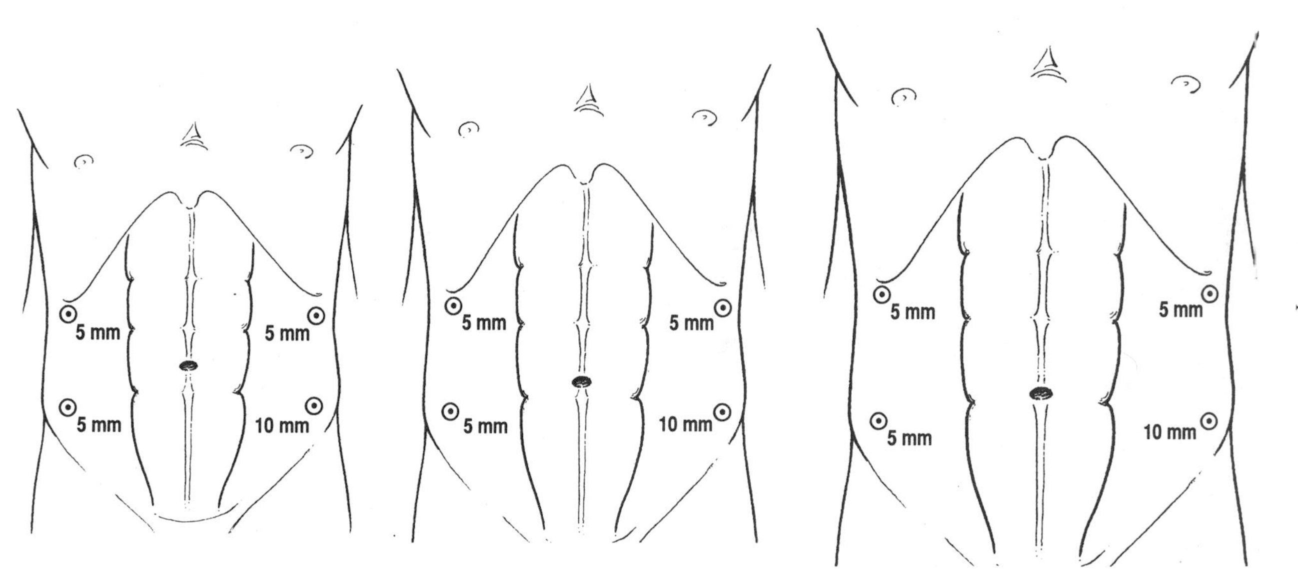

Figure 12.2.5. Alternate port scheme for ventral hernia repair.

2. With laparoscopic visualization, another 5-mm port is placed laterally and inferior to the defect.
3. After adhesiolysis, two mirror-image ports are placed on the opposite side of the abdomen, as far lateral to the defect as possible.
4. One of the four ports must be changed to a 10- or 12-mm port for introduction of the prosthesis. However, the other three ports may be 5 mm if the laparoscope is 5 mm.
5. This placement allows the use of the camera and tacker on the same side for tacking the opposite side of the mesh.

Brief Operative Description

1. After establishing laparoscopic access and placing ports, the first portion of the operation is to complete adhesiolysis between the viscera and the parietal peritoneum. This step includes reduction of all contents of the hernia sac.
2. The edges of the defect(s) are identified and marked on the abdominal wall. The combined size of all the defects is measured and the size of the mesh is chosen and cut, if necessary.
3. Sutures are placed at 5- to 6-cm intervals around the periphery of the mesh.
4. The mesh is rolled and placed into the abdominal cavity through the largest port.
5. The sutures are pulled through the abdominal wall muscles and tied over a bridge of muscle and fascia (through multiple 1- to 2-mm stab wounds in the skin).
6. The circumference of the mesh is tacked or stapled to the abdominal wall at 1-cm intervals between the sutures.

E. Selected References

Crawford DL, Phillips EH. Totally extraperitoneal laparoscopic herniorrhaphy. In: Zucker KA, ed Surgical Laparoscopy. Philadelphia: Lippincott Williams & Wilkins, 2001:571–584.

Fallas MJ, Phillips EH. Laparoscopic near-total preperitoneal hernia repair. In: Phillips EH, Rosenthal RJ, eds. Operative Strategies in Laparoscopic Surgery. New York: Springer-Verlag, 1995:88–94.

Heniford BT, Park A, Ramshaw BJ, Voeller G. Laparoscopic ventral and incisional hernia repair in 407 patients. J Am Coll Surg 2000;190(6):645–650.

Memon MA, Fitzgibbons RJ. Laparoscopic inguinal hernia repair: transabdominal preperitoneal (TAPP) and totally extraperitoneal (TEP). In: Scott-Conner CEH, ed. The SAGES Manual. New York: Springer-Verlag, 1999:364–378.

13.1. Spinal Access Operating Room Setup and Patient Positioning

Namir Katkhouda, M.D., F.A.C.S.
Sharan Manhas, M.D.

A. Equipment

1. Laparoscope, camera, and imaging equipment
   a. Advanced laparoscopic surgery cannot be performed without excellent instrumentation. This procedure is best performed with a three-chip digitally enhanced camera.
   b. The angle at which spinal surgery is performed is not usually straightforward, and therefore a 30° (or even 45°) scope is required to allow adequate visualization.
   c. Imaging equipment
      i. Fluoroscopic C-arm and fluoroscopy monitor
      ii. Radiolucent table (this is required for fluoroscopic guidance during cage implantation)
      iii. Two video monitors
2. Instrumentation: specific laparoscopic equipment required for spinal surgery
   a. Atraumatic graspers (in particular, a needle-nose grasper with an atraumatic tip is recommended)
   b. A 10-mm rotating right-angled dissector with an atraumatic blunt tip
   c. Laparoscopic Kittner dissectors
   d. Sharp scissors
   e. Medium and large clips
   f. Vessel retractor
   g. Vessel loops
   h. Atraumatic retractor (e.g., five-finger fan retractor)
   i. We recommend 5-mm ultrasonically activated shears because they limit lateral thermal damage
   j. A total of five ports
      i. Three 10-mm ports
      ii. One 5-mm port
      iii. One 15- to 18-mm port (for introduction of spinal instruments)

B. Preoperative Preparation

1. Mechanical bowel preparation to decrease bowel distension is optional
2. Foley catheter
3. Orogastric tube

C. Patient Positioning and Operating Room Setup

1. The patient is placed supine on a radiolucent operating table when operating on the L4–L5 or L5–S1 disk spaces (Figure 13.1.1). The modified lithotomy position can be used when performing higher-level spine cases such as L3–L4 or higher (Figure 13.1.2).
   a. The patient is either placed on a beanbag or is sufficiently padded to avoid any pressure injuries.
   b. The arms must be placed across the anterior chest to avoid interference with fluoroscopic imaging of the lumbar spine. The upper arms remain beside the torso, but the elbows are flexed, and the forearms are padded and laid transversely across the anterior chest. A foam pad can be placed between the arms and the chest as well as between the arms and the tape. It is important that the tape does not impede chest excursion and that the xiphoid process remain exposed.
   c. A roll is placed transversely under the patient's lumbar area.
   d. Steep Trendelenburg positioning must be used to facilitate exposure of the lumbosacral spine by displacing small bowel from the pelvis. The bean bag, stirrups, or tape are helpful in preventing the patient from sliding. If shoulder pads or shoulder table braces are used, great care must be used to avoid brachial plexus injury.
   e. The patient's head should be placed on a foam ring or pad and be strapped to avoid hyperextension of the neck.
   f. The patient must be positioned in such a way that the fluoroscopic C-arm can rotate around the patient to allow anteroposterior and lateral X-rays to be taken by the spine surgeon. Specifically, the patient must be placed on the table so that the lumbar spine is not overlying the post of the bed. This part of the bed must be free above and below for passage of the C-arm.
2. The laparoscopic surgeon stands on the right side of the patient facing the video monitor positioned at the foot of the operating table when performing L4–L5 or L5–S1 cases.
3. For higher-level spine cases, when the patient is in the modified lithotomy position, the laparoscopic surgeon stands between the legs and views the monitor to the left of the head of the table. Alternatively, if the patient is in the supine position for cases higher on the spine, the surgeon should stand on the patient's right side looking at the left cephalad monitor.

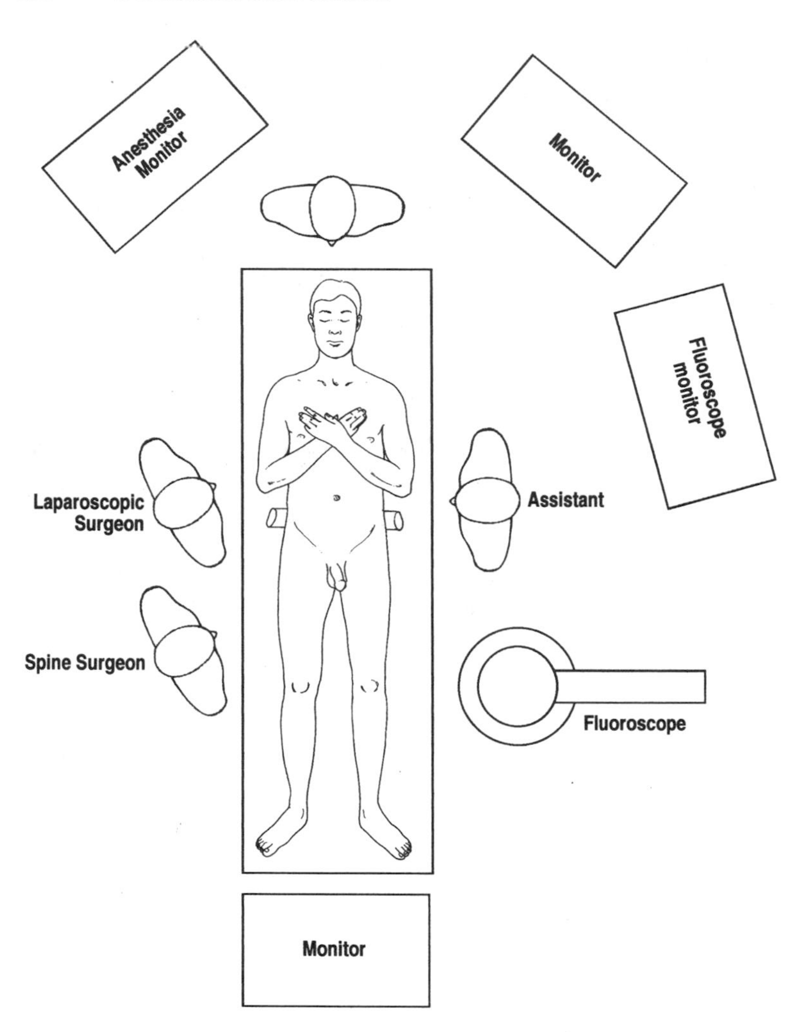

Figure 13.1.1. Supine patient position for spinal fusion.

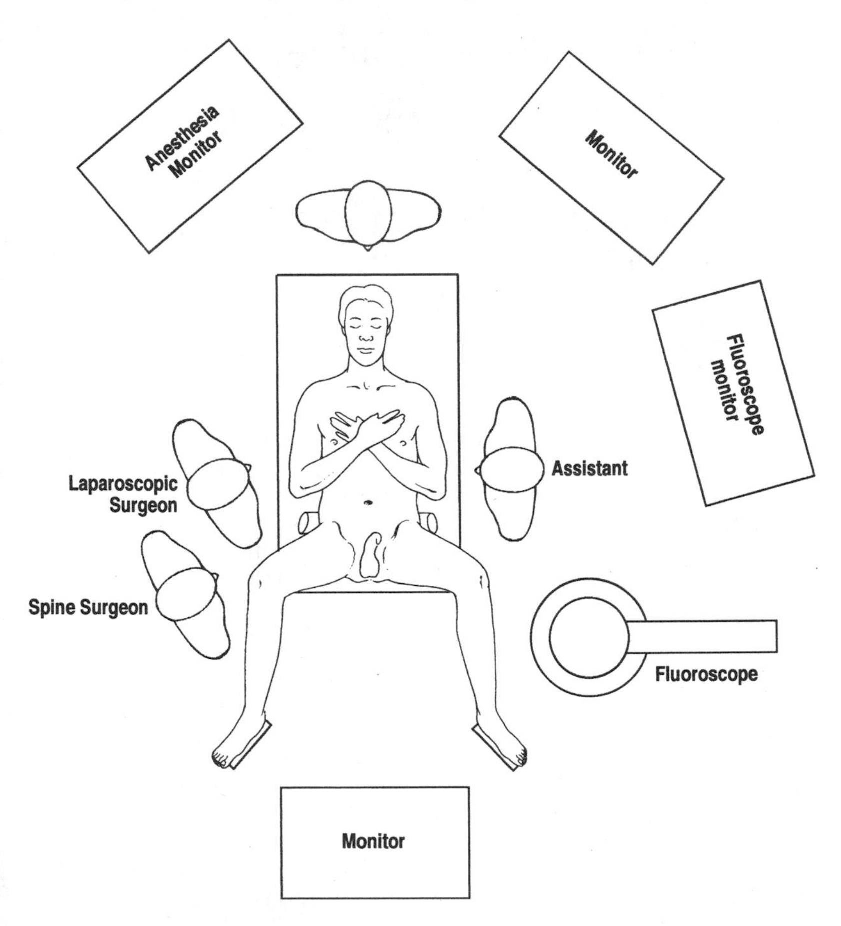

Figure 13.1.2. Modified lithotomy position for spinal fusion.

4. The spine surgeon stands on the patient's right side (if right handed) by the patient's legs and faces the video monitor and fluoroscopy machine placed behind the patient's left shoulder.
5. The assistant (who runs the camera) stands on the patient's left side and views the video monitor placed at the foot of the operating table. The assistant drives the camera and, in rare cases, may work through an optional port to retract the small bowel if exposure is difficult.

13.2. Spinal Access Surgery Port Placement Arrangements

Namir Katkhouda, M.D., F.A.C.S.
Sharan Manhas, M.D.

A. Port Placement

What follows are general guidelines; final selection of port sites is appropriately guided by the patient's anatomic variations. Thus, the surgeon should be forewarned that the port arrangements presented may need to be modified somewhat to accommodate a given patient. (Figure 13.2.1)

1. A 5- or 10-mm port (depending on size of laparoscope used) is placed at or just below the umbilicus (for patients with average or large body habitus) via the Veress needle method or via placement of a Hasson-type port after open cutdown (for large body habitus below, for petite body above). This will be primarily used as the camera port.

2. Two additional 10-mm trocars are next inserted under direct vision at the level of the left and right iliac crest just lateral to the border of the rectus muscle. Care must be taken to avoid the epigastric vessels. These are the operating ports for the laparoscopic surgeon. These trocars together with the camera port form a triangular configuration that minimizes "sword fighting" and helps avoid the "needle knitting" effect. (The availability of 5-mm clip appliers make it possible to use 5-mm ports instead of 10-mm ports at these locations.)

3. A 15- to 18-mm port is placed in the lower midline after the annulus has been laparoscopically exposed from side to side. This port is positioned in the lower midline superior to the bladder and is used for spinal instrumentation. It is often placed using fluoroscopic guidance to ensure a correct entry angle for working in the diseased disk space. Its location will be higher for L4–L5 than for L5–S1.

4. Occasionally, an additional 5-mm port may be needed in the left upper abdomen for the purpose of introducing an instrument to retract the small bowel with a fan retractor to provide better exposure of the spine.

5. For higher-level lumbar fusion, such as L3–L4 or rarely L4–L5, it may be desirable to place the camera port three fingers above the symphysis pubis and still maintain a triangular arrangement between this port and the lateral ports. This configuration allows the spinal instrumentation port to be inserted farther cephalad, even at the umbilicus, if necessary, and thus closer to the spinal target area.

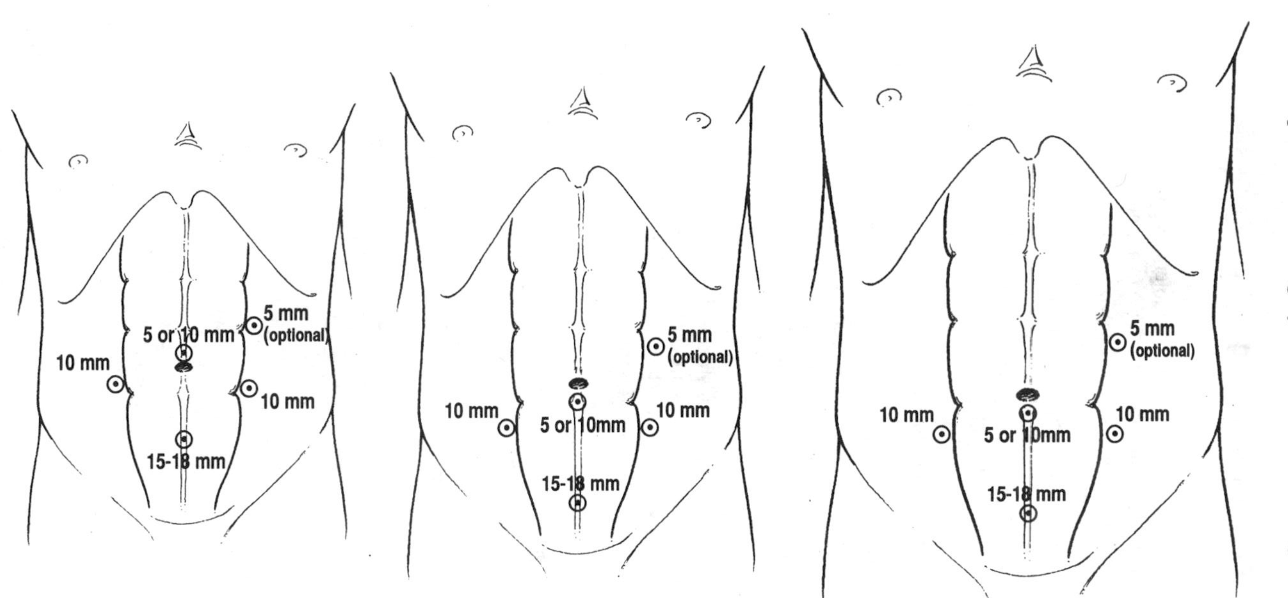

Figure 13.2.1. Port placement for spinal fusion.

B. Brief Description of Exposure Procedure

1. The patient is placed in steep Trendelenburg position. The surgical team member's locations about the table have been explained above. Dissection begins after sweeping the small bowel out of the pelvis. The sigmoid colon with its associated mesocolon is elevated and retracted to the left of the patient by the camera assistant. This exposes the sacral promontory. The sigmoid colon can be tacked in place by stapling the appendices epiploicae to the abdominal wall or by stapling the pericolic fat to the abdominal wall to hold the colon out of the way. This step can be accomplished with a hernia stapler. Two to three staples are usually sufficient to provide adequate tension on the mesocolon.
2. The posterior peritoneum is incised longitudinally over the sacral promontory.
3. The ureters are identified and avoided. The right ureter courses over the right iliac vessels and can usually be identified via visible peristalsis whereas the left ureter lies deep to the sigmoid colon in the retroperitoneal space.
4. Monopolar electrocautery should be avoided during the dissection to avoid injuring the presacral parasympathetic plexus, which can result in retrograde ejaculation.
5. Disk exposure is accomplished with a Kittner wand.
6. The middle sacral vessels are isolated, clipped, and divided.
7. The iliac artery and vein (left or right or both) are carefully dissected and retracted laterally with an endoscopic vascular retractor. The iliac vein represents the most hazardous part of the operation and should be protected during the spinal portion of the operation with a dental pledget.
8. At the L4–L5 level the left iliac artery must be formally dissected and retracted with a vessel loop. The vessel loop can either be held by the grasper of the camera assistant or exteriorized through a separate small skin incision. Next, the left iliac vein is exposed. The iliolumbar vein must be ligated to allow full mobilization of this vein. An alternative is to dissect the artery and vein as described before and then retract both vessels to the right medially in the event of a low bifurcation to expose L4–L5. To expose higher lumbar levels, the lumbar arteries and veins are exposed at the left side of the aorta and ligated. The big vessels are then retracted medially.
9. The dissection space should be large enough to allow the spinal surgeon to insert, through an 18-mm suprapubic port, the instruments needed to perform the spinal work.
10. Correct disk identification is accomplished by placing a Kirschner (K)-wire into the intervertebral space (intraoperatively or preoperatively from the back). The position of the K-wire is checked on anteroposterior and lateral fluoroscopic views. This localization also helps optimize positioning of the suprapubic working portal by ensuring that the docking trocar is perpendicular to the intervertebral disk space.

C. Selected References

Cloyd DW, Ovenchain TG, Savin M. Transperitoneal laparoscopic approach to lumbar discectomy. Surg Laparosc Endosc 1995;5(2):85–89.

Goldstein JA, McAfee PC. Minimally invasive surgery of the spine. J South Orthop Assoc 1996;5(4):251–262.

Katkhouda N. Advanced Laparoscopic Surgery: Techniques and Tips. London: Saunders, 1998.

Katkhouda N, Campos G, Vavor E, Mason RJ, Hume M, Ting A. Is laparoscopic approach to lumbar spine fusion worthwhile? Am J Surg 1999;178(6):458–461.

Lieberman IH, Willsher PC, Litwin DE, Salo PT, Kraetschmer BG. Transperitoneal laparoscopic exposure for lumbar interbody fusion. Spine 2000;25(4):509–515.

Mahvi DM, Zdeblick TA. A prospective study of laparoscopic spinal fusion. Techniques and operative complications. Ann Surg 1996;224(1):85–90.

Maun RA. Laparoscopic L5-S1 diskectomy: a cost-effective, minimally invasive general surgery-neurosurgery team alternative to laminectomy. Am Surg 1996;62(6):516–517.

McAfee PC, Regan JJ, Zdeblick T. The incidence of complications in endoscopic anterior thoracolumbar spinal reconstructive surgery. Spine 1995;20:1624–1632.

McAfee PC, Regan JJ, Geis WP, Fedder IL. Minimally invasive anterior retroperitoneal approach to the lumbar spine. Spine 1998;23:1476–1484.

Obenchain TG. Laparoscopic lumbar discectomy: case report. J Laparoendosc Surg 1991;1:145–149.

Olsen D, McCord D, Law M. Laparoscopic discectomy with anterior interbody fusion of L5-S1. Surg Endosc 1996;10(12):1158–1163.

Regan JJ, McAfee PC, Guyer RD, Aronoff RJ. Laparoscopic fusion of the lumbar spine in a multicenter series of the first 34 consecutive patients. Surg Laparosc Endosc 1996;6(6):459–468.

Regan JJ, Hansen Y, McAfee PC. Laparoscopic fusion of the lumbar spine: Minimally invasive spine surgery: a prospective multicenter study evaluating open and laparoscopic lumbar fusion. Spine 1999;24(4):402–411.

Slotman GJ, Stein SC. Laparoscopic lumbar diskectomy: preliminary report of a minimally invasive anterior approach to the herniated L5-S1 disk. Surg Laparosc Endosc 1995;5(5):363–369.

Slotman GJ, Stein SC. Laparoscopic L5-S1 diskectomy: a cost-effective, minimally invasive general surgery-neurosurgery team alternative to laminectomy. Am Surg 1996;62(1):64–68.

Tiusanen H, Seitsalo S, Osterman K, Soini J. Retrograde ejaculation after anterior interbody lumbar fusion. Eur Spine J 1995;4:339–342.

Zelko JR, Misko J, Swanstrom L, Pennings J, Kenyon T. Laparoscopic lumbar discectomy. Am J Surg 1995;169(5):496–498.

Zucherman JT, Zdeblick TA, Baily SA, Mahvi D, Hsu KY, Kohrs D. Instrumented laparoscopic spinal fusion. Preliminary results. Spine 1995;20(18):2029–2034.

14.1. Operating Room Setup and Patient Positioning for Laparoscopic Adrenalectomy and Donor Nephrectomy

Michael Edye, M.D., F.R.A.C.S., F.A.C.S.

A. Introductory Concepts

A. Both the adrenal gland and kidney can be approached transperitoneally or retroperitoneally. Retroperitoneal access is often used by surgeons with a background in urology or past experience with the lumbar approach to the adrenal gland. The prone position is used for the laparoscopic posterior approach to the adrenal. Positioning for the more common transperitoneal access is described in this chapter, with reference to the special needs of laparoscopy.

B. Patient positioning and OR setup are essential components for technical success because they ensure a stable and reproducible operative environment, which eliminates surprises.

C. For each procedure, accurate identification and dissection of *one* key structure facilitates rapid exposure of the target to be removed and successful completion of the procedure:
   1. Right adrenal: the lateral aspect of the vena cava
   2. Right kidney: the right renal vein
   3. Left adrenal: the left renal vein
   4. Left kidney: the left renal artery (or arteries)

D. As a rule, the laparoscope port should be sited so as to best visualize the key structure. From the list above, it is apparent that the patient position for transabdominal nephrectomy and adrenalectomy should be the same; however, some port positions and the location of the extraction site will vary depending on the target organ.

B. Operating Room Setup for Transabdominal Approach

A. The patient is placed in the lateral decubitus position (see positioning section below).

B. One surgeon and one assistant perform these procedures. In the transperitoneal approach, both surgeon and assistant stand facing the patient's abdomen, watching a monitor placed on the far side of the patient behind the patient's back (Figure 14.1.1).
C. The second monitor is placed on the surgeon's side of the table, behind the operative team. If the scrub nurse stands opposite the surgeons, on the far side of the table, she will be able to view the operation via this monitor (see Figure 14.1.1).
D. During procedures such as nephrectomy that require exposure, ligation, and division of large vessels, a scalpel with a large blade for rapid

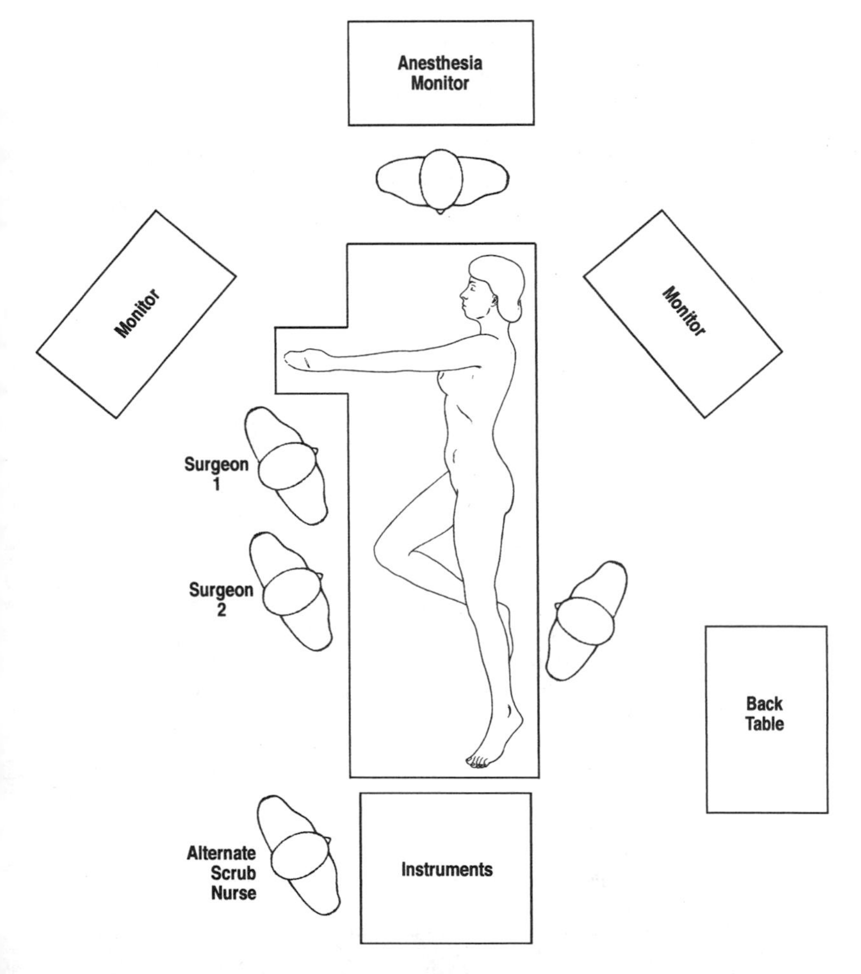

Figure 14.1.1. Operating room set up for left adrenalectomy or nephrectomy with patient in left lateral decubitus position.

laparotomy should be on the table and available at all times. Vascular instruments, self-retaining retractors, and other equipment necessary for a laparotomy should also be available in the room.

E. The kidney rest should be lowered or table flexion reduced, or both, before closing any muscle incisions, especially if it has been necessary to convert to an open procedure.

C. Transabdominal Approach: Patient Positioning

A. Lateral decubitus position: This is the recommended patient position. The full lateral decubitus position allows the mobile viscera (transverse colon, small intestine) to fall toward the midline, thus exposing the retroperitoneum. Other fixed organs such as spleen and colon will follow suit as they are freed from their attachments.

B. Extraction site: The extraction site should be planned in advance. Mark the proposed incision with an indelible pen after induction of anesthesia, while the patient is still supine. Once the patient is rolled into the decubitus position it is impossible to judge the midline and skin creases with accuracy; if the incision is chosen in this position, asymmetric and unsightly scars will often result. There are several possible incision locations through which a bulky structure such as the kidney can be removed.

   i. A Pfannenstiel transverse suprapubic incision is one option; the incision length is determined by the narrowest dimension of the kidney. The aponeurosis is incised transversely, after which a vertical incision is made between the rectus muscles, which are retracted laterally. This approach minimizes the trauma to the musculature such that, in many cases, little or no analgesic is required in the postoperative period.

   ii. A short (2-cm) muscle-splitting flank incision over the lateral border of the rectus is also well tolerated and gives ample room for removal of a small adrenal mass.

   iii. When hand-assisted methods are used, the kidney is usually extracted through the hand incision.

C. Conversion incision (contingency): Anticipate the need for a prompt conversion and plan accordingly before starting the case. The routine use of a kidney rest together with table flexion facilitates exposure should it be necessary to open the patient. A subcostal incision 3 cm from the costal margin can be made rapidly if the patient is properly positioned and provides good access to the vascular pedicle and the upper abdomen. It is wise to choose and mark the location of the conversion incision while the patient is supine.

D. Necessary operating table and positioning equipment: The following items should be available when performing these cases.

   1. Operating table that will flex in the middle, centered on a kidney rest
   2. Cushion to separate the legs
   3. Broad cloth tape (4 inches/10 cm wide, nonelastic)

4. Arm board and arm support
5. Axillary roll (I.V. fluid bag, molded silicone gel, or equivalent)
6. A bean bag for holding the patient
7. Pads to cover and protect bony prominences

E. Positioning the patient: sequence of events.
   1. Before turning the patient:
      a. Antithromboembolic leggings are fitted and activated.
      b. The patient is anesthetized and a urinary catheter inserted.
      c. The endotracheal tube is securely fastened to the patient's face. At all times great care is taken to ensure that the endotracheal tube remains intact, especially during position changes.
      d. The extraction site incision and the conversion incisions are clearly marked before repositioning.
      e. An assistant is delegated to hold the upper arm during the repositioning of the patient.
   2. Turning and positioning the patient
      a. A bean bag is placed on the table directly under the patient's trunk.
      b. The patient is next placed in the lateral decubitus position such that the side to be operated on is uppermost (see Figure 14.1.1). The patient's flank should be centered over the kidney rest. Once in position, the kidney rest is elevated. If a kidney rest is not available, a large bag of fluid should be placed under the flank.
      c. The bean bag, after being molded to the patient's body contour, is next suctioned, thus helping to secure the body position.
      d. The dependent limb is flexed at the knee and thigh while the upper leg is kept straight. The legs are separated by a cushion.
      e. The patient's abdomen should be close to the edge of the operating table (the reverse of the position used for conventional nephrectomy).
      f. An axillary roll is placed under the dependent axilla, which elevates the axillary contents. This should prevent compression of the brachial plexus.
      g. The table is placed in slight Trendelenburg position and then flexed at its center. A table flexion angle of 30° should be adequate (Figure 14.1.2).
      h. The head must be supported from below to keep the cervical and thoracic spines roughly axial without lateral flexion.

F. Securing the patient in position.
   1. Lower body:
      i. While the patient's back is maintained at right angles to the mattress, the lower trunk is securely but NOT tightly taped to the table. Broad adhesive cloth tape is recommended. The tape is attached to the table below the level of the hips (toward the feet) and is then run obliquely over the greater trochanter of the hip (yet below the pubis) before being attached to the opposite side of the table below hip level.

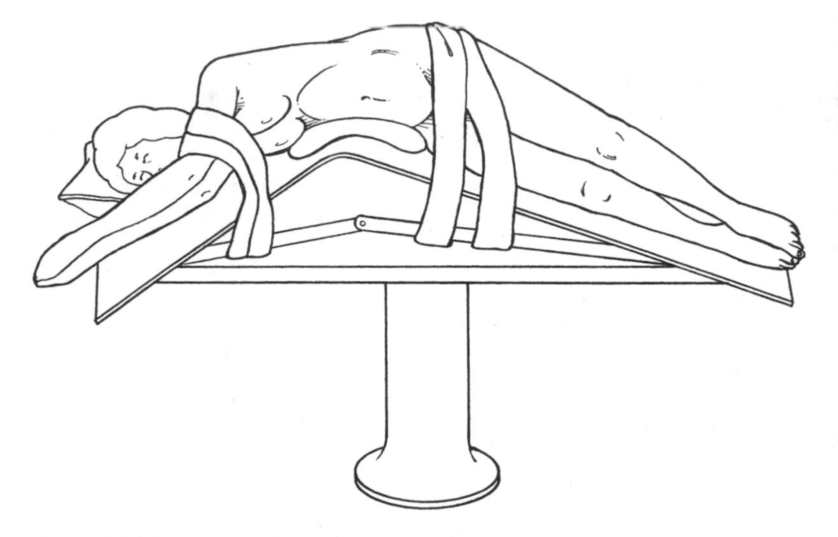

Figure 14.1.2. Lateral view of patient in lateral decubitus position with table flexed.

ii. When taped in this manner, access for a Pfannenstiel incision is preserved.
iii. This fixation prevents side-to-side displacement of the trunk. Care should be taken to ensure that the urinary catheter tubing is free of kinks and that it runs via gravity drainage to a reservoir at the anesthetist's end of the table.

2. Upper body:
   i. Bean bag as described above.
   ii. The lower arm lies on an arm board and is flexed at the shoulder and elbow so the hand is roughly level with the face.
   iii. The upper arm is supported on a stack of padding with about 90° of shoulder flexion. This will prevent the patient's arm from limiting the surgeon's access to the uppermost abdominal port.
   iv. The upper trunk is fixed in position with cloth tape that extends from the far end of armboard, over the upper shoulder, to the table on the opposite side.
   v. Note that although the patient should not be tightly taped, it is important that the adhesive should be in contact with the arm, shoulder, and trunk, unless the skin is in poor condition (as in renal failure, Cushing's syndrome, or the elderly) to prevent movement of the patient under the strapping. Removal of the tape at the case's end should be done gently. A solvent should be used to soften the adhesive in patients whose skin is in poor condition.

14.2. Port Placement in Laparoscopic Adrenalectomy and Donor Nephrectomy

Samer G. Mattar, M.D.
C. Daniel Smith, M.D., F.A.C.S.

A. Laparoscopic Adrenalectomy

A variety of laparoscopic approaches for adrenalectomy have been described. Each technique is associated with particular attributes that influence access strategy decisions. The selection of the optimal approach is based on patient characteristics, lesion factors, and surgeon experience. Each approach requires specific patient positioning, operating room setup, and port placement. This section presents the port placement arrangements for various approaches for laparoscopic adrenalectomy.

Although, strictly speaking, laparoscopy indicates entry into the abdominal cavity, the term has been used to describe the endoscopic access to other body regions, such as the retroperitoneum, for which the correct term would be "retroperitoneoscopy" or "lumboscopy." For the sake of simplicity, videoscopic retroperitoneal adrenalectomy is also described as "laparoscopic" retroperitoneal adrenalectomy.

1. **Port placement 1:** transabdominal lateral approach

The lateral decubitus position takes advantage of gravity as a facilitator of adrenal exposure. Additionally, by entering the abdominal cavity, the surgeon is afforded the opportunity to systematically assess abdominal contents before proceeding with dissection of the adrenal gland. (See Chapter 14.1.1 for details of positioning and operating room setup.)

a. **Left adrenalectomy** (Figure 14.2.1)
   i. Initial access is through an infraumbilical stab incision through which pneumoperitoneum is established with a Veress needle. Alternatively, the Veress needle may be inserted at the site of the first port, which is just below the costal margin along the anterior axillary line. A 5- or 10-mm cannula (depending on size of the laparoscope to be used) is inserted at this latter site, which is used for the laparoscope.
   ii. A second port (10 mm) is placed anteriorly, below the costal margin along the midclavicular line.
   iii. A third port (5 mm) is inserted below the costal margin along the midaxillary line.

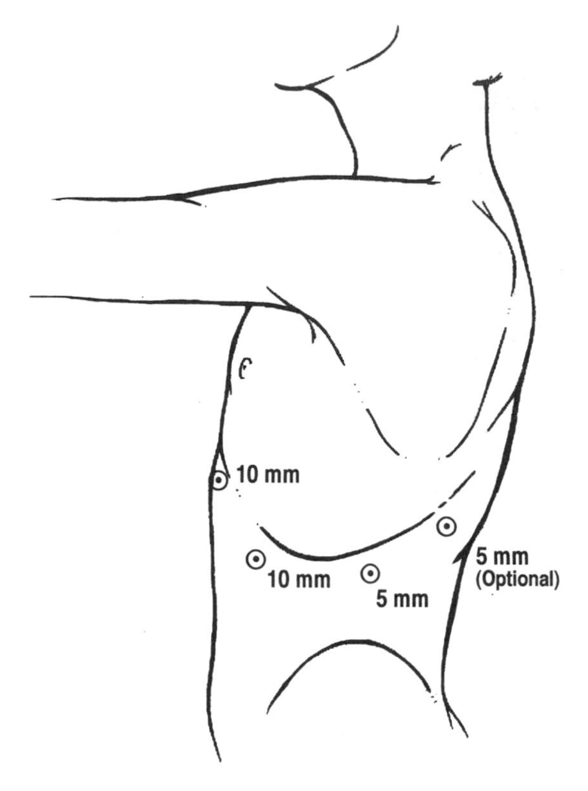

Figure 14.2.1. Port-placement for transabdominal lateral approach left adrenalectomy.

iv. Occasionally, a fourth port (5 mm) is necessary. This port is placed beneath the costal margin at the posterior axillary line.

b. **Right adrenalectomy** (Figure 14.2.2)

i. The port site locations for right adrenalectomy are similar to the arrangement described above. The ports in the anterior axillary line, midclavicular line, and posterior axillary line are all moved slightly anterior compared to the left side. However, a fourth port is invariably needed.

ii. The fourth cannula is placed in the epigastrium several centimeters below the costal margin. This port is dedicated for liver retraction. This port must be positioned so that a 5-mm retractor inserted through it will be parallel to the undersurface of the right lobe of the liver. Thus, the position and size of the liver determines the precise location (i.e., how far off the midline) of this fourth port.

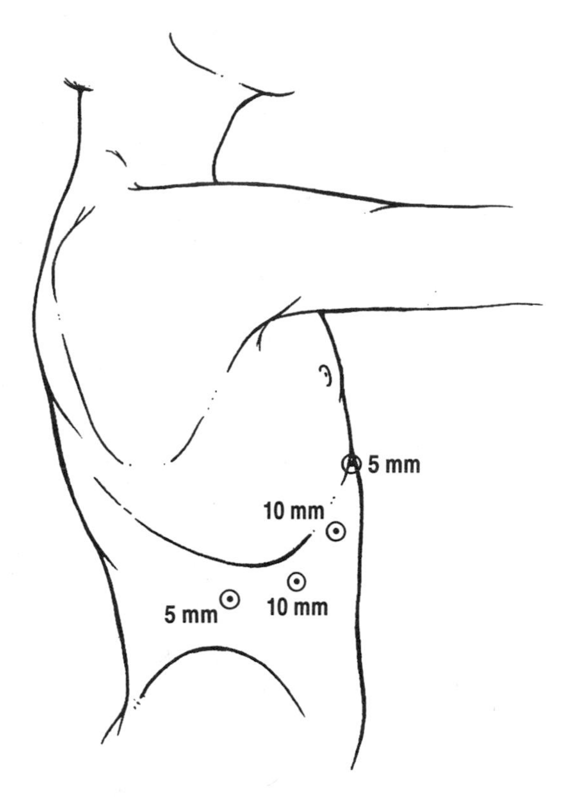

Figure 14.2.2. Port-placement for transabdominal approach lateral right adrenalectomy. The epigastric cannula is for the use of a 5-mm liver retractor.

2. Port placement 2: **retroperitoneal lateral approach**

This approach is occasionally favored in patients who have had previous intraabdominal operations and who possess small (<5 cm) adrenal lesions, most typically aldosteronoma. Proponents of this technique claim reduced discomfort and a shortened ileus secondary to the fact that the peritoneum is not breached; however, this has not translated into reduced morbidity rates. Liver displacement and retraction are not necessary in right adrenalectomy. Similarly, for left adrenalectomy, splenic dissection and colon retraction are avoided. However, thorough familiarity, on the part of the surgeon, with the retroperitoneal anatomy and perspective is mandatory. Other disadvantages include a limited working space, a paucity of identifying landmarks, and an abundance of retroperitoneal fat in obese patients. Figure 14.2.3A,B demonstrates overall layout for retroperitoneal approaches to the adrenal gland. The following port placement description applies to both left and right adrenalectomy.

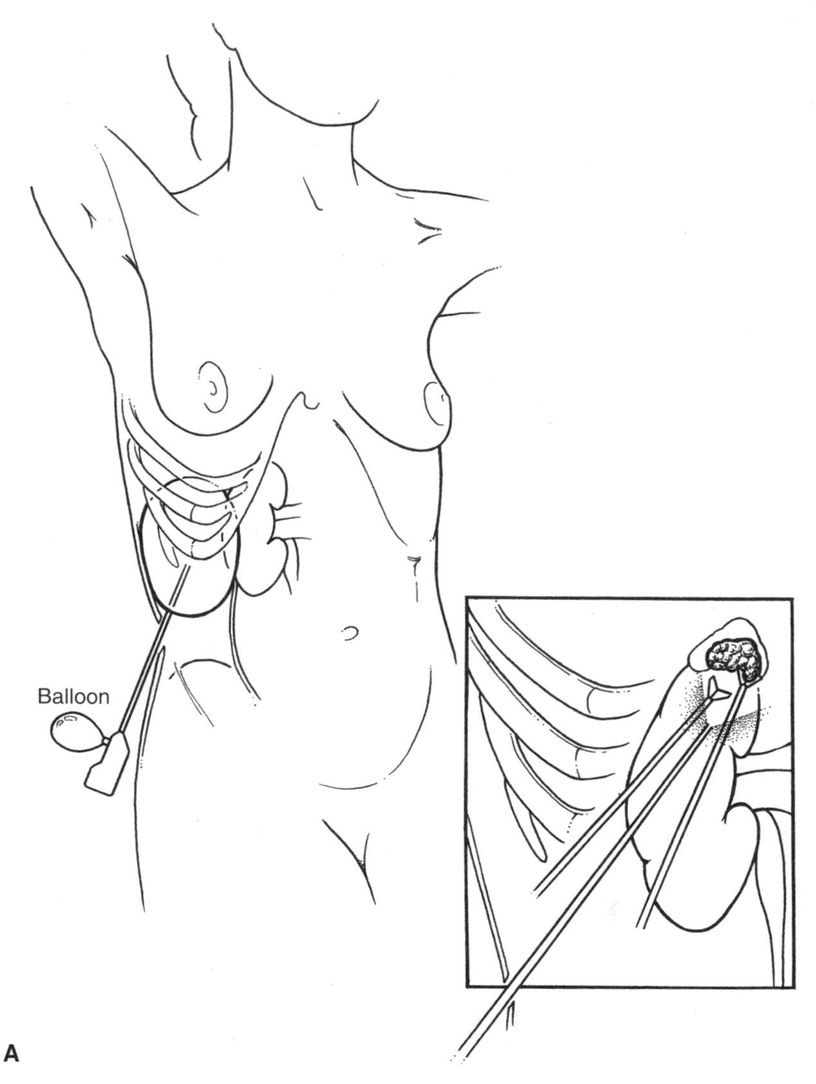

Figure 14.2.3. (A) Spatial relationships in the port-placement for retroperitoneal adrenalectomy. Inset demonstrates the position of instruments after creating the potential working space with the balloon dissector. (B) Port-placement for retroperitoneal lateral approach adrenalectomy.

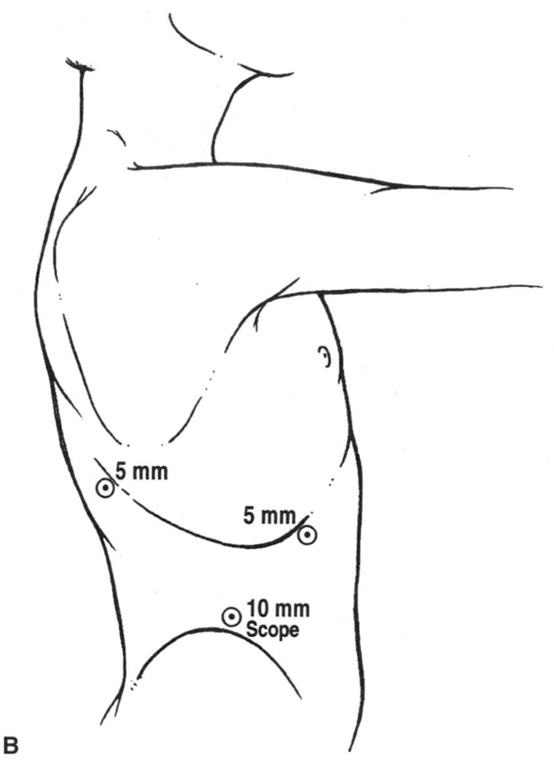

Figure 14.2.3. *Continued*

a. The patient is placed in the lateral decubitus position.
b. The laparoscope is placed through a 10-mm cannula situated above the iliac crest at the midaxillary line. The working space is developed initially by digital dissection, followed by balloon dissection and then gas insufflation. The remaining ports are placed after balloon dissection has been carried out.
c. A 5-mm trocar is placed below the costal margin at the posterior axillary line. Through this port, a forceps is used to reflect the peritoneum medially and to enlarge the working space such that an additional port can be accommodated.
d. A second 5-mm trocar is next inserted below the costal margin along the anterior axillary line.
e. If necessary, a third 5-mm port is placed above the iliac crest along either the anterior or the posterior axillary line.
f. Specimens are retrieved through the 10-mm cannula after replacing the 10-mm laparoscope with a 5-mm laparoscope.

3. Port placement 3: **transabdominal anterior approach**

This approach was commonly employed during the early years when the endoscopic methods and approaches to the adrenal gland were being developed. It has been largely abandoned in favor of the lateral approach. The anterior approach is occasionally utilized today for bilateral lesions. In these cases, the surgeon works against gravity. The adrenal gland, being positioned posteriorly in the retroperitoneum, is difficult to expose and visualize due to the overlying structures or submersion in a pool of blood or irrigation fluid. These drawbacks result in a need for additional port sites to provide adequate retraction and frequent application of a suction device to achieve optimal exposure. The port site arrangements are demonstrated in Figure 14.2.4.

a. The patient is placed in the supine position (or modified lithotomy position).
b. Abdominal insufflation is carried out either via the umbilicus (open Hasson technique) or via a Veress needle inserted about 2 cm superior to the umbilicus. The laparoscope is inserted via a cannula placed at this site.
c. Under direct vision, three additional 10-mm ports are inserted subcostally. The first is placed in the subxiphoid area to provide access for a retractor.
d. A second 10-mm port is placed about 2 cm below the costal margin in the midclavicular line.
e. The third 10 mm port is placed along the anterior axillary line about halfway between the iliac crest and the costal margin.

4. Port placement 4: **posterior approach**

As with the lateral retroperitoneal method, the posterior approach, carried out with the patient in the prone position, eliminates the need to deal with and retract the intraabdominal organs. Gravity pulls the liver, spleen, and splenic flexure of the colon away from the operative field. The first organ that is encountered with this method is the adrenal gland; therefore, minimal dissection is required. Further, the rib cage provides a rigid canopy that requires no retraction and results in the need for only a minimal amount of insufflation. Furthermore, the patient does not need to be repositioned in cases of bilateral adrenal lesions, minimizing anesthesia time. However, this approach also shares the disadvantages associated with lateral retroperitoneal access. The working space is small, and thus this method is not appropriate for large lesions. Additionally, the surgeon is unable to conduct an operative assessment of the intraabdominal organs, should this be necessary (e.g., malignancy). Finally, the prone position may not be attainable in some patients. Placing the operating table in the jackknife, flexed position helps widen the gap between the costal margin and the pelvis.

a. Port placement is preceded by transcutaneous ultrasonography to accurately delineate the position of the adrenal lesion and the kidney, particularly in relation to the 12th rib (Figure 14.2.5).
b. The outline of the 12th rib is drawn by palpation. An 11-mm port with a 0° laparoscope already inserted is advanced under direct vision through a 1.5-cm incision made 2 cm inferior and parallel to the 12th rib. The trocar is temporarily replaced with a dissecting balloon and then reinserted to insufflate.

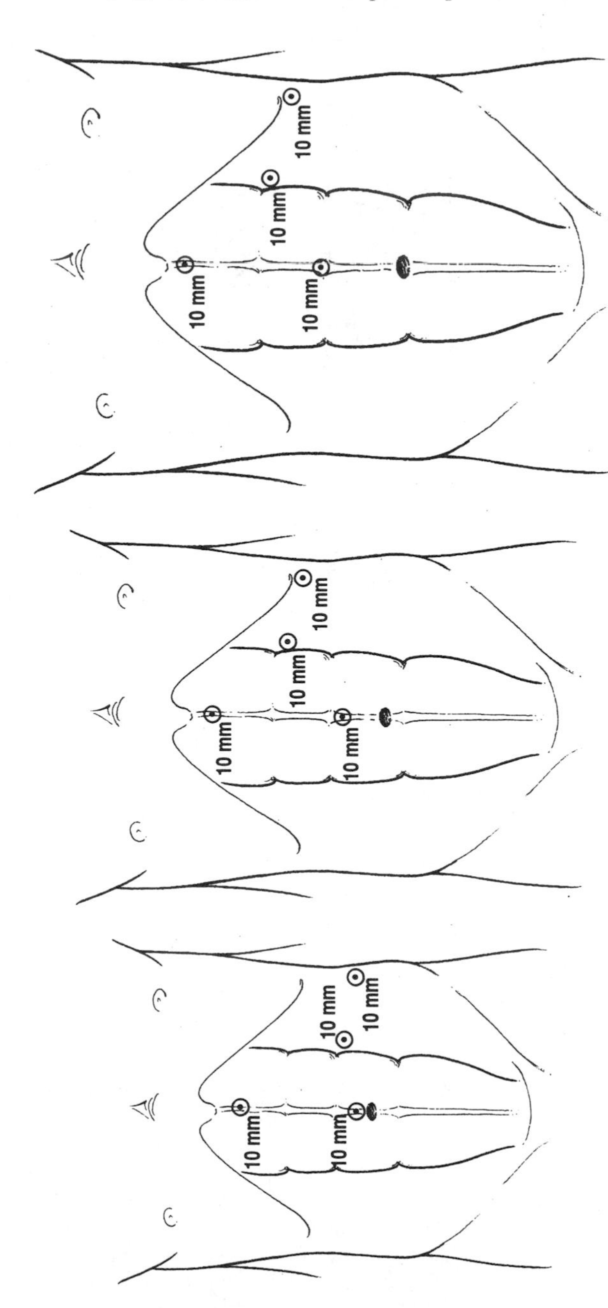

Figure 14.2.4. Port placement for transabdominal anterior bilateral adrenalectomy.

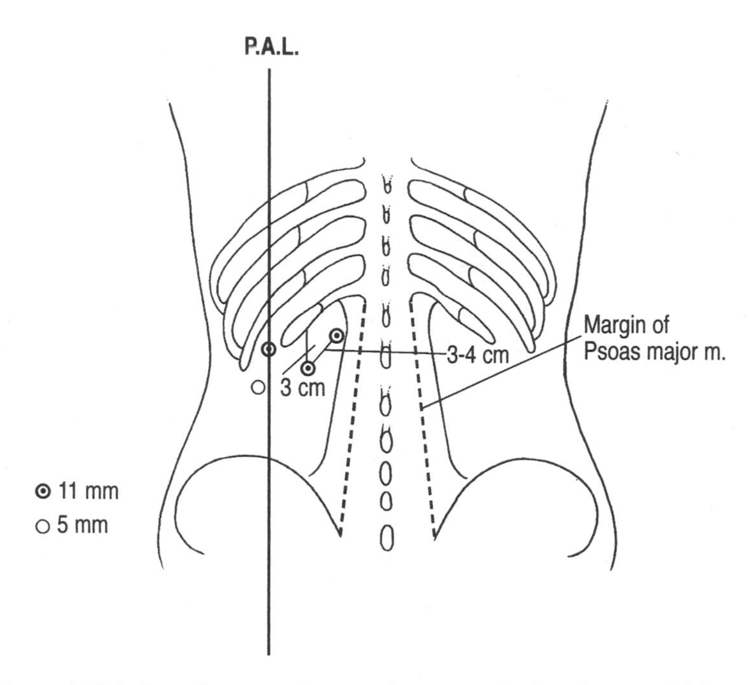

Figure 14.2.5. Port placement for posterior approach adrenalectomy. PAL, posterior axillary line.

c. Two additional ports are placed a few centimeters on either side of the initial port as the patient's body habitus allows. These ports may be either 11 or 5 mm.
d. Port sites are the same in relation to anatomic structures on each side.

B. Donor Nephrectomy

The main benefit from the application of laparoscopic principles to donor nephrectomy has been the greater acceptance of kidney donation and the overall expansion of the pool of kidney donors. This is particularly important in communities where cadaveric kidneys are not available. This goal was accomplished by following two basic surgical tenets. First, the safety and level of comfort of the donor is paramount. Second, the delivered kidney should be in pristine condition, ready to function immediately upon reperfusion and maintain a graft survival rate that is at least equal to that of open live donor nephrectomy.

Minimally invasive access, associated with the expeditious retrieval of the graft, has resulted in favorable clinical outcomes for both the volunteering donor and the recipient. Initial concerns regarding the safety of donors and the suitability of kidneys obtained through this method have largely been allayed as a result of experience and outcomes research. Laparoscopic approaches offer reduced patient discomfort, improved organ visualization, reduced hospitalization, and accelerated resumption of regular activities. Retroperitoneoscopic approaches can, in addition, avoid abdominal adhesions. As for the recipient, recent modifications, such as the incorporation of the hand-assist device, have produced grafts that have been subjected to warm ischemia times of only about 1 minutc. This fcat, in addition to the minimal manipulation of the kidney and the cautious dissection of the ureter, has resulted in graft function that is similar to that obtained after open nephrectomy.

Inherent to any operative strategy is the delivery of an intact kidney. For this purpose, any approach to the kidney will incorporate an extraction incision that must be adequately planned, and aptly considered when positioning and preparing the patient.

1. Port placement for hand-assisted donor nephrectomy (lateral decubitus position)
   a. The patient is placed in the lateral decubitus position. Then, the table is widely flexed and the kidney rest elevated.
   b. After the pneumoperitoneum has been created via a Veress needle introduced through an infraumbilical incision (note that this site for insufflation will later become incorporated into the incision for the hand-assist device), the locations for the hand-assist device and trocars are determined (Figure 14.2.6). The hand-assist device is ideally situated so that the umbilicus is at the center of the device, and a 7- to 8-cm vertical midline incision is planned. The hand device can also be inserted via a Pfannenstiel incision, which is more cosmetic. However, this is further away from the kidney and makes the procedure more difficult.
   c. The initial port, 5 or 10 mm depending on size of laparoscope to be used, is inserted immediately below the costal margin along the anterior axillary line.
   d. An optional 5-mm port is placed below the costal margin along the midclavicular line.
   e. A 10-mm port is situated below the costal margin along the midaxillary line, midway between the costal margin and the iliac crest. The surgeon uses this port and the midclavicular port until the hand-assist device is inserted, after which the first assistant takes over the 5-mm port.
   f. Hand-assisted right donor nephrectomy is more difficult for right-handed surgeons, and requires placement of the hand incision in the right lower quadrant or as a Pfannenstiel incision.
2. Port placement for laparoscopic donor nephrectomy

The totally laparoscopic approach uses the same port placement scheme that is described above before the placement of the hand-assist device; however, the extraction incision is not made until the end of the procedure. The extraction incision can be either a muscle-splitting incision in the left lower quadrant lateral to the rectus abdominus or a short Pfannenstiel incision. A hand-assist device is not utilized.

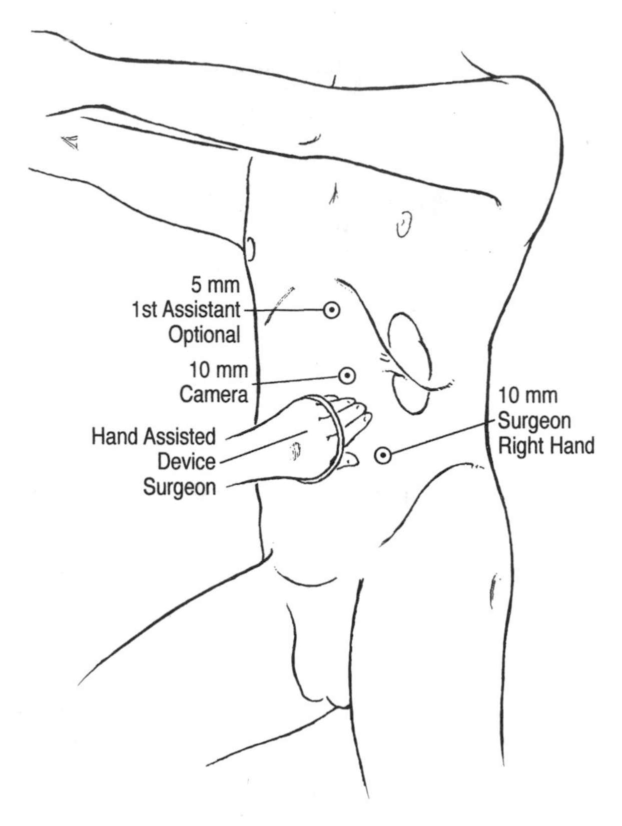

Figure 14.2.6. Port-placement for hand-assisted transperitoneal donor nephrectomy.

C. Selected References

Buell JF, Edye M, Johnson M, et al. Are concerns over right laparoscopic donor nephrectomy unwarranted? Ann Surg 2001;233:645–651.

Flowers JL, Jacobs S, Cho E, et al. Comparison of open and laparoscopic live donor nephrectomy. Ann Surg 1997;226:483–490.

Gagner M, Lacroix A, Prinz RA, et al. Early experience with laparoscopic approach for adrenalectomy. Surgery 1993;114:1120–1125.

Jacobs JK, Goldstein RE, Geer RJ. Laparoscopic adrenalectomy: a new standard of care. Ann Surg 1997;225:495–502.

Jacobs SC, Cho E, Dunkin BJ, et al. Laparoscopic live donor nephrectomy: the University of Maryland 3-year experience. J Urol 2000;164:1494–1499.

Linos DA, Stylopoulos N, Boukis M, et al. Anterior, posterior, or laparoscopic approach for the management of adrenal disease? Am J Surg 1997:173:120–125.

Siperstein AE, Berber E, Engle KL, Duh Q, Clark OH. Laparoscopic posterior adrenalectomy. Arch Surg 2000;135:967–971.

Slakey DP, Wood JC, Hender D, Thomas R, Cheng S. Laparoscopic living donor nephrectomy. Advantages of the hand-assisted method. Transplantation 1999;68:581–583.

Smith CD, Weber CJ, Amerson JR. Laparoscopic adrenalectomy: new gold standard. World J Surg 1999;17:389–396.

Suzuki K. Laparoscopic adrenalectomy: retroperitoneal approach. Urol Clin N Am 2001; 28:85–95.

15.1. Colorectal Resections: Patient Positioning and Operating Room Setup

Tonia M. Young-Fadok, M.D., M.S., F.A.C.S.

A. Room Layout: General Consideration

1. **Is the operating room large enough to accommodate the equipment necessary for a minimally invasive procedure?** This is a basic consideration when a laparoscopic case is assigned to an operating room (OR) not usually used for laparoscopic procedures or when performing an advanced procedure for the first time. Compared to an open case, laparoscopic procedures require considerably more space to accommodate the towers, monitors, and other specialized equipment.

2. **Positioning of the OR table.** In most minimally invasive colorectal resections, a portion of the procedure is carried out extracorporeally. To ensure optimal visualization for this part of the case, it is important that the operating table be well positioned beneath the OR lights. The orientation of the operating table (obliquely, longitudinally, or transversely) in relation to the anesthesia equipment, the shape of the room, and the OR doors also needs to be carefully considered because of the large amount of equipment that must be arrayed about the OR table. A poor table position may impede the repositioning of TV monitors or other equipment or hamper the circulating nurse's ability to move about the room.

3. **Two basic body positions** are utilized for colorectal resections, the supine position and the modified lithotomy position. The choice of body position affects the subsequent OR setup. Surgeon preference and the type of procedure to be performed dictate the position choice.

4. **The supine position** may be used for simpler procedures where limited colonic mobilization is required and when access to the perineum for circular stapling or colonoscopy is not necessary. Examples of such procedures are creation of ileostomy or colostomy, small bowel resection, ileocecectomy, and right hemicolectomy. In contrast, some laparoscopic surgeons nearly always utilize the modified lithotomy position, regardless of the specific operation to be performed, because it permits the surgeon or assistant to stand between the legs to dissect or retract when working in the upper abdominal quadrants. This spot is ideal for flexure takedown and separation of the omentum from the transverse colon.

5. **The modified lithotomy position** is uniformly used for left-sided colorectal resections and for subtotal colectomy. This position provides access to

the perineum for stapling or colonoscopy and, as described above, provides an excellent vantage point from which the surgeon can carry out portions of the procedure. For these reasons, some experts utilize this position for all colorectal resections.

6. **Bilateral arm tuck.** Most laparoscopic surgeons place and tuck both arms at the patient's sides when performing colorectal resections regardless of which body position is used. This arrangement provides the surgical team full access to both the left and the right sides. The arms are tucked only after the anesthesia team has had the opportunity to place intravenous and arterial lines as well as a blood pressure cuff, pulse oximeter, and the rest of their equipment. The inside and the outside aspects of the arms must be well padded before tucking.

7. Most equipment should be in position or in the room ready to be moved into position before the patient is brought into the room. This will expedite the commencement of the operation. Depending on the room size, it may be necessary to keep certain pieces of equipment that are required for a single aspect of the case or that may not be needed at all in the corridor immediately outside the room. Examples of this type of equipment include the ultrasound machine and the colonoscopy/endoscopy tower.

8. This chapter is concerned with body position on the table and OR setup. The figures also illustrate where the surgeon, first assistant, and, if utilized, the cameraperson would likely stand during the procedure. Port placement options are discussed in the next chapter. Most port placement schemes can be utilized in conjunction with either the supine or the modified lithotomy position. However, the left lateral decubitus position for sigmoid colectomy requires a unique port arrangement that is briefly mentioned in that section.

9. Methods of securing the patient to the OR table are discussed in a separate section. The issue is not revisited in subsequent sections. The approaches to a variety of other operating room setup and patient positioning issues are the same regardless of which colorectal segment is being removed. Rather than repeat the discussion in each section devoted to a different type of resection, the information is given once and the reader is referred back to the earlier section.

10. Utilizing the figures. All but one of the following sections concern one or several different types of segmental colorectal resections. Right hemicolectomy is considered separately whereas sigmoid colectomy, low anterior resection, and abdominoperineal resection are discussed together. Finally, the OR setup and port arrangement for distal transverse, splenic flexure, and proximal descending segmental colectomy are presented.

11. **Scrub nurse position.** There are two basic strategies in regard to the position of the scrub nurse. The first is to place the scrub nurse, the instrument table, and the mayo stand at the foot of the table, either directly below the table or off the left or right foot (see Figures 15.1.2, 15.1.3). It is often possible, depending on the specific operation, to place the elevated mayo stand over the draped legs. The alternate approach, which is the preference of the author, is to position the scrub nurse at the head of the table (see inset in Figure 15.1.5). In this case the elevated mayo stand is placed over the head of the patient and the scrub nurse stands off the patient's right shoulder. The instrument table is positioned behind the nurse toward the right-hand corner of the room. The anesthesia machine and equipment should be placed behind the anesthetist and to the left of the patient's head. This approach can be used for any segmental colec-

tomy. In this chapter, in all but one of the figures the scrub nurse has been placed at or to the side of the foot.

B. Methods of Securing the Patient to the Operating Table

1. A number of methods can be used to help secure the patient's position on the OR table. This is especially important because steep or "radical" body positions are often needed during laparoscopic bowel cases. Surgeon custom and preference largely determine which method(s) are utilized. It is important to note that there is controversy regarding the efficacy and safety of some of these methods. Some surgeons feel very strongly that one or another of these methods is quite dangerous and should be avoided. No systematic study of these positions in the setting of minimally invasive procedures has been carried out. Some methods can be used regardless of whether the patient is in the supine or the modified lithotomy position; others apply to one or the other position. A brief description of each method follows.

   a. **Ankle straps:** These can be used to prevent patient movement. The ankles must be well padded and the straps placed so that the blood flow to the feet is not restricted (*for supine position*).
   b. **Stirrups:** These are necessary when placing the patient in the modified lithotomy position. The stirrups serve to anchor the patient as well as to suspend the legs in an abducted position. There are a variety of stirrup designs to choose from on the market today. These stirrups cradle the lower legs below the level of the knee. Venodyne stockings should be placed on the legs before placing the legs into the stirrups. The legs are secured in the stirrups either with the attached straps or with Ace bandages that are wrapped around the stirrup and leg. The stirrups should be adjusted so that no pressure is placed on the lateral aspect of the leg near the knee to avoid a nerve injury.
   c. **Bean bag:** This device is placed beneath the patient's trunk. Suction is applied to this device after the sides of the bag have been rolled up around the arms and the bag has been molded about the patient. It is important to note that the bean bag works best if it is itself anchored to the table (not the cushions) via Velcro or some other means (*for both supine or modified lithotomy position*).
   d. **Chest taping:** The patient can be further secured by placing a 3-inch piece of tape across the chest from table to table to keep the bean bag from giving way. The tape is placed at the level of the manubrium. It is important to place a pad between the tape and the chest wall so as to protect the skin (*for both supine or modified lithotomy position*).
   e. **Table strap:** Standard for almost all cases done in the supine position, Velcro table straps are attached to the sides of the table

and wrapped over the legs to secure the lower extremities (*supine position only*).

f. **Shoulder braces:** Most surgeons agree that shoulder braces are potentially quite dangerous (potential for brachial plexus or shoulder injury) and, therefore, do not recommend their use.

g. The efficacy of each of these methods can be tested before prepping and draping the patient by briefly placing the patient in steep Trendelenburg or sharp lateral tilt.

C. Right Hemicolectomy

1. **Equipment setup** (Figure 15.1.1)

   a. An orderly approach, commencing at the head of the table, is useful to ensure appropriate positioning of equipment.

   b. The **anesthesiologist** needs sufficient space for the anesthesia equipment and for the I.V. poles to which the cephalad end of the OR drapes are attached. The latter should be positioned as close to the head of the table as possible so as not to limit the surgeon's or assistant's ability to situate themselves ideally for the various operative tasks.

   c. It is necessary to work in the right upper and the right lower quadrants of the abdomen. The main video monitor needs to be placed on the patient's right side facing the surgeon. For most of the case this monitor is ideally located toward the head of the table. The video slave is positioned on the left side behind the surgeon.

   d. The laparoscopic insufflator, light source, energy sources (cautery, ultrasonic shears, or other), recording devices, Venodynes, and other equipment are usually placed on a ceiling-mounted boom or cart(s) or tower. For a right colectomy, the tower or boom is best positioned beneath or adjacent to the main video screen on the patient's right side (see Figure 15.1.1). In this way, most, if not all, of the cables, tubing, and wires are passed off to the right side, which frees up the left side of the patient such that the surgeon can easily change his position to facilitate the various steps of the procedure. The equipment should be positioned so as not to interfere with table position changes (Trendelenburg or side-to-side airplaning).

   e. One member of the surgical team needs to move to the right side of the table to carry out the extracorporeal portion of the operation. This fact should be kept in mind when arranging the connecting cables, tubing, and other equipment so that an access path is provided for the surgeon.

   f. The **surgical nurse/technician** stands at the foot of the table, usually on the patient's right side, with a mayo stand positioned over the patient's feet. It is important that the scrub nurse elevate the mayo stand when the patient is placed in steep Trendelenburg.

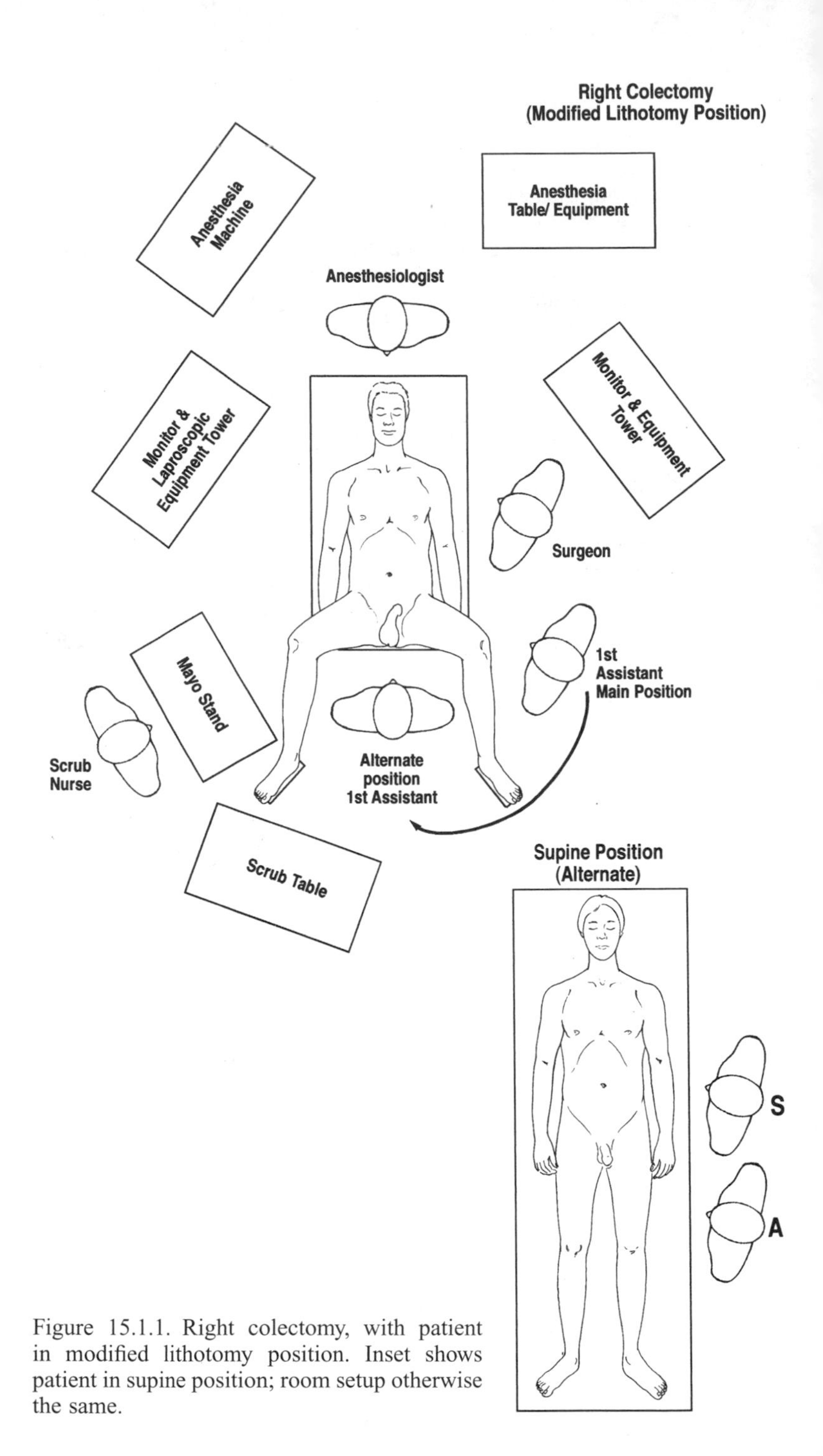

Figure 15.1.1. Right colectomy, with patient in modified lithotomy position. Inset shows patient in supine position; room setup otherwise the same.

2. **Patient position for right colectomy**
   a. Supine position (see Figure 15.1.1, inset)
      i. The patient is situated on the OR table so as to provide the anesthesiologist adequate exposure to the patient. Ideally, the patient's knees are positioned over the knee break in the OR table.
      ii. When utilizing the supine position, the surgeon and camera assistant will both be standing on the patient's left side during the laparoscopic portion of thc case. During the open portion of the case, either the surgeon or the first assistant moves to the right side of the table.
      iii. Pneumatic compression stockings should be utilized as for any major case.
   b. **Modified lithotomy position** (see Figure 15.1.1)
      i. The patient is positioned so that the buttocks are at the edge of the table break. The legs must be placed in stirrups and secured.
      ii. If the operation is to be done with three surgeons, the surgeon would stand on the patient's left side. The camerperson would also stand on the left, for the majority of the case. The first assistant would stand between the legs or on the left side with the surgeon (for ileocolic mobilization). For the open part of the case, the surgeon or assistant would go to the patient's right side.
      iii. If the operation is to be completed with two surgeons, then the first assistant would stand either on the patient's left side or between the legs for the laparoscopic part of the case.
   c. **Table positioning for right colectomy**
      i. The OR table is placed in the reverse Trendelenburg position with the right side tilted upward for the hepatic flexure takedown.
      ii. To mobilize the terminal ileum and the cecum, the patient is placed in the Trendelenburg position with the right side inclined upward. The surgeon and cameraperson are either both positioned on the patient's left side or one of them stands between the legs.
      iii. To separate the midtransverse colon from the omentum and to enter the lesser sac, the patient should be in a mild reverse Trendelenburg position without lateral tilt.

D. Sigmoid Resection, Low Anterior Resection, and Abdominoperineal Resection (APR)

1. **Equipment setup**
   a. With few exceptions, the modified lithotomy position is used for sigmoid and low anterior resections. (See discussion in preceding section.)
   b. **Scrub nurse position.** Sigmoid resection and low anterior resection require two different laparoscopic monitor positions and several alterations in the position of the surgical team. The scrub nurse must shift position when the operative team moves. When the lower abdominal and pelvic mobilization of the colon and rectum is taking place (Figure 15.1.2), the scrub nurse can stand between the legs. During the splenic flexure takedown (Figure 15.1.3), the first assistant will move to between the legs. The scrub nurse can reposition just below the patient's right or left foot after pulling back the scrub table. During the perineal portion of an APR, the scrub nurse must also reposition further away from the table to provide access to the perineal operative team. Another option is to position the scrub nurse at the head of the table (Figure 15.1.4). The scrub nurse can position themselves to the side of either lower leg *or* stand at the head of the table. Regardless of the RN's position, the instrument stand and nurse must be far enough away that they do not block access to the patient for the surgeon or assistant.
      i. If the scrub nurse is to be off the **foot of the table** the RN must not prevent someone from standing between the legs or block access to the side of the patient.
      ii. Similarly, if at the **head of the table** the nurse must not block a surgeon from standing at the patient's shoulder to get a particular vantage point during the case or prevent a monitor from being repositioned off the patient's shoulder during flexure takedown. The instrument stand should not be positioned over the patient's face but rather away from the patient. It is important when using this position that both the surgical and anesthesia team be aware of the distance between the endotracheal tube and the anesthesiologist (Figure 15.1.5). It is prudent to place a foam rubber ring or pad over the face to prevent accidental injury.
   c. For subtotal colectomy or proctocolectomy, dissection will be carried out in **all four quadrants** of the abdomen. In this case it is important that all monitors can be moved freely on each side of the OR table to facilitate either flexure takedown or pelvic dissection. At a minimum, two monitors are required, one on the left and one on the right side of the patient. For left colectomy and low anterior resection (LAR), the left monitor must be shifted from a position at the foot of the table to a new location off the

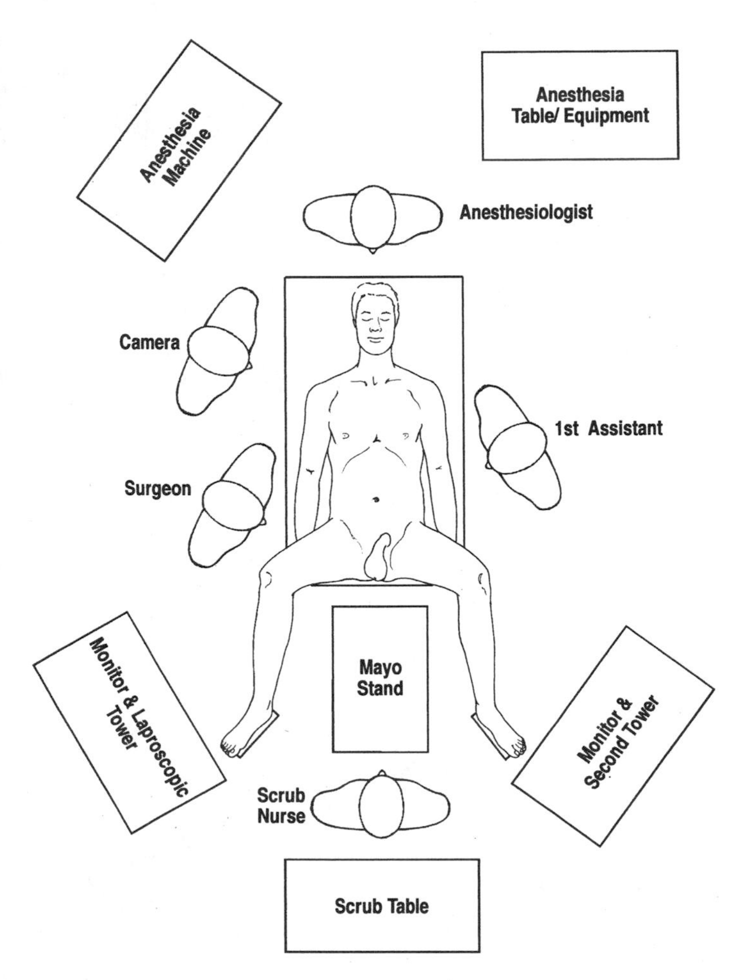

Figure 15.1.2. Sigmoid colectomy, low anterior resection, and abdominoperineal resection. Patient in modified lithotomy position. Staff and equipment positioned for pelvic dissection.

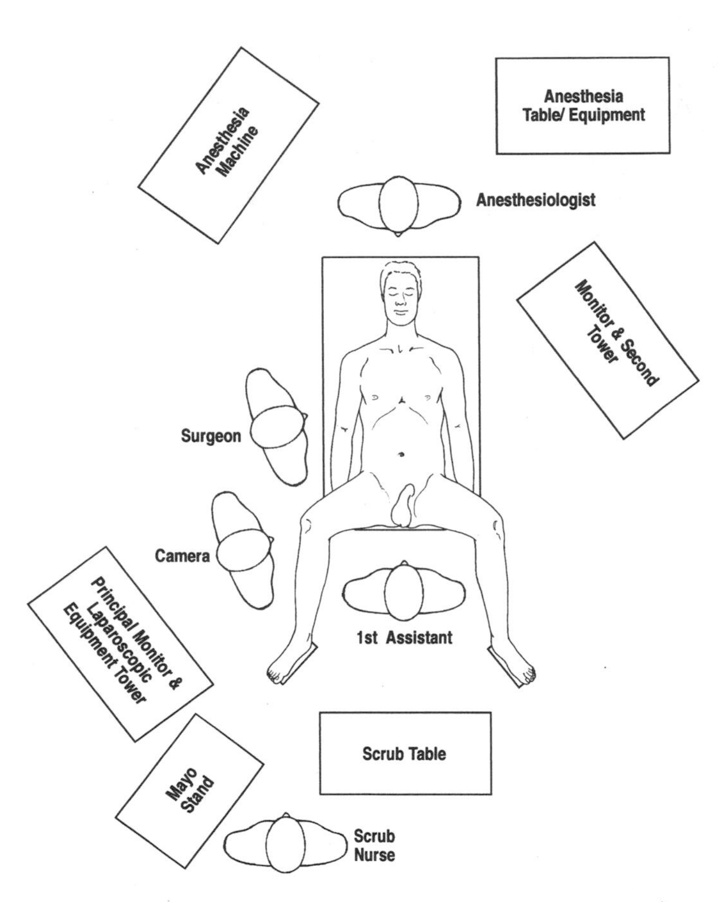

Figure 15.1.3. Sigmoid colectomy for low anterior resection and abdominoperineal resection. Arrangement of equipment and position of OR staff for splenic flexure mobilization.

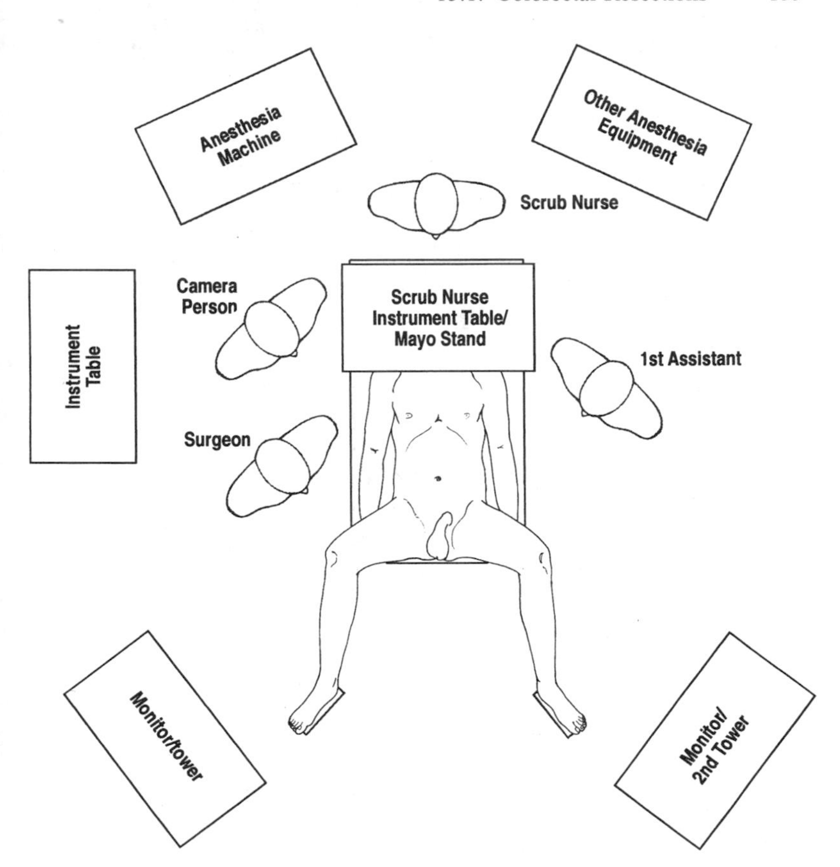

Figure 15.1.4. Alternate scrub nurse position for sigmoid or low anterior resection. The scrub nurse is positioned at the head of the table, off the patient's right shoulder, with an elevated mayo stand placed above the patient's head. The main instrument table is placed behind the nurse. The surgeons and laparoscopic monitors are positioned for a sigmoid colectomy or low anterior resection.

left shoulder to facilitate splenic flexure takedown (for these procedures the right monitor can remain stationary off the right leg). If a third monitor is available, one can be placed opposite the left shoulder and the other at the level of the left foot.

d. **Cables, tubing, and wires.** It is best to pass all cables and tubes off the same side of the table, if possible. Furthermore, ideally, they should all be passed off toward either the head or the foot of the table. This allows the surgeon or assistant access to that side of the patient without having to climb over cables or requiring the circulating nurse to unplug one or more devices to make

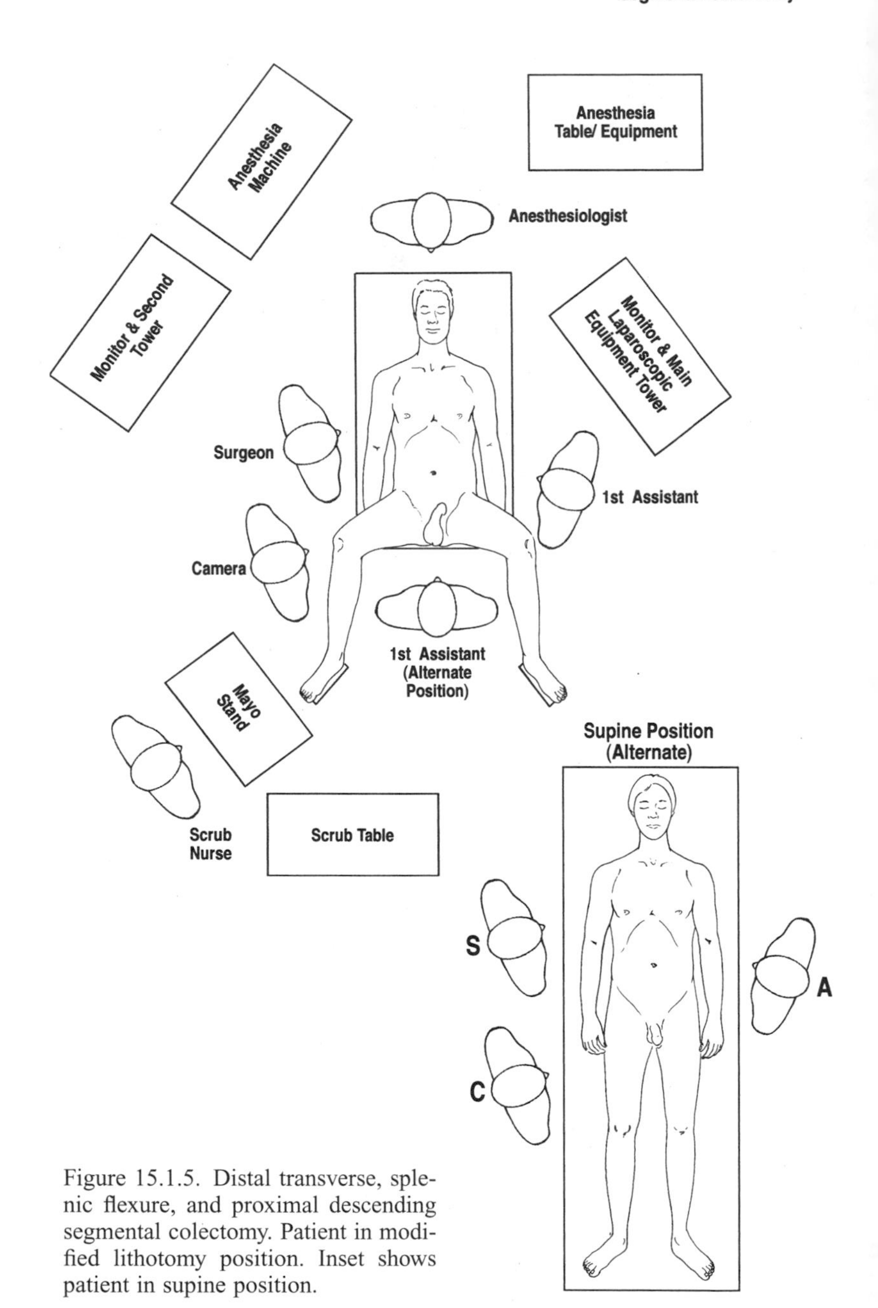

Figure 15.1.5. Distal transverse, splenic flexure, and proximal descending segmental colectomy. Patient in modified lithotomy position. Inset shows patient in supine position.

a path for the surgeon. The side chosen for the cables and tubing should be the one whose monitor will remain stationary during the case. In the case of LAR or left colectomy, the cables should be passed off the right side of the patient so that the left monitor can be shifted from the foot to the left shoulder when mobilizing the splenic flexure.

2. **Patient position**
   a. The modified lithotomy position is almost exclusively used for sigmoid and distal left. The patient's legs must be placed in well-padded stirrups (e.g., Welch-Allen, Lloyd-Davies, or other similar device) after the pneumatic compression stockings have been put on the lower legs. The legs must be secured in the stirrups using the straps provided or by wrapping Ace bandages around the lower leg and stirrup. Once secured, the compression stockings must be fully inflatable. Lateral pressure on the lower leg at the knee level must be avoided to prevent a nerve compression injury.
   b. The stirrups need to be positioned such that the thighs are parallel to the abdominal wall. This will allow full use of the lower abdominal ports, especially when working in the upper quadrants. If the thighs are angled upward the port cannot be sharply torqued caudad to provide access to the flexures or transverse colon.
   c. **Bilateral arm tuck.** As mentioned, both arms should be padded and tucked at the patient's side. Before taking the patient out of the lithotomy position, when elevating the foot of the table after completing the operation it is important to make sure that the hands are well away from the table break to avoid injury.
   d. In general, the surgeon stands on the side of the patient opposite the segment of colon being mobilized, with a video monitor in the line of vision. The camera operator stands adjacent to the surgeon and the first assistant stands across the table or between the legs. Each operation can be approached in numerous ways. It is useful for the surgeon to select a logical sequence for the operative tasks at hand. The chosen order of dissection will determine the initial positioning of the monitor on the left side of the patient. What follows is a list of the components of a left colectomy or LAR with brief mention of the best monitor and surgeon location for each part of the operation.
   e. **Proximal descending colon and splenic flexure mobilization (Figure 15.1.3):** The patient is placed in the reverse Trendelenburg position with the left side inclined upward. The left-sided monitor is best placed off the left shoulder of the patient. The surgeon and camera operator stand on the patient's right. The first assistant should stand between the legs.
   f. **Sigmoid colon, distal descending colon, and rectal mobilization (Figure 15.1.2):** The OR table is placed in the Trendelenburg position with the left side upward. The left-sided monitor should be located off the patient's left lower leg or foot. The surgeon and camera operator stand on the patient's right while the first assistant stands on the left side.

E. Transverse, Splenic Flexure, and Proximal Descending Segmental Colectomy

As mentioned above, the modified lithotomy position can be used for all types of colon resections; however, some surgeons prefer to carry out transverse colectomies, splenic flexure, and proximal descending segmental colectomies with the patient in the supine position (see inset, Figure 15.1.4).

F. Selected References

Darzi A, Lewis C, Menzies-Gow N, et al. Laparoscopic abdominoperineal excision of the rectum. Surg Endosc 1995;9:414–417.

Geis WP, Coletta AV, Jacobs M, et al. Benefits of complexity scales in laparoscopic colectomy. Int Surg 1994;79:230–232.

Marcello PW, Milsom JW, Wong SK, et al. Laparoscopic restorative proctocolectomy: case-matched comparative study with open restorative proctocolectomy. Dis Colon Rectum 2000;43:604–608.

Nelson H, Young-Fadok T. Laparoscopic colectomy. In: Baker RJ, Fischer JE, eds. Mastery of Surgery, 4th edition. Philadelphia: Lippincott Williams & Wilkins, 2001;1581–1588.

Senagore AJ, Luchtefeld MA, Mackeigan JM. What is the learning curve for laparoscopic colectomy? Am Surg 1995;61:681–685.

Thibault C, Poulin EC. Total laparoscopic proctocolectomy and laparoscopy-assisted proctocolectomy for inflammatory bowel disease: operative technique and preliminary report. [see comments]. Surg Laparosc Endosc Percutan Tech 1995;5:472–476.

Young-Fadok TM. Laparoscopic colorectal surgery. In: Zuidema GD, Yeo CJ, eds. Shackelford's Surgery of the Alimentary Tract, 5th edition. Philadelphia: Saunders, 2002; 204–217.

Young-Fadok TM, Nelson H. Laparoscopic right colectomy: a five-step procedure. Dis Colon Rectum 2000;43:267–273.

Young-Fadok TM, Hall-Long K, McConnell EM, Gomez Rey G, Cabanela RL. Advantages of laparoscopic resection for Crohn's disease: improved outcomes and reduced costs. Surg Endosc 2001;15:450–454.

Zucker KA, Pitcher DE, Martin DT, Ford RS. Laparoscopic-assisted colon resection. Surg Endosc 1994;8:12–17; discussion 18.

15.2. Port Placement Arrangements: Laparoscopic-Assisted Colorectal Resections

Patrick Colquhoun, M.D., M.Sc.
Steven D. Wexner, M.D.

A. Importance

The success of any operation is predicated upon adequate visualization of the surgical field and facilitated by appropriate amounts of traction and countertraction along the planes of dissection. Port placement in minimal access surgery affects each of these factors and is thus of paramount importance for any minimally invasive procedure.

B. Factors Affecting Port Placement in Colorectal Surgery

As per the general introductory remarks concerning port placement, a wide variety of port arrangements have been utilized for minimally invasive colorectal resection. The number of ports required varies from three to five depending on which expert you ask. With very few exceptions, these are laparoscopic-assisted procedures in which a portion of the procedure is done extracorporeally. The proportion of the case that is done laparoscopically varies considerably from surgeon to surgeon. In general, the greater the proportion of the case done with the abdomen closed the greater the likelihood that four or five ports will be needed. Certainly, in teaching situations five ports are needed if both the first assistant and the surgeon are to each have two ports. In rare cases, a sixth port may prove necessary. In general, the operating surgeon stands opposite the pathology he intends to operate on.

In the text that follows, a number of port placement patterns are provided for each type of colorectal resection. These patterns and approaches are the opinions and recommendations of numerous laparoscopic colorectal experts that were polled. Although some surgeons routinely use three ports for certain colorectal resections, only four- and five-port arrangements are presented in this chapter.

The port placement scheme for a given case is influenced by a number of factors including body habitus, past laparotomy or laparoscopy scars, and, most importantly, the location of the pathology to be resected as well as the extent of resection planned. If a temporary or permanent stoma is anticipated, the ostomy location should be marked preoperatively. The site might be suitable for a port. Adjacent ports should be placed so as to fall outside the baseplate of a stoma appliance. If reasonable, one of the port sites can be placed so that it can be extended to permit specimen removal. The brief outline below lists the pertinent factors and variables that should be taken into account.

1. Patient factors
   - Body habitus
   - Prior scars
   - Cosmesis (Langer's lines)
2. Technical factors
   - Ostomy site
   - Drain site
   - Specimen extraction site
3. Pathology
   - Tissue diagnosis
   - Size of lesion

The goals of the operation should be clearly delineated. The order of operation should be decided preoperatively as this will guide the operating room setup (i.e., monitor placement). The general port placement scheme can be selected preoperatively; however, the final port positions should be chosen while examining the patient in the supine or lithotomy position after the patient has been anesthetized. It is at this point that the surgeon can best select the port sites that will permit the widest access to the quadrants in question. The surgeon must also be flexible as it may prove necessary to deviate from the original plan.

C. Port Placement for Laparoscopic Ileocolic Resection or Right Hemicolectomy

Experienced surgeons use between three and five ports when carrying out a right colectomy. Many different arrangements have been described; three will be discussed in this chapter. Most surgeons agree on the location of three of the ports: a periumbilical site as well as a left upper and left lower quadrant site. The location of the fourth and, if utilized, the fifth port, however, varies from surgeon to surgeon (lower midline, or right lower or right upper quadrant). There is also one arrangement that makes use of midline ports only. Regardless of the port scheme, the patient is placed in either the supine or the modified lithotomy position. The operating room setup is reviewed in the preceding chapter. (See Figure 15.2.1 and Chapter 15, Section C.) Separate descriptions of the port placement scheme for each of the three port arrangements follow. A brief description of the actual procedure is given after the first port arrangement is explained. This description, with some exceptions, applies to the other two port arrangements as well.

I. Port arrangement 1 for right colectomy (Figure 15.2.1)
   a. Port positioning

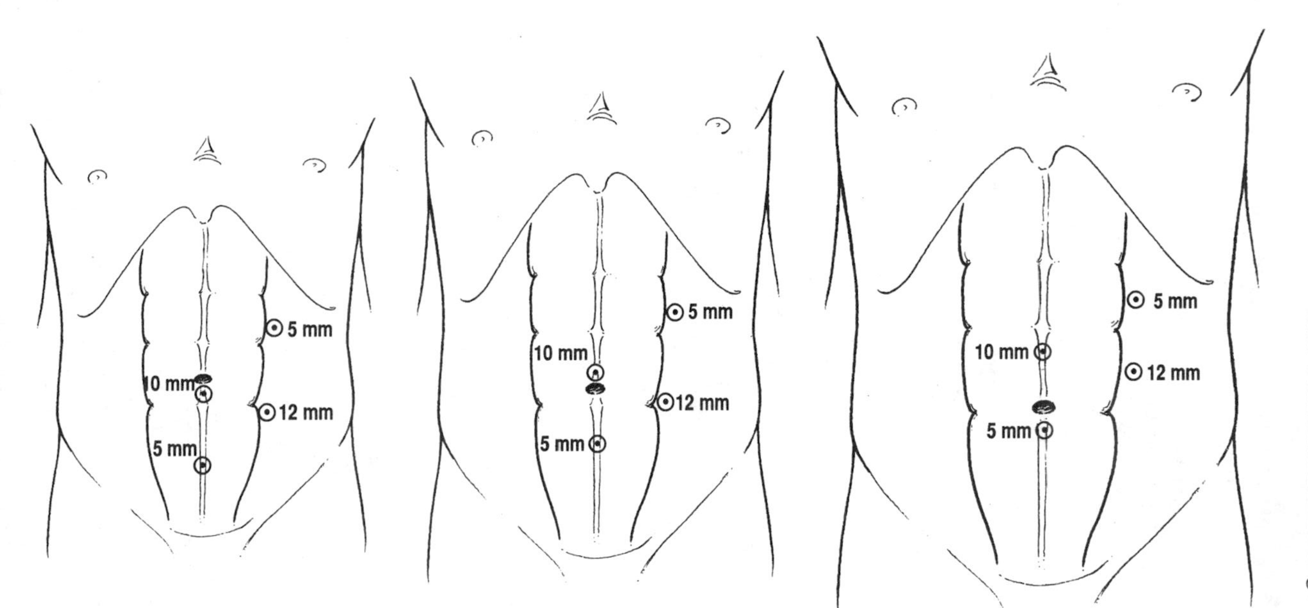

Figure 15.2.1. Port arrangement 1 for right hemicolectomy (four-port method). Umbilical site is used for exteriorization of specimen and extracorporeal resection and anastomosis. This site is therefore orientated vertically and placed in the midline fascia to facilitate the subsequent incision.

1. A 10- to 12-mm (assuming that a 10-mm telescope will be used) periumbilical port is placed that is primarily used for the laparoscope.
    a) Commonly, this is enlarged later in the case to permit specimen extraction and anastomosis.
    b) Vertically oriented (if midline periumbilical extraction site is planned).
    c) Supra- or infraumbilical location. In most patients with a small body habitus, an infraumbilical location is best to minimize or avoid working directly beneath the camera port. In patients with an average-sized abdomen, the port can go either immediately above or below the umbilicus, depending on its precise position (low- or high-riding). In patients with a broad and lengthy abdomen, the camera port should be placed 2–5 cm above the umbilicus; if an infraumbilical site is chosen in lengthy patients, parts of the case may prove more difficult because of poor reach of the telescope.
2. A 10- to 12-mm port is placed in the left lower quadrant lateral to the rectus muscle via a transverse or vertical incision (transversely for best cosmetic result).
    a) Depending on the body habitus, the best location for this port ranges from 2 to 3 cm below the level of the umbilicus to a point several centimeters above the umbilicus. In general, the larger the anterior abdominal wall surface area the more cephalad this port should be placed.
    b) To a certain extent, the position of the left upper quadrant port dictates the position of this port. The latter port must be at least two fingerbreadths below the costal margin and the left lower quadrant port four fingerbreadths below the upper port.
    c) If the bowel is to be divided, or a laparoscopic stapling device is to be used via this location, then a 12-mm port should be placed in this location.
3. A 5-mm port is placed in the left upper quadrant, lateral to the rectus muscle and at least two fingerbreadths below the costal margin. A transverse incision is recommended.
4. A 5-mm port is placed in the lower midline about four fingerbreadths below the periumbilical port. This is the fourth and final port. Either a transverse or vertical incision can be used.

b. Brief description of procedure
    1. Most surgeons position the 10-mm camera in the periumbilical port. The principal surgeon can use either the two left-sided ports or the left lower port and the lower midline port. The surgeon stands on the patient's left side for most of the procedure but may move between the legs for portions of the case if the patient is in lithotomy position. The first assistant stands either on the left side of the patient or between the

legs (if the modified lithotomy position is used). The first assistant holds the camera with one hand and a retractor or cutting instrument inserted via the remaining port in the other hand. Alternately, the surgeon can hold the camera in order to give the first assistant 2 ports to work with. This operation can usually be carried out without a second assistant; however, if a third person is involved they can stand on the patient's right side or, if the modified lithotomy position is used, on the patient's left side alongside the surgeon.

2. **Medial to Lateral Approach:** Right hemicolectomy can be approached via a lateral to medial or a medial to lateral mobilization approach. The lateral to medial approach follows the same order as utilized for an open case and is not reviewed here. The medial to lateral method permits very early devascularization, which some consider important for cancer cases; a brief description of this technique follows. The omentum is first flipped above the transverse colon. The ileocolic mesentery is identified then elevated and retracted in a caudad and right lateral direction. This tents up or "bowstrings" the ileocolic blood vessels, which can be easily dissected from the surrounding tissues and then ligated. The stapler, if used, is usually inserted via the left lower quadrant 12-mm port. (Note: The precise order of the next several steps varies from surgeon to surgeon.) The ileocolic pedicle is then lifted up and laterally, after which the dissection plane between the posterior mesocolon and the anterior Gerota's fascia is established and developed. The right branch of the middle colic vessels is next identified and divided. The ileocolic attachments are next divided at the level of the pelvic brim after they have been exposed by retracting the terminal ileum and cecal mesentery upward, cephalad, and medially. The dissection is continued beneath the mesentery toward the head until the previous medial to lateral plane is joined. The lateral attachments (line of Toldt) are next divided up to hepatic flexure. The omentum is then separated from the right half of the transverse colon by dividing the avascular plane between the two structures exposed by reflecting the omentum cephalad and lifting it upward. At this point, the still-attached right colon and terminal ileum can be exteriorized via the enlarged periumbilical port through a wound protector. Alternately, the bowel can be divided intracorporeally after choosing the proximal and distal points of division and dividing the remaining mesentery. After being fully detached, the specimen is placed in a bag, the umbilical port enlarged, and the specimen extracted. The end of the ileum and the transverse colon are next exteriorized and the anastomosis constructed.

II. Port arrangement 2 for right colectomy (Figure 15.2.2)

a. Port positioning

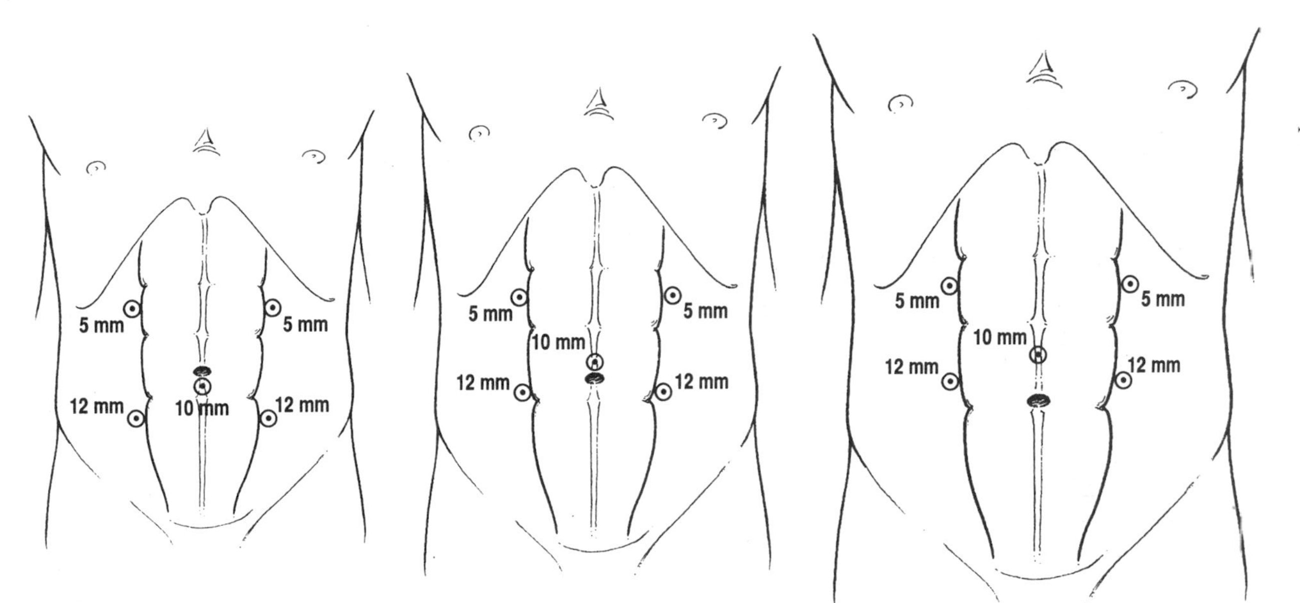

Figure 15.2.2. Port arrangement 2 for laparoscopic-assisted right colectomy (four- or five-port method). Main difference is that a right lower quadrant port is used instead of a lower midline port. Optional right upper quadrant 5-mm port as well.

1. The periumbilical and two right-sided ports are placed in the same location as for port arrangement 1 described immediately above (same port sizes).
2. Instead of a lower midline port, a right lower quadrant port, lateral to the rectus muscle, is utilized (5–12 mm). This port is usually placed just above or below the level of the umbilicus depending on the body habitus.
3. A fifth port, usually 5 mm in diameter, if needed, is placed in the right upper quadrant lateral to the rectus muscle and at lease two fingerbreadths below the costal margin.

b. Brief procedure description
   1. If the five-port scheme is used then a separate cameraperson will be needed; depending on the part of the case they are best situated on the patient's left or right side or between the legs. For hepatic flexure takedown and omental separation, the first assistant may stand on the patient's right side. The procedure description for the first port arrangement applies here as well. The big difference is that the second assistant has two ports and thus can use both hands all the time.

III. Port arrangement 3 for right colectomy (Figure 15.2.3)
   a. Port positioning
      1. A supraumbilical 12-mm port is placed.
      2. A second 12-mm port is placed in the midline 7 cm caudad to the supraumbilical port.
      3. A third port, 5 mm in diameter, is placed 7 cm beneath the second port, also in the midline.
      4. The final port is an epigastric 5-mm midline port.
   b. Both the surgeon and the first assistant stand on the patient's left side. The camera goes in the more cephalad 12 mm port. The surgeon utilizes the two caudal ports (5 mm and 12 mm) while the first assistant holds the camera and retracts/assists with the most cephalad 5 mm port. Either a medial to lateral or a lateral to medial mobilization can be accomplished with this port arrangement. When the intracorporeal portions of the operation have been completed, an incision is made connecting the two central ports (on either side of the umbilicus) and the specimen is delivered and the anastomosis constructed. If deemed necessary, after the anastomosis, the incision can be closed, the pneumoperitoneum reestablished, after which the abdomen can be laparoscopically inspected for bleeding or to check the orientation of the bowel.

D. Port Placement for Laparoscopic-Assisted Sigmoid Colectomy and Anterior Resection

Most surgeons utilize a five-port approach for left-sided segmental resections although some use only four ports. Here, a single five-port scheme is

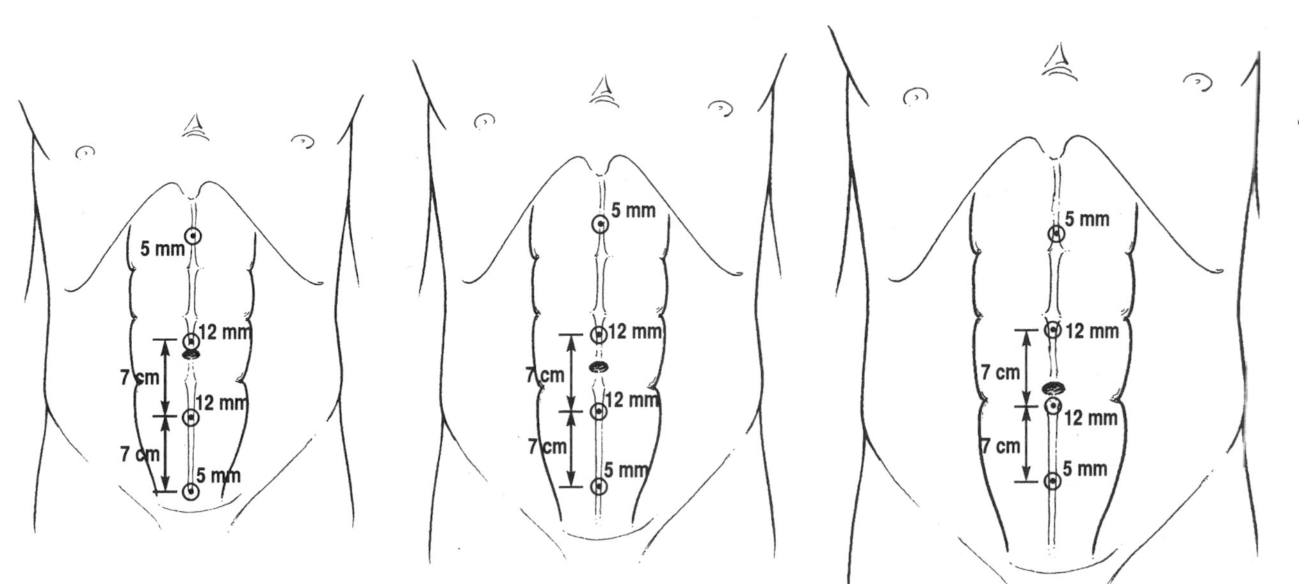

Figure 15.2.3. Port arrangement 3 for laparoscopic-assisted right colectomy (four-port method). A midline port scheme. All ports placed at least 7 cm apart.

described. The standard "box" arrangement with the camera port in the center is the most common pattern (Figure 15.2.4). Some surgeons utilize a midline suprapubic port instead of a left lower quadrant port. The suprapubic port facilitates linear stapling of the distal rectum during low anterior resection but is of little to no use during splenic flexure takedown. In the "box" arrangement that is to be presented, a lateral port is placed in each of the four quadrants. The camera port again is located periumbilically; the decision to place it supra- or infraumbilically is made based on the location of the tumor, the body habitus, and the relative vertical position of the umbilicus. Depending on the colon segment to be removed (proximal rectum versus splenic flexure), the whole port arrangement must be shifted either cephalad or caudad, as dictated by the body habitus. A caudally oriented port scheme facilitates the lower abdominal and pelvic portions of a distal sigmoid resection or anterior resection; however, such an arrangement makes splenic flexure takedown more difficult.

I. Port positioning (five-port "box" method)
   1. A 10- to 12-mm port is placed in a periumbilical location (assuming that a 10-mm telescope is to be used). This port is used mainly for the laparoscope. A vertical or transverse incision can be utilized.
   2. A 10- to 12-mm port is placed in the right lower quadrant, via a transverse incision, preferably lateral to the rectus muscle.
   3. A 5-mm port is placed in the right upper quadrant lateral to the rectus via a transverse incision.
   4. A second 5-mm port is placed in the left upper quadrant through a transverse incision and lateral to the rectus muscle (not utilized by some surgeons who employ a three- or four-port method).
   5. A 5- to 10-mm port is inserted in the left lower quadrant, again lateral to the rectus muscle, via a transverse incision (not utilized by surgeons who use a three-port scheme).

II. Brief procedure description
   1. The patient is placed in the modified lithotomy position with both arms tucked. As is true for most operations, there are several ways to approach this procedure. What follows is a description of the medial to lateral approach in which proximal mesenteric devascularization is accomplished early in the case. The telescope is placed in the periumbilical port with surgeon and cameraperson on the patient's right side. The first assistant stands on the patient's left side. Two monitors are positioned off the foot of the table.
   2. The bowel is retracted via the left ports up and to the left. Via the right-sided ports, the peritoneum at the base of the rectosigmoid mesentery is scored starting at the sacral promontory down into the pelvis. The presacral plane is developed beneath the mesentery toward the left. The left ureter can usually be identified in this way.
   3. Dissection is continued cephalad and the proximal sigmoidal vessels, or inferior mesenteric artery (IMA) and inferior mesenteric vein (IMV), are dissected and isolated, after which they are divided (after finding the left ureter). By lifting the cut vascular bundle upward and dissecting from medial to lateral, the colonic

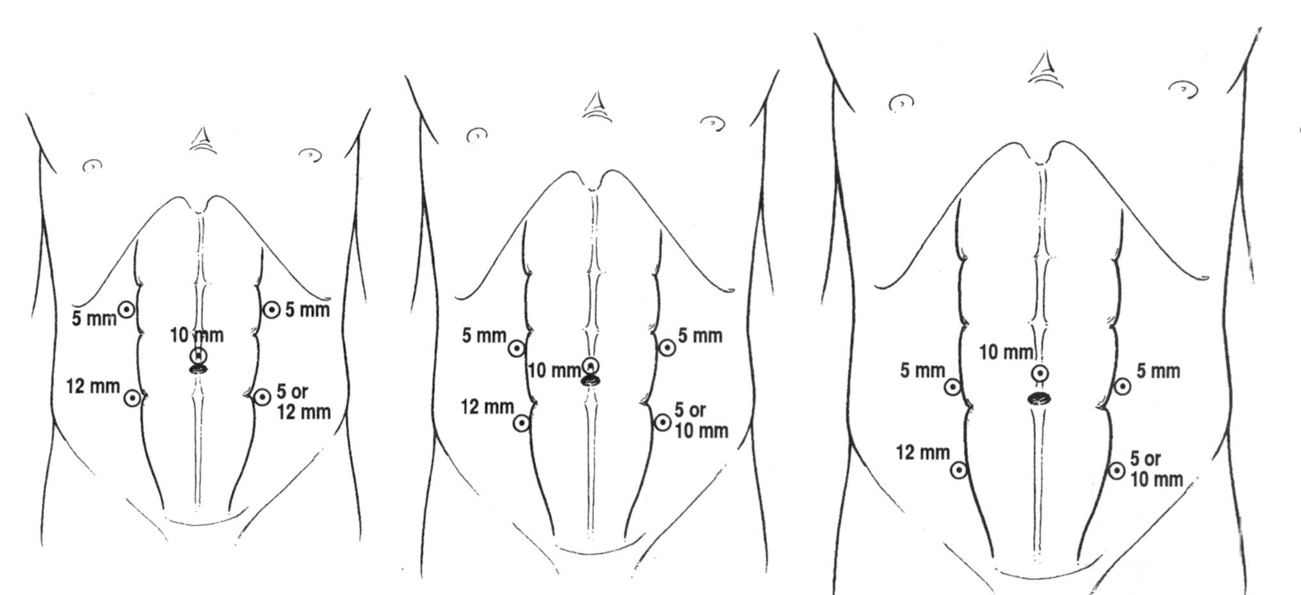

Figure 15.2.4. Port arrangement for laparoscopic-assisted sigmoid resection, left hemicolectomy, and anterior resection (five-port method).

mesentery can be separated from the ureterogonadal structures and kidney.

4. Next, the pelvic dissection is completed and the distal point of resection chosen. After developing a plane between the mesentery and rectum, the former is divided and the latter transected. The splenic flexure is then taken down (lateral dissection and omental peel), after moving the monitor on the patient's left to the head of the table. The surgeon stands between the legs with the first assistant and cameraperson on thc patient's right for flexure mobilization. A port wound is enlarged or an additional suprapubic transverse incision (either true Pfannenstiel or with muscle division) made, through which the specimen is delivered, the bowel divided proximally, the pursestring placed, and the circular stapler proximal anvil inserted. After closing the wound, pneumoperitoneum is reestablished and the anastomosis carried out.

E. Port Placement for Proximal Descending, Splenic Flexure, or Transverse Colectomy

I. **Port positioning**
   a. The same basic five-port scheme used for sigmoid resection is utilized; however, the entire arrangement is shifted cephalad, toward the target quadrants. The cephalad shift is more pronounced in patients with lengthy and broad anterior abdominal walls (Figure 15.2.5).
   b. Before committing to the locations for the final ports, it is important to laparoscopically explore the abdomen after the camera port and one or two other ports have been placed. The length (redundancy) and position of the transverse, sigmoid, and descending colon segments can be assessed. The colon anatomy may well influence the port positioning.
   c. The location of the base of the transverse mesentery and the origin of the middle colic vessels as well as the location of the takeoff of the ileocolic vessels may also mandate a shift in port positions.

II. Brief procedure description
   a. See the preceding chapter for the details of room set up and position of the surgical team. The monitors are placed at the head of the table. The patient is positioned in either the modified lithotomy or the supine position.
   b. Choosing which mesenteric vessels are to be divided and which spared is a unique aspect of resections in this region. The lesion's precise location will determine which vessels need to be divided.

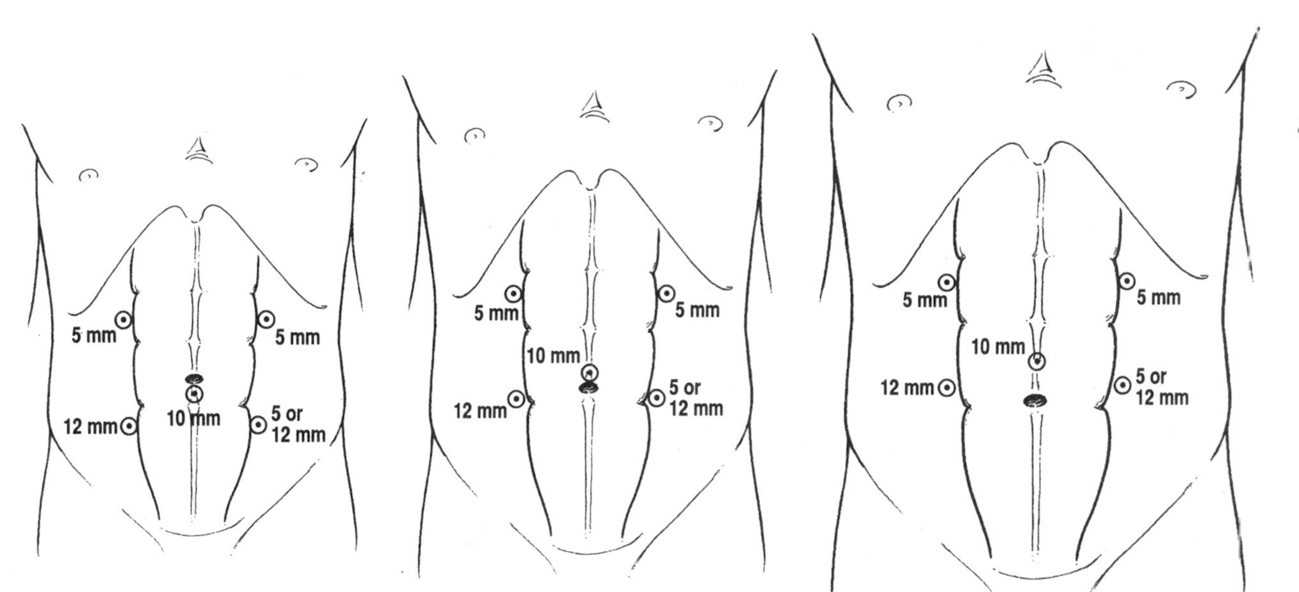

Figure 15.2.5. Port Arrangement for laparoscopically assisted splenic flexure, descending and transverse colectomy (five-port method).

In regards to a splenic flexure neoplasm, for example, division of the IMA at the origin will necessitate resection of most, if not all, of the left colon and results in an very long distal margin. Therefore, it is more logical to divide the left colic and, usually, the first sigmoidal branches of the IMA just distal to their takeoff for a flexure lesion. In this way, the sigmoid colon can be preserved. The surgeon may choose to also divide the left branch of the middle colic vessels for distal transverse and flexure lesions because these lesions usually fall between the middle colic and left colic vessels.

c. The descending, proximal sigmoid, and the distal transverse colon must be mobilized. In regard to the latter, the lesser sac is entered either by peeling the omentum off of the transverse, or, if the omentum is adherent to a tumor, the gastrocolic ligament is divided and the left omentum sacrificed. Once mobilized but before enlarging an incision and removing the specimen, the bowel may be divided intracorporeally (surgeon's choice). The anastomosis is usually accomplished extracorporeally.

d. In regard to a transverse colon neoplasm, attention is focused initially on the length of the transverse colon and the location of the base of the transverse mesocolon (also the origin of the middle colic vessels). Early devascularization is more difficult in this instance but can be carried out if done carefully. For a true mid-transverse colon lesion, both the splenic and hepatic flexures almost always need to be mobilized.

e. Either the midline port (if the initial incision was vertically oriented) or the left upper quadrant port site can be enlarged for specimen retrieval and anastomosis. If the latter port is enlarged, the transverse wound is extended and the underlying muscle either split (muscle-splitting approach that does not cut muscle) or divided. A wound protector should be used in all instances.

F. Port Placement for Laparoscopic Abdominal Perineal Resection

I. **Overview**

The same basic five-port scheme used for sigmoid resection is utilized (see Figure 15.2.4); however, the whole arrangement needs to be shifted toward the pelvis, regardless of body habitus, because otherwise it is very difficult, using standard instruments and telescope, to reach the distal pelvis. This port shift is more pronounced in patients with lengthy and broad anterior abdominal walls. Unlike sphincter-saving left-sided resections, access to the left upper quadrant is not an issue, because splenic flexure takedown is not required. The site chosen for the permanent end colostomy, selected preoperatively, is usually utilized as the location for the upper left lateral port. Except in patients with minimal anterior abdominal wall surface area, an infraumbilical location should be used for the camera port for the reasons already stated. This is the only type of colorectal resection that is routinely accomplished without enlarging a port wound for specimen retrieval.

II. Brief procedure description

a. See the preceding chapter for patient positioning and equipment details. The monitors remain at the foot of the table, off to the left and right, for the entire case. The camera person usually stands on the right side of the patient along with the surgeon. The first assistant stands on the patients left side. Most utilize a 30°, 10-mm telescope.

b. Order of operation: The mobilization of the rectosigmoid and sigmoid can be carried out in a medial to lateral or a lateral to medial approach. In either case the ureters are identified and the posterior plane established between the mesorectum and the presacral tissues. The mesentery is divided proximally at the sigmoidal or IMA level. The posterior, lateral, and anterior pelvic dissection is then carried out laparoscopically to the levator muscle level. Exposure is obtained by carefully retracting the rectum in one direction and the pelvic sidewall in the opposite direction. This maneuver can be very difficult in a narrow and deep pelvis. Nonetheless, superior visualization of the pelvis is obtained laparoscopically in the opinion of most minimally invasive surgeons. After completing the transabdominal pelvic dissection, the proximal colon is divided. The perineal portion of the operation is carried out in the usual manner and the specimen is removed via the perineal wound. In preparation for the stoma, several ellipses of skin are excised from the left upper port wound, and the fascial and peritoneal openings are enlarged, after which the proximal colon end is exteriorized. The wounds are closed and the stoma matured.

G. Selected References

Franklin ME. Laparoscopic low anterior resection and abdominal perineal resections. Semin Colon Rectal Surg 1994;5:258–266.

Metcalf AM. Laparoscopic colectomy. Surg Clin North Am 2000;80(4):1321–1326.

Phillips EH, Rosenthal RJ. Operative Strategies in Laparoscopic Surgery. New York: Springer, 1995.

Young-Fadok TM, Nelson H. Laparoscopic right colectomy: five-step procedure. Dis Colon Rectum 2000;43(2):267–271; discussion 271–273.

Wexner SDW. Laparoscopic Colorectal Surgery. New York: Wiley-Liss, 1999.

15.3. Port Placement Arrangements for Hand-Assisted Colorectal Resections

Jeffrey L. Cohen, M.D.

A. General Considerations

1. Hand-assisted laparoscopic techniques should be viewed as a tool in the armamentarium of minimal access surgeons that can be used in a variety of ways. Hand-assisted methods can be utilized as the primary technique to be used throughout a colorectal resection (right colectomy) or they can be used as a salvage method in the midst of a standard laparoscopic operation. These methods can also be used solely for a particular portion of a laparoscopic operation in a planned manner [sigmoid or low anterior resection (LAR)].

2. Perceived advantages include restoration of tactile sense and spatial relationships, improved ability to retract the colon or other organs, and added control and confidence when dissecting and dividing inflamed tissue or vascular structures. These methods are easier to learn than standard laparoscopic techniques and may save time as well. Finally, the incision required for a hand-assisted operation is just slightly larger than that required for a standard laparoscopic colectomy.

3. There are a growing number of commercially available hand-assisted devices on the market presently. The latest generation of devices available at the time of publication were: the Lap Disc (Ethicon) and the Gelport (Applied Medical). These are, for the most part, third-generation devices that are far superior to the original devices. Most will maintain the pneumoperitoneum and the laparoscopic exposure with the hand outside of the abdomen. Further, it is possible to insert a laparoscopic port through several of these devices, instead of the hand, which greatly increases their versatility. For a short-duration application (e.g., mobilization and transection of a diverticular phlegmon) it may not be necessary to use a device at all. Provided the hand incision is small enough, the forearm, that has a larger diameter than the hand and wrist, will occlude the opening and prevent the leakage of gas.

4. A basic principle of hand-assisted operations is that the hand incision must be located well away from the quadrant(s) where the hand-assisted dissection is to take place. Dissection immediately beneath or adjacent to the hand incision is usually quite difficult, if not impossible, because the bulk of the hand obstructs both the view of and access to the underlying structures. It is for this reason that some surgeons, for sigmoid and low anterior resection, make the hand incision well into the case, after the sigmoid and rectosigmoid mobiliza-

tion have been completed using standard laparoscopic methods. In contrast, the lower midline hand port can be placed at the start of a right colectomy because the dissection is, for most of the case, well lateral to the hand port location.

5. The size of the ports utilized in a given case will vary depending on the surgeon's choice of (1) camera (5 or 10 mm diameter), (2) the diameter of the tissue-cutting and division device chosen for the operation (5, 10, or 12 mm), and (3) whether a linear stapler is to be used (12 mm diameter).

B. Right Colectomy

I. Lower midline hand incision location: port placement scheme (Figure 15.3.1)

1. The patient is placed in the modified lithotomy position with the thighs parallel to the anterior surface of the abdominal wall. The supine position is also an option, however, this position eliminates an excellent working position, mainly the between the legs vantage point. (For operating room setup, see Chapter 15.1, Sections B and C, and Figure 15.1.1.)
2. A 12-mm port is placed supraumbilically in the midline.
3. A port is placed in the midline in the midepigastric region. Either a 5-mm or a 10-mm port can be placed (Figure 15.3.1 shows a 5-mm port).
4. In the teaching setting, a third port is inserted into the left side of the abdomen just lateral to the rectus abdominus muscle at or a bit above the level of the umbilicus. Either a 5-mm or a 10-mm port can be placed in this location (10-mm port shown in Figure 15.3.1).
5. A lower midline incision is made to accommodate the surgeon's left hand. The cephalad extent of this incision should be at least 7 cm beneath the supraumbilical port. The selected hand-assisted device is then inserted or applied, after which the hand is inserted.

II. Lower midline hand incision location: brief summary of procedure

1. The surgeon stands on the left side of the patient. The first assistant/cameraperson stands on the patient's left cephalad to the surgeon. The laparoscope is placed through the midepigastric port; the scissor or harmonic scalpel are inserted through the upper midline port.
2. A description of both the lateral to medial and the medial to lateral approaches follows.
   a. Lateral to medial: The surgeon inserts the left hand into the abdomen and retracts the right colon medially. The patient is rotated steeply to the left. The ileocolic attachments and the white line of Toldt are incised. The dissection is continued up the ascending colon and around the hepatic flexure.

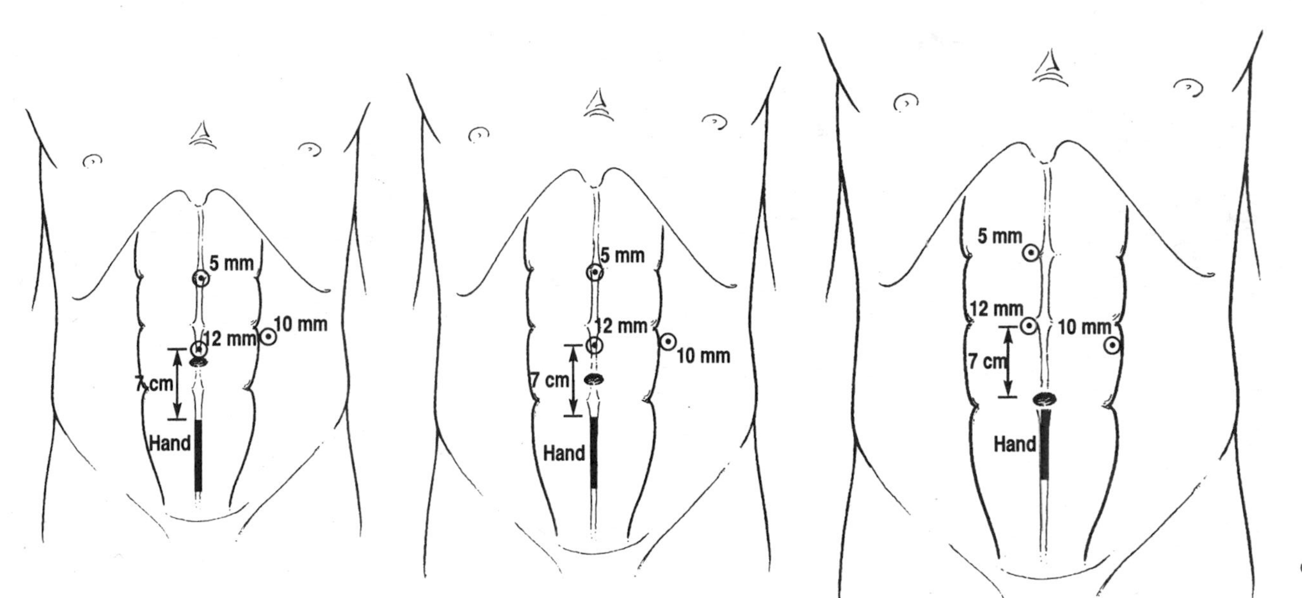

Figure 15.3.1. Right colectomy port and hand incision arrangement 1 (infraumbilical midline hand incision location). Note: there should be at least 7 cm distance between the 12-mm midline camera port and the hand incision.

b. Medial to lateral approach: To expose the origin of the ileocolic vessels, the ileocecal portion of the mesentery is grasped and lifted upward and laterally. This maneuver reveals the location of the ileocecal bundle by bowstringing these vessels. A window is made on either side of the vessels, after which a stapler or tissue-cutting device, inserted via the supraumbilical port or the left lateral port, is used to transect the vessels.

3. The omentum is next separated from the transverse colon sharply, using the left hand to expose the plane between the omentum and the underlying transverse colon. Here the third port is useful in retracting the omentum cephalad and upward while the hand retracts the transverse colon downward.
4. Further mesenteric division can be carried out once the points of transection have been chosen.
5. The terminal ileum and transverse colon can be divided intra- or extracorporeally using a linear stapling device. If performed intracorporeally, extra care must be taken to avoid twisting the small bowel on its mesentery when delivering the specimen.
6. The resection is completed and the anastomosis carried out extracorporeally.
7. Pneumoperitoneum can be reestablished to permit inspection of the operative field and the abdominal wounds after removal of the ports.

III. Right lower quadrant hand incision location: port placement (Figure 15.3.2)

1. The patient's body position on the operating table and the room set up are the same as for the lower midline hand incision location described above.
2. A 12-mm port is placed supraumbilically in the midline.
3. A 5- or 10-mm port is placed in the midepigastric region (5 mm shown).
4. The third laparoscopic port, for teaching cases or difficult dissections on the left side, is placed lateral to the rectus muscle at or above the level of the umbilicus. A 5-mm or 10-mm port can be used in this location (10 mm shown).
5. The hand incision is placed transversely in the right lower quadrant at least 7 cm caudad to the supraumbilical port location. The incision should not be made so low as to prevent the hand from reaching the hepatic flexure of the colon (Figure 15.3.2). As shown in Figure 15.3.2, for patients with large and broad abdominal walls the port arrangement is shifted in a cephalad direction.

IV. Right lower quadrant hand incision location: brief summary of procedure

1. Same as described above.

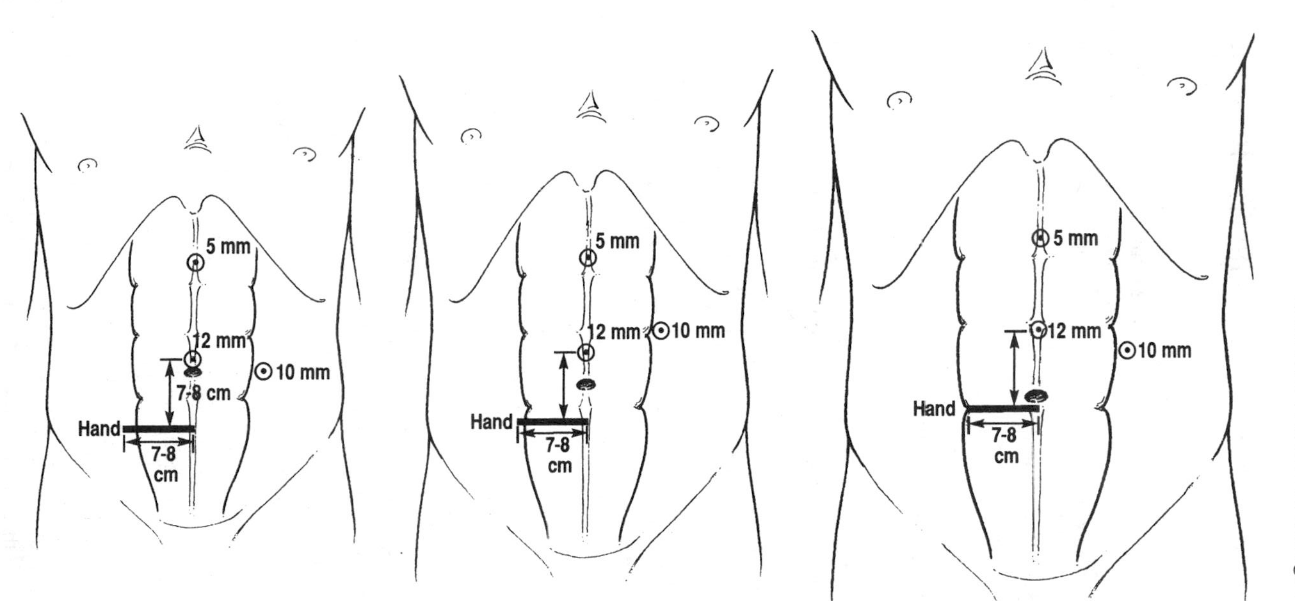

Figure 15.3.2. Right colectomy port and hand incision arrangement 2 (right lower quadrant hand incision location). Note: there should be at least 7 cm distance between the 12-mm midline camera port and the hand incision.

C. Sigmoid Colectomy/Low Anterior Resection

Two different hand-assisted approaches are presented next. The first utilizes a left lower quadrant oblique incision whereas the second calls for a lower midline incision location. The initial dissection and first several steps of the procedure are done using the laparoscopic ports alone before making the hand-assisted incision for both port/hand schemes.

I. Left lower quadrant oblique hand incision location: port placement (Figure 15.3.3)
   1. The patient is placed in the modified lithotomy position with thighs parallel to the abdomen (see Chapter 15.1, Figures 15.1.2, 15.1.3, and text of Section D).
   2. As for right colectomy, a 12-mm port is placed supraumbilically (Figure 15.3.3). The use of a 10-mm, 30° laparoscope is advised.
   3. A 5-mm port is placed on the right side, lateral to the rectus muscle, about at the level of the umbilicus (Figure 15.3.3).
   4. A 12-mm port is placed to the right of the midline, again lateral to the rectus muscle, low enough to permit intracorporeal transection of the rectum (Figure 15.3.3).
   5. To fully mobilize the splenic flexure and to retract, in general, it is usually necessary to insert a fourth port. A 5-mm port will suffice and is best placed in the midline midway between the xiphoid process and the umbilicus (Figure 15.3.3).
   6. Laparoscopic dissection and mobilization of the rectosigmoid and proximal rectum is done before adding the hand incision (using the older devices) because the intracorporeal hand obscures this area. The hand-assisted device is inserted via a muscle-splitting, oblique, left lower quadrant oblique incision. This incision is usually placed just above the groin area; however, the location may vary based on the extent of mobilization accomplished laparoscopically before making the incision.
   7. If one of the latest generation of hand devices is used, then the hand port can be placed earlier in the case because it is possible to work with the hand outside of the abdomen. If need be, a port can be introduced via the hand port device.

II. Left lower quadrant oblique hand port location: brief description of procedure (sigmoid/LAR)
   1. Initial mobilization of the sigmoid and upper rectum can be performed laparoscopically before making the left lower quadrant incision for the hand. The patient should be placed in steep Trendelenburg and rotated to the right to facilitate dissection. Either a lateral to medial or a lateral to medial approach can be used.
      a. Lateral to medial approach: Retract the left colon and sigmoid colon to the right, then sharply incise the white line of Toldt. Extend this lateral dissection caudally into the left iliac fossa down to the pelvic cul-de-sac. The ureter and gonadal vessels are identified from the left and swept laterally. Next, the peritoneum overlying the medial aspect of the

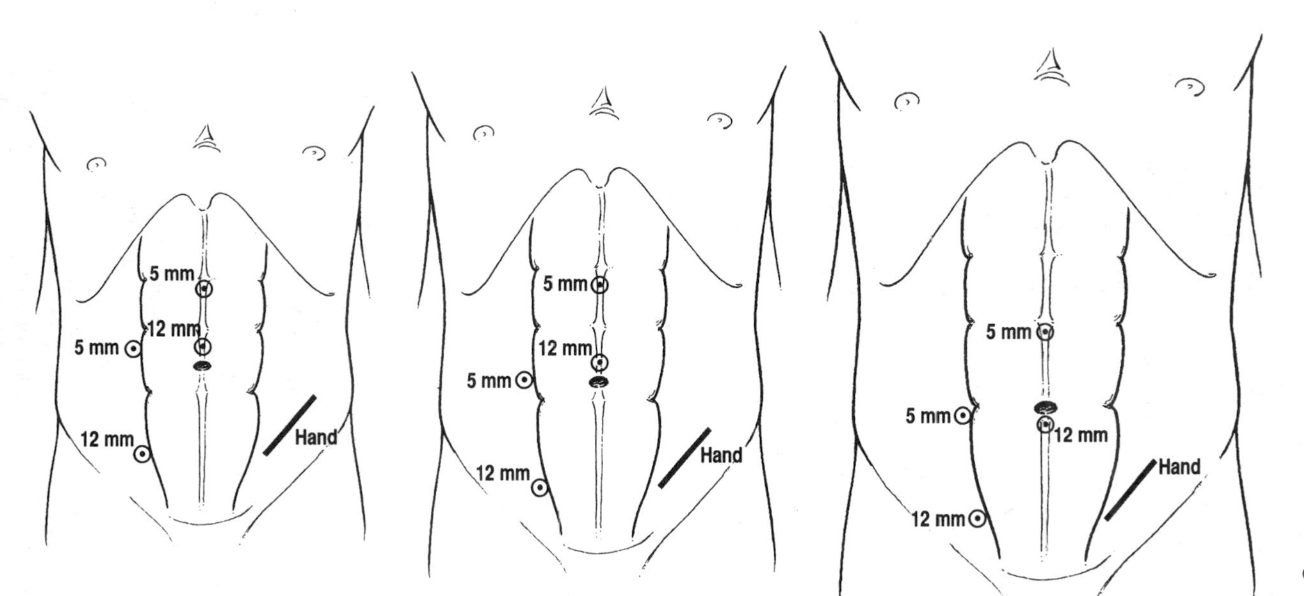

Figure 15.3.3. Sigmoid and low anterior resection port and hand incision arrangement 1 (left lower quadrant oblique hand incision location).

rectosigmoid mesocolon is scored down to the anterior peritoneal reflection and the presacral plane established.

b. Medial to lateral approach: Dissection is begun at the right base of rectosigmoid mesocolon and extended into the pelvis. The left ureter can usually be identified from the right as the presacral plane is developed. The lateral attachments are next divided.

2. The left lower quadrant incision is next made and the left hand inserted into the abdomen. Regarding the pelvic dissection, the surgeon stands on the patient's right and inserts the left hand through this incision into the abdomen toward the pelvis.
3. The point of distal resection is chosen and a window created between the mesentery and the rectum utilizing hand-assisted techniques. Next, the mesentery and bowel are divided using a laparoscopic linear stapling device inserted via the right lower quadrant port. Multiple applications of the stapler will be necessary. The surgeon's hand can thin out the mesentery as well as guide and position the stapler.
4. The proximal blood supply can be next isolated and then transected at the desired level using a linear stapler or other device.
5. If necessary, the splenic flexure would next be mobilized: the surgeon stands between the patients leg's and again inserts the left hand into the abdomen in a cephalad direction. The hand is first used to retract the descending colon medially, thus exposing the lateral attachments. The hand is then used to retract the transverse colon down and toward the feet while the midepigastric port is used to reflect the omentum up and cephalad. The avascular attachments between omentum and colon are then divided and the lesser sac entered.
6. The proximal colon can be transected extracorporeally, via the hand incision, with a linear stapler. The proximal EEA (End to End Anastomosis) anvil and pursestring are next placed, after which pneumoperitoneum is again established.
7. The anastomosis is constructed. The intracorporeal hand can be used to guide the stapler through the Hartmann pouch, to reattach the stapler and the proximal anvil and to keep other pelvic structures out of the stapler. When checking for an anastomotic leak via rectal air insufflation, the intracorporeal hand can be used to occlude the proximal colon.

III. Suprapubic midline hand incision location for sigmoid or LAR: port placement (Figure 15.3.4)

1. Rationale: This port/hand scheme offers advantages for middle and distal rectal neoplasms when a sphincter-saving operation is planned. This arrangement can also be used for more proximal rectosigmoid resections, although for these lesions the left lower quadrant hand incision (discussed above) may be advantageous.
   a. In the case of middle or distal rectal neoplasms, it is usually difficult to transversely divide the rectum distally, especially in a narrow pelvis. It is easier to divide the rectum and

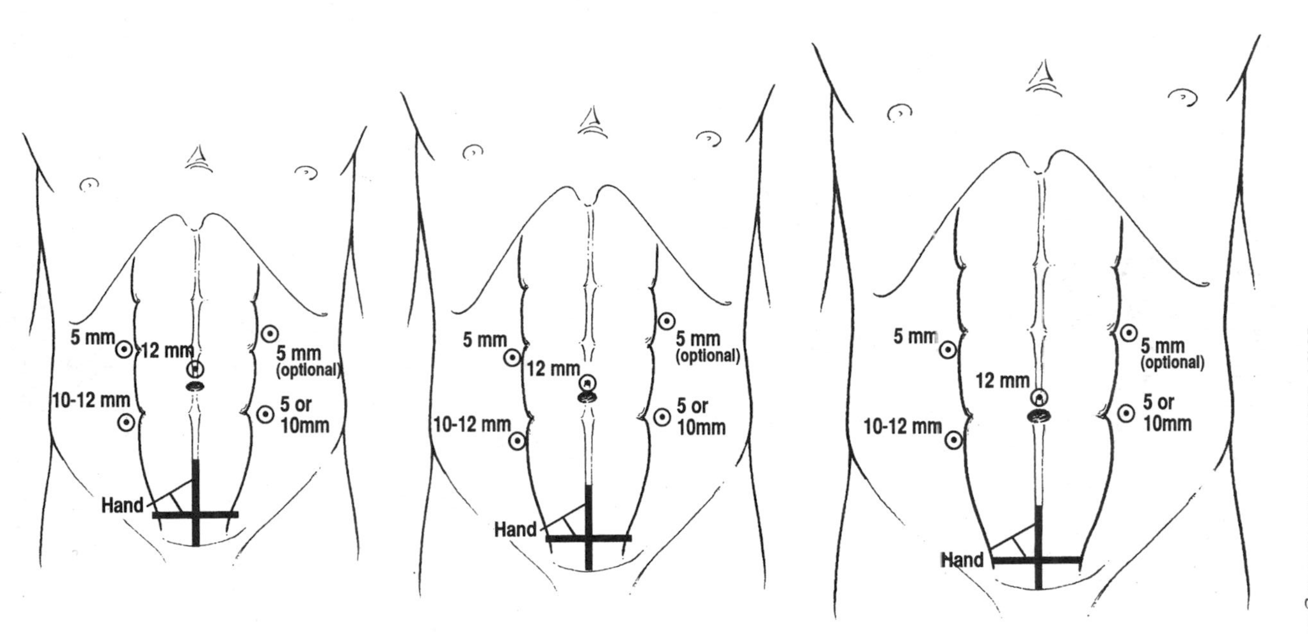

Figure 15.3.4. Sigmoid and low anterior resection port and hand incision arrangement 2* (infraumbilical hand incision location). Note: Either a midline or a transverse hand incision can be utilized. The 5-mm left upper quadrant port is optional. Care must also be taken to ensure that the lower abdominal ports are not placed too close to the hand incision. (*This arrangement can also be used for total abdominal colectomy and ileal pouch-anal procedures.)

construct the anastomosis using open methods via an incision centered on the lower midline than through a left lower quadrant oblique incision. Therefore, unlike the method discussed immediately above, pneumoperitoneum is not reestablished after the specimen has been removed.

b. With the older hand devices the disadvantage of having the hand incision in the midline was that, with the hand inside, the hand usually blocked and obscured the view of the pelvis. Therefore, the pelvic dissection and mobilization that was to be done laparoscopically had to be completed before inserting the hand. The intracorporeal hand was used primarily to facilitate the mobilization of the splenic flexure. However, with the latest generation of hand devices it is possible to work laparoscopically with the hand outside of the abdomen. Further, it is possible to put a laparoscopic port through the hand device and, thus, to add a standard laparoscopic port. Thus, the current hand devices can be placed at the start or early in the procedure and the hand can be utilized in the abdomen where it is useful or removed when it is in the way.

c. This method can also be used for proximal rectal resections, although as already mentioned, the left lower quadrant oblique hand incision method is preferred in that situation.

2. Four ports are usually sufficient (a fifth can be added if necessary). Modified lithotomy position with thighs parallel to the abdomen is utilized (see Chapter 15.1, Figures 15.1.2, 15.1.3, and text of Section D).
3. A supraumbilical 10- or 12-mm port is used mainly for the telescope (10 mm shown). A 10-mm, 0° or 30° laparoscope is recommended.
4. Three lateral ports are placed (5, 10, or 12 mm, surgeon preference): one on the left and two on the right. All are placed lateral to the rectus muscle. One right-sided port is placed in the lower right upper quadrant while the other right port is placed in the upper right lower quadrant. The lone left-sided port is placed almost at the level of the umbilicus at the lateral border of the rectus muscle. A right-sided 12-mm port must be used if the bowel is to be divided intracorporeally (Figure 15.3.4).
5. Although usually not necessary for sigmoid or low anterior resection, an additional 5-mm port can be placed in the left upper quadrant (optional port in Figure 15.3.4).
6. If one of the latest generation of hand devices is used, then the hand port can be placed at the start of the case. If a first-generation device is being used, then, as discussed above, the hand incision is not made at the start of the case. Either a vertical midline incision starting at the pubic symphysis or a transverse incision two fingerbreadths cephalad from the pubic symphysis can be used. If a transverse skin incision is made, then the surgeon can either transversely divide the rectus muscle

bilaterally or utilize the Pfannenstiel approach, which avoids rectus muscle division by dissecting the muscle from beneath the anterior rectus fascia and then entering the abdomen via a midline incision made in the midline. The Pfannenstiel is recommended as it is less traumatic; however, if there is an above-average chance that conversion will be necessary, then it is best to utilize a midline incision, which can easily be extended cephalad to provide access to the upper abdomen.

IV. Brief description of procedure for lower midline or suprapubic transverse hand incision port scheme
   A. Using a first-generation hand device (which do not easily permit laparoscopic dissection with the hand outside of the abdomen):
      1. The rectosigmoid and sigmoid mesenteric dissection and bowel mobilization is carried out laparoscopically. Depending on the level of rectal transection, the mesentery is then divided either distally or proximally.
         a. If a proximal rectal transection is planned then the rectal dissection is carried out, after which a window is made between the mesorectum and the bowel. The rectum and mesentery are then divided intracorporeally with a linear stapler.
         b. If a mid- or low rectal transection is planned (via open methods) then the rectum is mobilized as far as possible into the pelvis; however, neither rectum nor mesorectum is divided. Next, the proximal point of bowel transection is chosen, after which the proximal bowel and the remaining mesentery is fully divided.
      2. Splenic flexure mobilization: The lower midline or transverse incision is made and the hand device placed. The surgeon stands between the legs and after inserting the left hand into the abdomen retracts the colon medially. The surgeon's right hand, working via one of the left lateral ports, divides the lateral attachments toward and around the flexure. The omentum is then "peeled" off the transverse colon as described immediately above.
      3. Medial to lateral splenic flexure mobilization: This is best done laparoscopically either before the hand incision is made or with the hand out of the hand-assisted device. The colon mesentery cephalad to the inferior mesenteric artery takeoff is incised medially just beneath or just above the inferior mesenteric vein (IMV), depending on whether the IMV is to be divided or preserved. While lifting up the mesentery the dissection between the anterior Gerota's fascia and the posterior aspect of the colonic mesentery is continued laterally and in a cephalad and caudad direction. The remaining thin lateral attachments are next divided from lateral to medial after pulling the descending colon medially and upward. The omentum is then peeled off the distal transverse colon to complete the flexure takedown.

4. The case is then completed via the hand incision (it may be necessary to enlarge this incision to final length of 9–11 cm) using open methods. For mid- and low rectal resections (where the rectum is still intact distally), the rectal mobilization to the levator floor is completed and the rectum via the hand incision, after which the rectum and mesentery are divided using open methods. For more proximal lesions, where the distal bowel transaction has been done intracorporeally, the bowel is divided proximally via open methods, the pursestring placed, and the proximal EEA anvil inserted.
5. A standard double-stapled circular transanal anastomosis.

B. Procedure description using latest generation hand devices (which allow for fully laparoscopic dissection with hand outside of the abdomen):
1. The hand device can safely be placed at the start of the case. In fact, it can be placed before establishing the pneumoperitoneum. With a hand inside the abdomen (passed via the device) protecting the viscera, the first port can be safely introduced (provided a trocar-less port system is used). Next, the pneumoperitoneum is established and the other ports placed.
2. Depending on the order of dissection, the hand can be left inside or withdrawn to permit fully laparoscopic dissection in the pelvis. If the flexure is to be taken down first, then the hand is best left in. The intracorporeal hand can assist during either medial to lateral approach or lateral to medial flexure mobilization. The hand can also be useful when dissecting, mobilizing, and dividing the proximal sigmoid vessels or inferior mesenteric artery and vein. If the pelvis is wide enough the hand, introduced by the first assistant standing on the patient's left and facing the foot of the bed, can be used to elevate and retract the rectosigmoid and rectum. If not, the hand can be removed and that portion of the case can be done laparoscopically.
3. Please see the section immediately above for the remainder of the procedure description which is, for the most part, the same.

D. Total Abdominal and Subtotal Colectomy and Ileal Pouch–Anal Procedures

I. Port location (Figure 15.3.5)
1. Modified lithotomy position with both arms tucked. (Initial operating room set up as per Chapter 15.1, Sections B and C, and Figures 15.1.2 and 15.1.3)

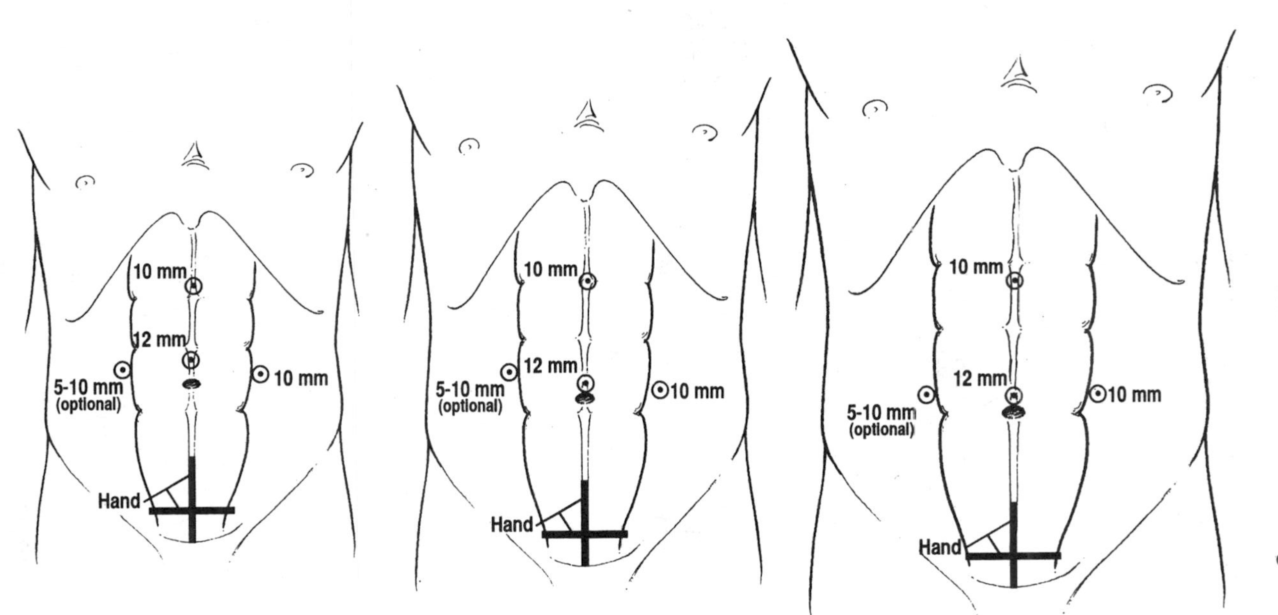

Figure 15.3.5. Total abdominal colectomy and ileal pouch-anal procedures port and hand incision arrangement 1.

2. A 12-mm port is placed supraumbilically. This port will be utilized for both the camera and for dissection. The use of a 10-mm, 30° laparoscope is advised.
3. A 10-mm port is placed in the midline in the midepigastric region (if a 5-mm camera can be used, then a 5 mm port can be utilized in this position).
4. An additional 10-mm port is placed laterally in the left midabdomen, positioned such that it will provide access to the splenic flexure.
5. If a fourth port is necessary for the mobilization of the transverse or left colon, it can be placed on the right side, lateral to the rectus muscle just above or below the level of the umbilicus. This port can be either 5 or 10 mm in diameter (surgeon preference).
6. Hand incisions: The two most commonly used incisions are a lower midline and a suprapubic transverse incision.
   a. A lower midline incision is made at the start of the case to accommodate the surgeon's nondominant hand from both the right and left sides of the operating table.
   b. Alternatively, a Pfannenstiel incision (via a suprapubic transverse skin incision) can be made. Proponents believe that, in addition to being more cosmetic, there is less pain associated with this approach. It may be difficult to reach the flexures via this approach in patients with a lengthy and broad abdominal wall. When in doubt it is best to use the midline incision because, if conversion is needed, it is a simple matter to extend the incision cephalad. Gaining access to the upper abdomen via a true Pfannenstiel is problematic and might require making a midline incision that joins the suprapubic transverse incision (forming a "T").

II. Brief description of procedure

1. The dissection is begun on the right colon. This can be done from lateral to medial or vice versa.
   a. Lateral to medial approach: The patient is rotated steeply to the left. The surgeon stands on the patient's left. The cameraperson is also on the left, cephalad of the surgeon. The laparoscope is inserted through the midline midepigastric port. The surgeon inserts the left hand into the abdomen to retract the right colon medially. The surgeon's right hand manipulates a scissor, harmonic scalpel, or other cutting tool via the supraumbilical port.
   b. Medial to lateral: As described above in the right colectomy section (B.II).
2. Mobilization and devascularization of the right and proximal transverse colon is carried out as per the above description for right colectomy.
3. Omental separation is continued from the right to the left transverse colon. Next, the middle colic vessels can be isolated and divided along with the base of the mesentery.

4. After reaching the splenic flexure the surgeon will need to move to the right side of the patient or between the patient's legs, inserting the left hand, once again, into the abdomen. The patient is rotated steeply to the right and placed in steep Trendelenburg. The left colon is next mobilized.
5. With the surgeon's left hand retracting the left colon medially and the right hand controlling the cutting instrument placed via the left lower quadrant port, the white line of Toldt is divided sharply and the left colon is mobilized. Additionally, the remaining splenic flexure attachments are divided.
6. The peritoneum overlying the lateral aspect of the sigmoid mesentery is incised sharply, allowing the left ureter to be identified and swept laterally away from the base of the mesentery.
7. The left colic, proximal sigmoidal branches, and the intervening mesentery can be divided intracorporeally at this point.
8. Next, the abdomen is desufflated and the entire colon is delivered via the hand incision. If not already divided, the mesenteric vessels can be transected extracorporeally. (Of note, when a Pfannenstiel incision is utilized, devascularization is best accomplished intracorporeally.)
9. The specimen is exteriorized. It is possible to divide the sigmoid colon and mesentery extracorporeally via the hand incision. If an ileoanal pouch reconstruction is to be performed, it is generally preferable to divide the ileocolonic mesentery extracorporeally, so as to preserve the ileal branches of the ileocolic vessels.
10. Resection is completed and an ileocolic or ileorectal anastomosis can be performed extracorporeally. If a total proctocolectomy and ileoanal pouch reconstruction is to be performed, the remaining rectal resection and anastomosis can be performed through the hand incision.

III. Alternate port arrangement for subtotal, total abdominal colectomy, or ileal pouch–anal anastomosis (Figure 15.3.4)
   1. The modified lithotomy position with both arms tucked is again utilized.
   2. This is the same basic arrangement depicted in Figure 15.3.4. A total of four ports, with a fifth optional port, in addition to the hand device is utilized to carry out the operation. The hand incision location or choices is the same as for the just described method.
   3. A supraumbilical 10-mm port is placed and serves as the main camera port.
   4. A 10- or 12-mm port is placed in the middle of the left abdomen just lateral to the rectus muscle. This is the main dissection port used when mobilizing and devascularizing the right colon.
   5. Two right-sided ports are placed, both lateral to the rectus muscle. The more cephalad port is placed in the lower right upper quadrant whereas the other is placed in the right lower quadrant. The upper right port is best placed after the right

colon and proximal transverse colon have been mobilized and devascularized. This port is used to retract and assist during the left transverse and descending colon mobilization and devascularization.

6. A fifth, optional port, can be placed in the left upper abdomen, lateral to the rectus muscle. This would be helpful when mobilizing a difficult hepatic flexure.

IV. Procedure description for alternate port placement scheme for subtotal, total abdominal colectomy, or ileal pouch–anal anastomosis

1. The order of dissection is the same and the intracorporeal hand utilized from the very beginning of the case. One commonly used approach is to mobilize the right colon initially followed by the transverse, descending, sigmoid, and rectum.
2. The camera is mostly situated in the supraumbilical port.
3. The surgeon stands either between the legs or on the patient's left side with the left hand inserted into the abdomen.
4. The surgeon's left hand mobilizes and cuts tissue via instruments inserted via the left lower quadrant port.
5. The left upper and right upper quadrant ports are mainly used to retract and expose.
6. Once the intraabdominal colon has been fully mobilized, the pneumoperitoneum is dropped and the case completed via open methods using standard open methods.

E. Selected References

Ballantyne GH, Leahy PF. Hand-assisted laparoscopic colectomy vs. open colectomy: a prospective randomized study. Surg Endosc 2004;18(4):577–581.

Clark D, Gerhart (eds). Procedure Manual of Hand-Assisted Laparoscopic Surgery.

Darzi A. Hand-assisted laparoscopic colorectal surgery. Surg Endosc 2000;14(11):999–1004.

Litwin OE, Darzi A, Jakimowicz J, et al. Hand-assisted laparoscopic surgery (HALS) with the hand port system: initial experience with 68 patients. Am Surg 2000;231(5): 715–723.

Loungnarath R, Fleshman JW. Hand-assisted laparoscopic colectomy techniques. Semin Laparosc Surg 2003;10(4):219–230.

Vithianathan S, Cooper Z, Betten K, et al. Hybrid laparoscopic flexure takedown and open procedure for rectal resection is associated with significantly shorter length of stay than equivalent open resection. Dis Colon Rectum 2001;44(7):927–935.

16.1. Patient Positioning and Operating Room Setup: Splenectomy

Joseph B. Petelin, M.D., F.A.C.S.

A. Operating Room Setup

1. The operating room (OR) is set up the same regardless of the position of the patient. The anesthesia machine is at the head of the bed. A monitor is placed at the shoulder of the patient on each side of the patient's head, regardless of patient position. The OR technician or nurse stands on the patient's left, toward the feet. The back table and mayo stand will be in that area.

   Most surgeons use a standard mayo stand at the foot to store the standard equipment for laparoscopic splenectomy (this is labeled MAYO 1 in the diagram). In addition, some surgeons find that a second mayo stand located on the patient's left at the level of the hip provides for efficient placement of the tools (scissors, harmonic dissector, graspers, and clip appliers) most frequently used during the procedure.
2. Equipment

   The general complement of laparoscopic and open equipment is needed for laparoscopic splenectomy. Most of this equipment is placed on the mayo stand at the foot of the table; less frequently used items may be stored on the back table.
   a. Special laparoscopic splenectomy equipment may be needed for laparoscopic splenectomy.
      i. It is wise to have a wide-mouthed (>4-cm-long jaws) grasper available, if possible, in the event that emergency vascular control is necessary.
      ii. An endovascular linear stapler is a very useful device for controlling and dividing the splenic hilum. It may also be used for division of the short gastric vessels. In the absence of a wide-mouthed grasper, it may be used for temporary control of the splenic hilum in an emergency.
      iii. Ligatures and/or sutures of "0" and "2-0" braided nonabsorbable material may used for control of the splenic vessels.
      iv. An automatic clip applier is useful for control of smaller vessels.
      v. Harmonic scissors have made a huge impact on the dissection around the spleen. The lienocolic ligament and the short

gastric vessels are effectively controlled and divided with this instrument.

b. Laparotomy equipment

This is usually placed on the back table for use in the case of an emergency.

B. Patient Positioning: Introduction

The importance of patient positioning for laparoscopic splenectomy cannot be overemphasized. Four alternatives are possible: supine, lithotomy, right lateral decubitus, and anterolateral (partial right lateral decubitus, 40°–50°). A bean bag greatly facilitates patient positioning in the latter three approaches.

The supine and lithotomy positions, initially reported in the early 1990s, have largely been replaced by the lateral and partial lateral positions. The former are currently only used for patients with massive splenomegaly (>20 cm length), pediatric or very thin patients, or those in whom concomitant surgery (e.g., laparoscopic cholecystectomy) is planned.

C. Supine Position

Presently, few surgeons prefer the supine position for adult laparoscopic splenectomy uncomplicated by massive splenomegaly or the need to perform concomitant procedures. The patient is placed supine on the operating table with lower extremities together and the upper extremities at the patient's sides (Figure 16.1.1). The surgeon stands on the patient's right side and the assistant on the patient's left. The assistant operates the camera and manipulates an instrument for retraction or to otherwise assist. (See Chapter 16.2, Figure 16.2.1, for port placement scheme.)

1. Advantages

Setup and positioning time is significantly shorter when the supine position is utilized. The location of the initial port (often periumbilical) is also more familiar to the surgeon than the sites used when the patient is in the lateral position. Exploration of the abdomen for accessory spleens is thought to be easier with the patient in the supine position. Conversion to laparotomy is also facilitated in this position. Concomitant surgery, for example, laparoscopic cholecystectomy, is easier to accomplish in this position.

2. Disadvantages

Exposure of the left upper quadrant, the spleen, the tail of the pancreas, the posterolateral ligaments, and the short gastric vessels is significantly more difficult when using the supine approach. These problems have been held responsible for the increased operative time and blood loss encountered in patients undergoing laparoscopic splenectomy in the supine position.

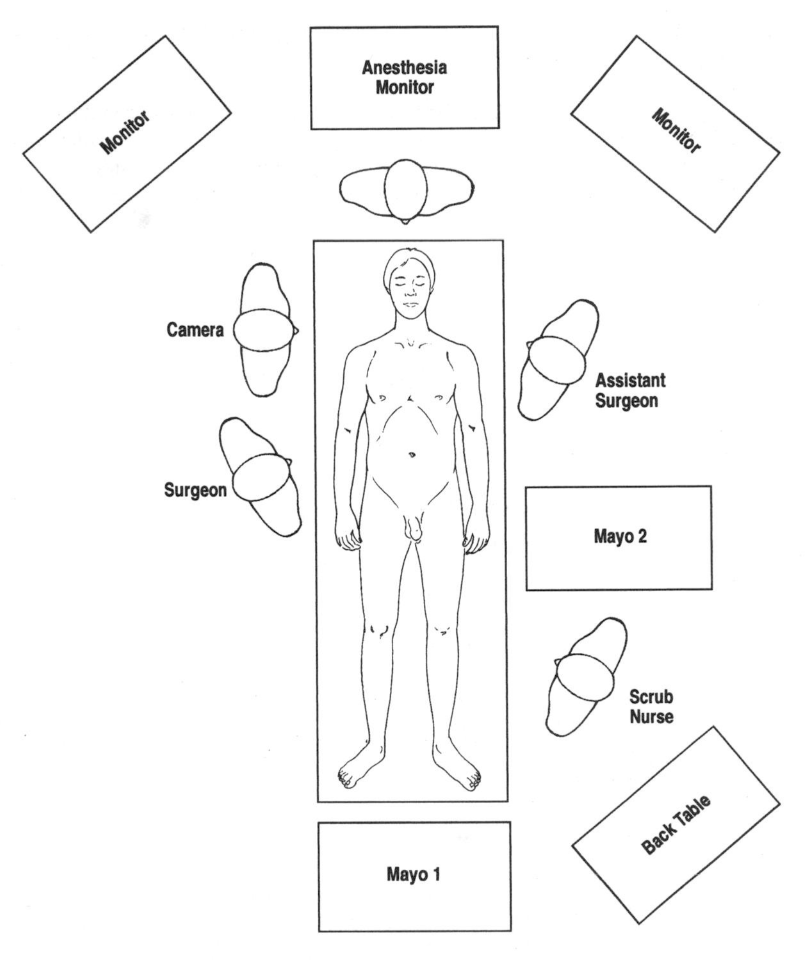

Figure 16.1.1. Supine position for splenectomy.

D. Modified Lithotomy Position

In the modified lithotomy approach, the legs are placed in stirrups such that the thighs are parallel to the anterior abdominal wall. The arms are tucked at the sides. Except for the positioning of the legs, this position is similar to the supine approach. The patient's left side can be elevated by placing a roll under it, thus achieving a partial lateral position. With the patient thus positioned, a space exists between the legs in which the surgeon can stand (Figure 16.1.2). The cameraperson is located on the right of the patient and the first assistant stands on the patient's left in most cases. The first assistant can also stand on the right side caudad to the camera person. (See Chapter 16.2, Figure 16.2.1, for accompanying port placement scheme.)

1. Advantages

Some surgeons feel more comfortable doing the case from between the legs. This approach also decreases the crowding at the operating table, by allowing the cameraperson and the first assistant to stand alone on opposite sides of the patient. Obviously, if a robotic camera holder is to be used, crowding is less of an issue.

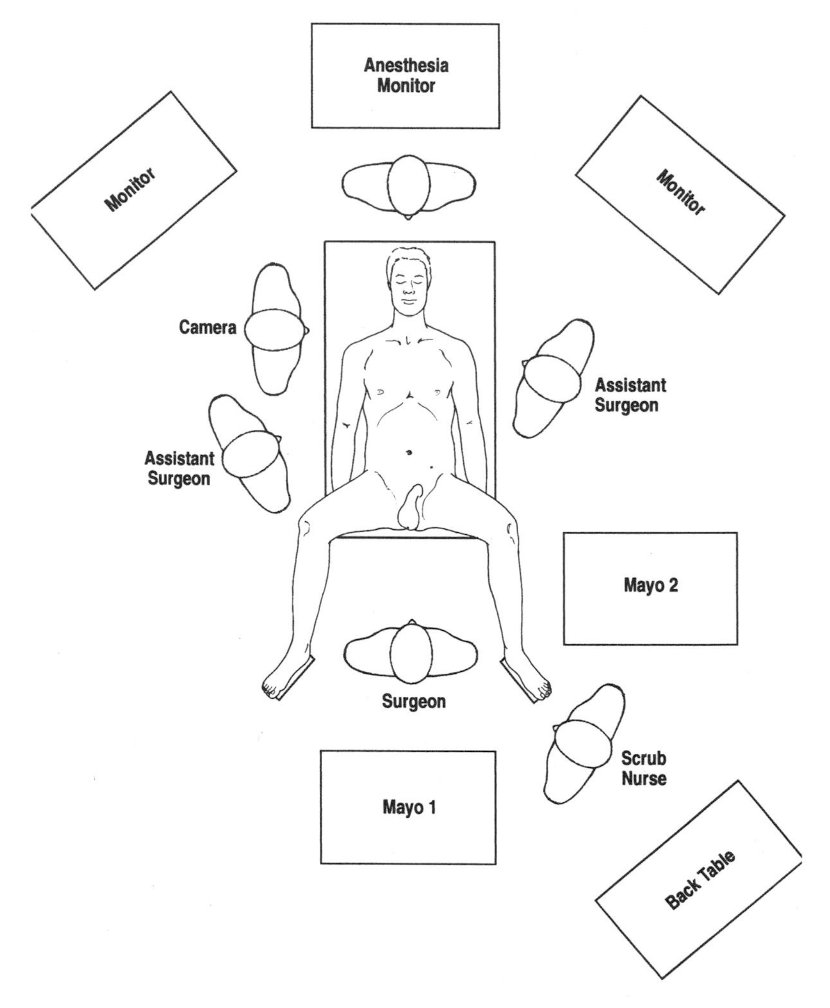

Figure 16.1.2. Modified lithotomy position for splenectomy.

2. Disadvantages

It takes more time to place the patient in this position compared to the supine, lateral, or anterolateral positions. The legs are placed into the stirrups and then secured, after which the "foot" of the table must be detached. There is also a low incidence of stirrup-related complications associated with this position. The latter can largely be avoided by carefully positioning and padding the legs.

E. Lateral Position

A full lateral position (right lateral decubitus) is often preferred for laparoscopic splenectomy (Figure 16.1.3). Here, the patient's left upper extremity is either suspended from an attached table support or is supported across the patient's chest with a pillow. A soft roll is placed under the right axilla in a transverse direction. The lower extremities are usually partially flexed with a pillow between the knees. The shoulders and lower extremities are strapped or taped to the table to prevent movement. The midportion of the OR table is flexed and the "kidney rest" is elevated to maximize the distance between the left costal margin and the left iliac crest.

When using the lateral position, the surgeon and one assistant both stand on the patient's right side. The assistant operates the camera while standing cephalad to the surgeon. A second assistant may stand on the patient's left in this situation. If needed, they may assist by using an instrument passed through a more posterior port in the flank. The anesthesia personnel are located at the head of the table. (For port placement schemes, see Chapter 16.2, Figures 16.2.3, 16.2.4.)

1. Advantages

The lateral position usually provides excellent exposure of the posterior ligaments, the hilar structures, the tail of the pancreas, and the short gastric vessels. Many authors have reported less blood loss and shorter operative times when this approach is used.

2. Disadvantages

Initial port placement is slightly more difficult and dangerous with the patient in the full lateral position. In this position, the spleen shifts to a more medial location where the risk of injury is greater. Extra care must be taken to ensure safe placement of the first trocar. The use of visually directed ports facilitates the insertion of the initial trocar. Left upper extremity suspension from a transverse rod has the potential disadvantage of obstructing instrument maneuvers during the case; therefore, placement of the left upper extremity on a pillow is preferred.

Exploration of the abdomen for accessory spleens, concomitant surgery (e.g., laparoscopic cholecystectomy), and conversion to laparotomy are more difficult from this position than from other positions. This position is nearly impossible to use in patients with massive splenomegaly because visualization of the vital structures is obscured by the splenic mass.

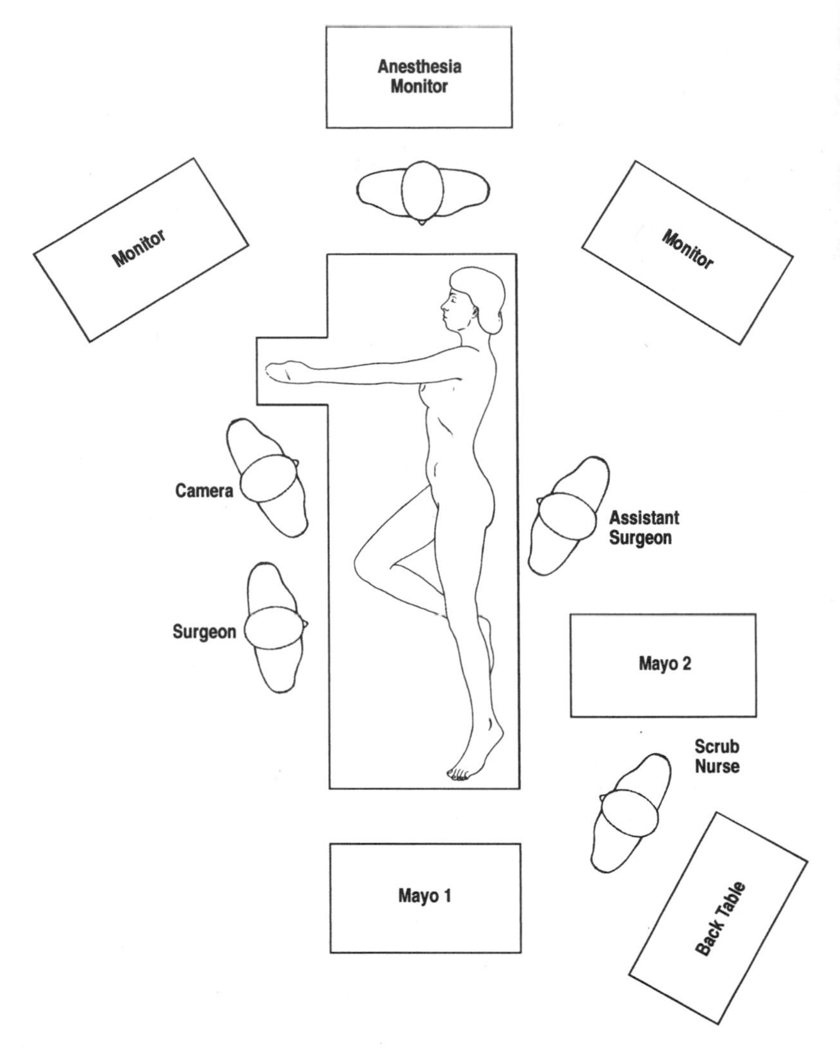

Figure 16.1.3. Lateral position for splenectomy.

F. Anterolateral (Partial Right Lateral Decubitus) Position

The anterolateral position represents an attractive compromise position that incorporates the benefits of both the supine and lateral approaches for laparoscopic splenectomy. A bean bag placed under the patient facilitates positioning.

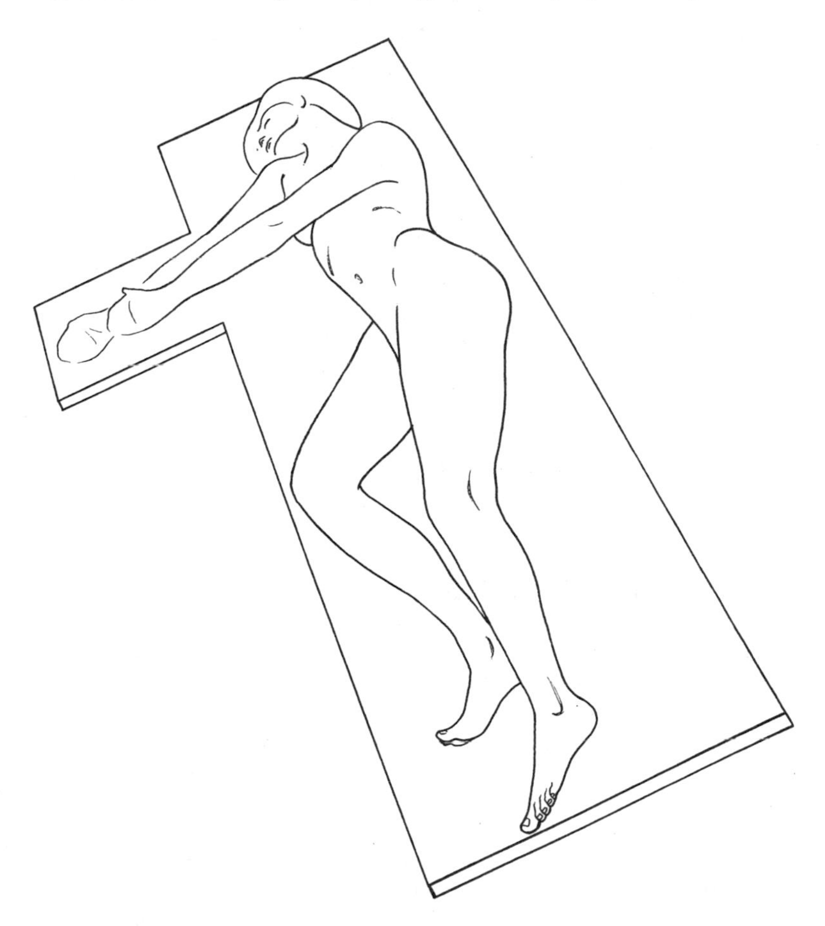

Figure 16.1.4. Right anterolateral decubitus position for splenectomy.

A shoulder roll is placed beneath the patient's right axilla. The patient is initially placed in the full lateral position, then laid back to a 45° position, and then the bag is deflated to harden it into position (Figure 16.1.4). Pillows are placed between the patient's upper and lower extremities. Straps are placed across the shoulders and the hips to secure the patient to the table. The kidney rest is elevated and the table is flexed to maximize the distance between the left costal margin and the left iliac crest. For this position, the surgeon and first assistant/camera operator both stand on the patient's right side. A second assistant could stand on the patient's left side. If it becomes necessary to tilt the patient to a more supine position, the first assistant/camera operator may move to the patient's left side.

1. Advantages

The partial lateral position usually provides excellent exposure of the posterior ligaments, the hilar structures, the tail of the pancreas, and the short gastric vessels. Initial access to abdomen is usually easier and less dangerous than a full lateral approach. Tilting the OR table to the right (counterclockwise, when viewed from the feet) will yield the equivalent of a full lateral position. Tilting the OR table to the left (clockwise) will yield the equivalent of a supine position, facilitating the search for accessory spleens, concomitant surgery (e.g., laparoscopic cholecystectomy), and conversion to laparotomy.

2. Disadvantages

There are no particular disadvantages associated with using this position unless the OR table cannot be rotated as described above.

G. Selected References

Bemelman WA, deWit LT, Busch ORC, et al. Hand-assisted laparoscopic splenectomy. Surg Endosc 2000;14:997–998.

Cadiere GB, Verroken R, Himpens J, et al. Operative strategy in laparoscopic splenectomy. J Am Coll Surg 1994;179:668–672.

Dexter SPL, Martin IG, Alao D, et al. Laparoscopic splenectomy: the suspended pedicle technique. Surg Endosc 1996;10:393–396.

Gigot JF, Lengele B, Gianello P, et al. Present status of laparoscopic splenectomy for hematologic diseases: certitudes and unresolved issues. Semin Laparosc Surg 1998; 5:147–167.

Gossot D, Fritsch S, Celerier M. Laparoscopic splenectomy: optimal vascular control using the lateral approach and ultrasonic dissection. Surg Endosc 1999;13:21–25.

Hebra A, Walker JD, Tagge EP, et al. A new technique for laparoscopic splenectomy with massively enlarged spleens. Am Surg 1998;64:1161–1164.

Hellman P, Arvidsson D, Rastad J. Handport-assisted laparoscopic splenectomy in massive splenomegaly. Surg Endosc 2000;14:1177–1179.

Katkhouda N, Mavor E. Laparoscopic splenectomy. Surg Clin N Am 2000;80(4): 1285–1297.

Klingler PJ, Tsiotos GG, Glaser KS, et al. Laparoscopic splenectomy: evolution and current status. Surg Laparosc Endosc 1999;9(1):1–8.

Kollias J, Watson DI, Conventry BJ, et al. Laparoscopic splenectomy using the lateral position: an improved technique. Aust N Z J Surg 1995;65:746–748.

Meijer DW, Gossot D, Jakimowicz JJ, et al. Splenectomy revisited: manually assisted splenectomy with the Dexterity Device™: a feasibility study in 22 patients. J Laparosc Endosc Adv Tech 1999;9(6):507–510.

Nishizaki T, Takahashi I, Onohara T, et al. Laparoscopic splenectomy using a wall-lifting procedure. Surg Endosc 1999;13:1055–1056.

Park AE, Gagner M, Pomp A. The lateral approach to laparoscopic splenectomy. Am J Surg 1997;173:126–130.

Park AE, Birgisson G, Mastrangelo MJ, et al. Laparoscopic splenectomy: outcomes and lessons learned from over 200 cases. Surgery 2000;128(4):660–667.

Poulin EC, Mamazza J. Laparoscopic splenectomy: Lessons from the learning curve. Can J Surg 1998;41:1:28–36.

Rege RV, Merriam LT, Joehl JJ. Laparoscopic splenectomy. Surg Clin N Am 1996; 76(3):459–468.

Smith CD, Meyer TA, Goretsky MJ, et al. Laparoscopic splenectomy by the lateral approach: a safe and effective alternative to open splenectomy for hematologic diseases. Surgery 1996;120(5):789–794.

Szold A, Sagi B, Merhav H, et al. Optimizing laparoscopic splenectomy: technical details and experience in 59 patients. Surg Endosc 1998;12:1078–1081.

Targarona EM, Espert JJ, Bombuy E, et al. Complications of laparoscopic splenectomy. Arch Surg 2000;135:1137–1140.

Trias M, Targarona EM, Balague C. Laparoscopic splenectomy: an evolving technique. A comparison between anterior and lateral approaches. Surg Endosc 1996;10:389–392.

16.2. Splenectomy: Port Placement Arrangements

William E. Kelley Jr., M.D.

The laparoscopic approach to splenectomy has gradually been embraced by the general surgery community over the past decade. As previously discussed, there are four positions in which the patient can be placed to undergo laparoscopic splenectomy. The patient position and the size of the spleen dictate where the ports should be placed. The port placement schemes need to be adjusted for very large spleens.

A. Port Placement 1

Supine and modified lithotomy position (see Chapter 16.1, Figures 16.1.1, 16.1.2)

A. **Description of port arrangement**

1. Refer to operating room (OR) set up in Chapter 16.1, Figures 16.1.1, 16.1.2
2. The anterior modified lithotomy position described by Flowers et al. places the patient supine or with the left side elevated by a roll beneath the left flank, with both arms tucked. Monitors are placed above and lateral to each shoulder. Exposure is enhanced by placing the table in moderate to steep reverse Trendelenburg position. Rotating the table slightly left brings the patient to a supine position to explore for accessory spleens and expose the splenic pedicle anteriorly. Rotating to the right facilitates exposure of the lateral attachments. (Some authors prefer a semilateral modified lithotomy position with the patient on a bean bag support at a 45° angle, right side down, with the left arm across the patient's chest. In the latter position, the table can be rotated left to approach the splenic pedicle anteriorly with the patient supine, or right to bring the patient almost to a lateral decubitus position to approach the splenic pedicle posteriorly. The port placement is essentially the same for both these positions.)
3. The first port (10 mm) is placed in a periumbilical location and is for the camera (Figure 16.2.1). For an average or short-waisted patient, the trocar is inserted at the upper rim of the umbilicus. In a tall patient, however, the first port must be inserted above the umbilicus, and sometimes to the left of midline to permit adequate exposure during dissection of the splenic pedicle and the

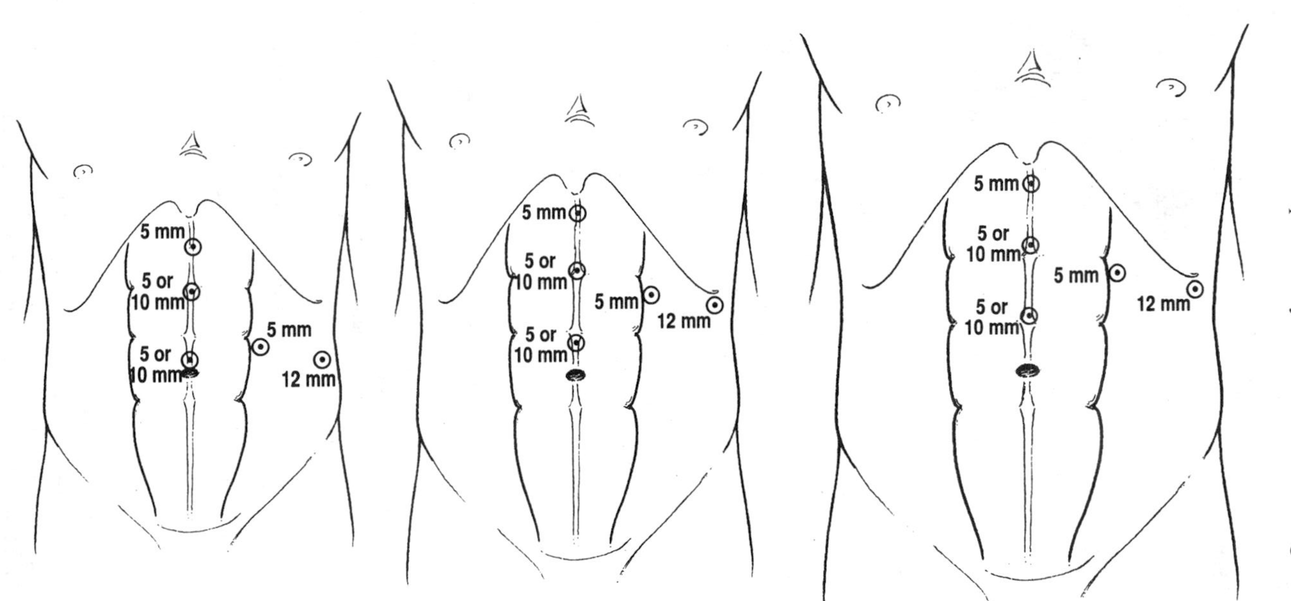

Figure 16.2.1. Port placements for supine or modified lithotomy position.

upper pole of the spleen. For larger spleens, the camera port may have to be positioned to the right of midline, but rarely below the level of the umbilicus, except in the case of a very large spleen. A 30° laparoscope is advised to optimally visualize the anatomy and to allow precise placement of the working and retracting ports.

4. The second port (10 mm) is inserted in the midepigastrium between the xiphoid process and the camera port in the midline for an average-size patient and spleen. For a small patient or a large spleen, this port is placed to the right of midline. The 30° scope may need to be moved to this port to improve visualization of the cephalad aspect of the splenic pedicle or of the upper pole of the spleen. (If a 5-mm, 30° laparoscope is available, then a 5-mm port can be placed in this location.)
5. The third port (5 or 10 mm) is inserted at the xiphoid process, angled to the left of the falciform ligament. This port is used to retract the stomach to expose the short gastric vessels, the splenic pedicle, and the lower pole vessels. If a reliable and atraumatic 5-mm grasper is available, a 5-mm port will suffice. If not, then a 10-mm port will be needed to accommodate a 10-mm Babcock or similar retractor.
6. The fourth port (12 mm) is placed in the left anterior axillary line near the left costal margin, but comfortably below the lower pole of the spleen. The linear stapler, assuming one is used, is passed via this port to staple the hilar vessels. This port placement affords the best angle of approach to the splenic pedicle.
7. The fifth port (12 mm) is inserted in the left upper quadrant in the left midclavicular line above the level of the camera port to allow the surgeon to reach the cephalad short gastric vessels comfortably. This trocar should not be placed too far cephalad, however, to prevent operating instruments from obscuring the camera view.
8. In the supine position the surgeon stands on the patient's right side and the assistant on the left. In the modified lithotomy position, the surgeon stands between the legs and an assistant stands on each side of the patient.

B. Brief description of procedure

1. The five-trocar placement described above allows maximum flexibility for the surgeon and assistants.
2. Some surgeons prefer to operate through the midepigastric and midclavicular left upper quadrant ports two and five, leaving the most lateral port for the assistant. With this approach the camera operator holds the laparoscope through the periumbilical port and maintains exposure with a retractor through the subxiphoid port.
3. Other surgeons prefer to operate via ports four and five, leaving ports two and three for the assistant and port one for the camera. Because the patient is positioned in a 40°–60° right lateral tilt, most of the lateral exposure is provided by gravity. Many surgeons use both these port strategies during splenectomy, depending upon the structures being dissected or divided.

4. The surgeon stands between the patient's legs and approaches the splenic pedicle anteriorly. The lower pole attachments of the spleen are mobilized and the caudal branches of the splenic pedicle are divided. We prefer next to divide the short gastric vessels, using an ultrasonic sheer or Ligasure (Valley Labs, Tyco, Inc.) to expose the splenic pedicle on its cephalad and anterior surfaces. The splenic pedicle is then mobilized posteriorly by careful blunt dissection from below and above, and the splenic vessels are divided using a linear stapler progressing in a cephalad direction. The table is then rotated to the right, the lateral splenic attachments are divided, and the posterior aspect of the spleen is dissected free.

B. Port Placement 2

Full lateral decubitus position (see Chapter 16.1, Figures 16.1.3, 16.1.4)

A. **Description of port arrangement** (method of Park, Gagner et al.)
   1. A 5- or 10-mm port is inserted along the costal margin medial to the midaxillary line (Figure 16.2.2). With insufflation, this trocar moves in a caudal and slightly medial direction, away from the costal margin. A 30° laparoscope is inserted through this port.
   2. The 12-mm port is inserted lower in the midaxillary line.
   3. Another 5- or 10-mm port is inserted posterior to the camera port, along the costal margin near the anterior axillary line.
   4. After mobilization of the splenic flexure, a fourth port (5 mm) may be inserted posteriorly in the flank near the costal margin, if necessary. This port is used by an assistant to elevate the lower pole of the spleen and to maintain exposure during dissection.
   5. When using the lateral decubitus approach for a very small patient or for resection of a large spleen, the port locations must be positioned in a more medial and caudal orientation (Figure 16.2.3). Port placement must allow adequate distance from the spleen to avoid inadvertent injury to the capsule and permit actuation of the instruments, especially the linear stapler. At the same time, the surgeon must be able to reach the cephalad short gastric vessels and the upper pole phrenic attachments.
   6. In this position, the surgeon and camera operator stand on the patient's right side. If an additional assistant is needed, they will stand on the patient's left.

B. **Brief description of procedure**
   1. The patient is positioned in the full right lateral decubitus position with the left arm supported by a sling. A kidney rest is raised and the table is flexed to open the left costophrenic angle. The assistant's monitor is placed next to the upper right border of the table at the 11 o'clock position. The surgeon's monitor is placed behind the patient's shoulders at the 2 o'clock position relative to

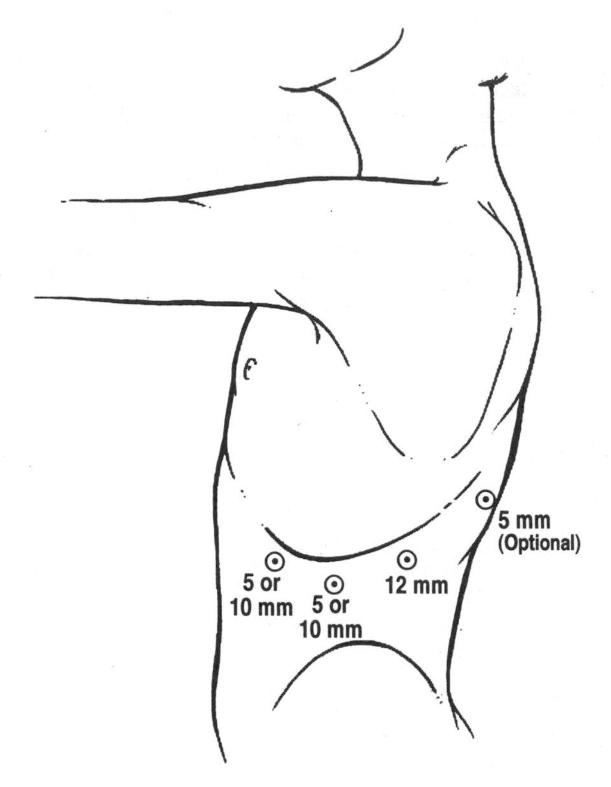

Figure 16.2.2. Port placement for lateral position.

the table. Many surgeons choose to work through the two lower ports with the laparoscope in the cephalad port. Other surgeons prefer ports two and three, while the camera assistant uses the middle port. The first assistant works via the fourth port.

2. The surgeon stands to the right side of the table, facing the patient. The camera operator stands on the same side, cephalad to the surgeon. The first assistant is positioned on the right side of the table, behind the patient.
3. In this position the dissection begins posteriorly, mobilizing the lateral attachments of the spleen, leaving a 1- to 2-cm border of parietal peritoneum to grasp for atraumatic manipulation of the spleen. The spleen is reflected medially, exposing the hilum. The splenic vessels are divided using the linear stapler from below, progressing cephalad, leaving the tail of the pancreas posteriorly. With the spleen elevated, the short gastric vessels are then divided with the ultrasonic shears, the Ligasure device, or sharply

between clips. The vascular upper pole lienophrenic attachments are then divided with the same technique that was used for the short gastric vessels.

C. Port Placement 3

Alternative lateral position arrangement (see Chapter 16.1, Figures 16.1.3, 6.1.4)

A. Description of port arrangement

1. The first port (5 or 10 mm) is inserted just medial to the anterior axillary line at the costal margin. A 30° laparoscope is inserted through this port. Thus, the camera port in this scheme is located to the left of the surgeon's right- and left-hand instrument ports (Figure 16.2.4).

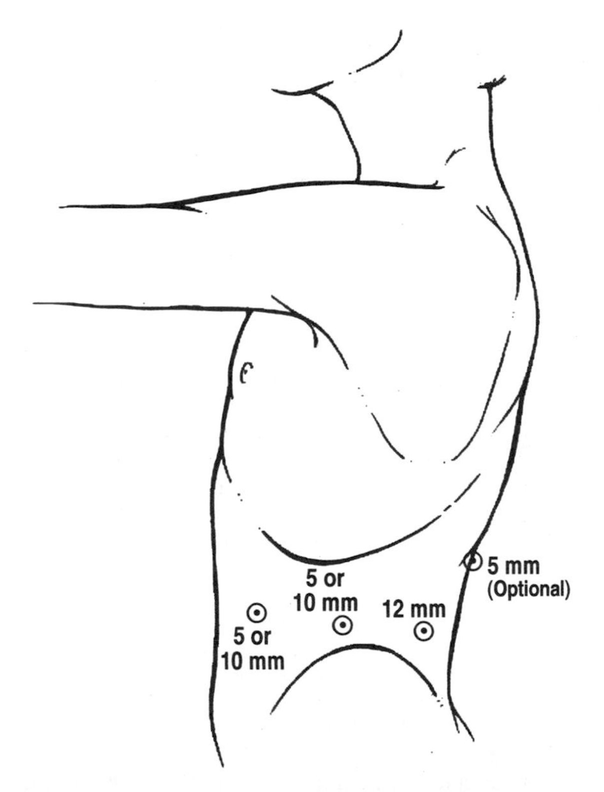

Figure 16.2.3. Port placement for lateral position in a patient with a large spleen.

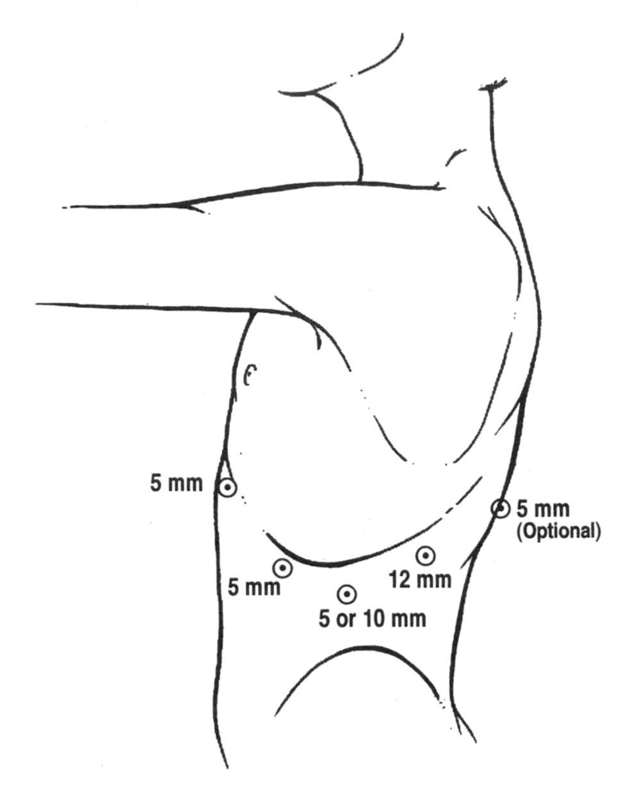

Figure 16.2.4. Alternate port placement for lateral position.

2. The second port (5 or 10 mm) is then inserted 2 cm below the costal arch in the midaxillary line.
3. The third port is introduced near the posterior axillary line near the costal margin. This is a 12-mm trocar to accommodate a linear stapler.
4. A fourth port, for the assistant, can be introduced posteriorly near the costal margin, just below the lower pole of the spleen after the splenic flexure has been mobilized.
5 In this position, the surgeon and camera operator stand on the patient's right side. If an additional assistant is needed, they will stand on the patient's left.
6. When using the lateral decubitus approach for resection of a large spleen, the trocars must be positioned in a more medial and caudal orientation (see Figure 16.2.4). Port placement must allow adequate distance from the spleen to avoid inadvertent injury to the capsule and permit actuation of the instruments, especially the linear stapler. At the same time, the surgeon must be able to

reach the cephalad short gastric vessels and the upper pole phrenic attachments.

B. Brief description of procedure

1. The room and operating team setup is the same as for the Park and Gagner technique.
2. The 30° laparoscope is initially inserted via the first port (in the anterior axillary line).
3. Later, the laparoscope is moved to the second port (in the midaxillary line). The surgeon then operates via the first and third ports. The assistant works through the fourth port.
4. The operation is conducted in the same fashion as in the Park and Gagner lateral decubitus scheme. This port placement is not appropriate for a large spleen wherein the lower pole would prevent insertion of the second and third trocars. Also, exploration for an accessory spleen is more limited.

D. Port Placement 4

Modified semilateral decubitus approach (see Chapter 16.1, Figure 16.2.5)

A. Description of port arrangement

1. Gigot has described a port placement scheme using a 45° semilateral decubitus position. When the table is rotated to the left or right, the patient will approach either the supine position or the full lateral decubitus position, respectively. Surgeons who prefer the semilateral decubitus position believe that they can make a better exploration for accessory spleens when the table is rotated to the left and that they have improved access anteriorly to the splenic pedicle. When the table is shifted to the full decubitus position (right side of patient down), excellent gravity-related exposure of the spleen is obtained.
2. The first port (5 or 10 mm) is inserted in the midaxillary line just below the costal arch and is the site where the 30° laparoscope is introduced (Figure 16.2.5).
3. The second port (5 or 10 mm) is inserted in the left subxiphoid location. This port is used by the cameraperson to retract and provide exposure.
4. The third port (12 mm) is inserted below the costal margin at or near the posterior axillary line. This port is used for dissection and for the linear stapler.
5. The fourth port (5 mm) is inserted between the first and second ports, near the costal margin and midclavicular line. The precise position depends on the size of the spleen and the anatomy of the gastrosplenic ligament.
6. If needed, a fifth port (usually 5 mm) can be introduced posteriorly for use by the second assistant.

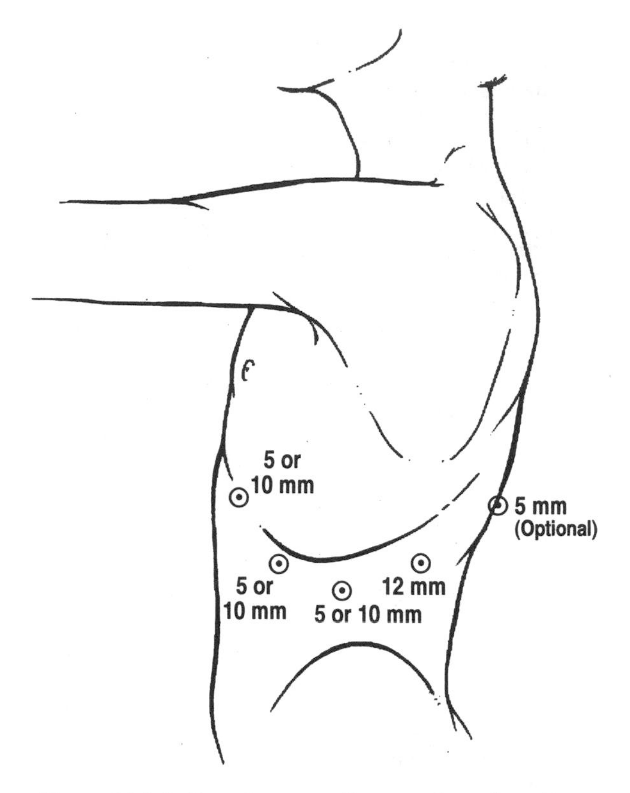

Figure 16.2.5. Port placement for anterolateral position.

7. In this position, the surgeon and camera operator stand on the patient's right side. If an additional assistant is needed, she will stand on the patient's left. If the patient is rotated to a more supine position, the surgeon and assistant positions are changed to those used for the supine position.

B. Brief description of procedure

1. The room and operating team setup is the same as in the full lateral decubitus position.
2. The table is rotated to the left, bringing the patient to a nearly supine position. An initial inspection is made for accessory spleens. The splenocolic ligament is divided and the lower pole vessels are divided.
3. The table is rotated to the right, bringing the patient to a full lateral decubitus position. At this point the dissection proceeds much the same as in the full lateral decubitus position. The spleen is mobilized laterally and the splenic vessels are exposed posteriorly. The hilar vessels are separated from the pancreas and the

dissection of the splenic vessels proceeds from below upward taking advantage of both anterior and posterior exposure. The patient can be rotated back toward a supine position again if necessary as the short gastric vessels are divided and the dissection of the upper pole attachment is completed. With the patient rotated toward the supine position at the end of the procedure, the exploration for accessory spleens is finished.

E. Selected References

Cadiere GB, Verroken R, Himpens J, et al. Operative strategy in laparoscopic splenectomy. J Am Coll Surg 1994;179:668–672.

Delataire B, Maignien B. Laparoscopic splenectomy: the "hanged spleen" technique. Surg Endosc 1995;9:528–529.

Flowers JL, Lefor AT, Steers J, et al. Laparoscopic splenectomy in patients with hematologic diseases. Ann Surg 1996;224:19–28.

Gigot JF. Present status of laparoscopic splenectomy for hematologic diseases: certitudes and un-resolved issues. Semin Laparosc Surg 1998;5:147–167.

Katkhouda N, Mavor E. Laparoscopic splenectomy. Surg Clin N Am 2000;80:1285–1297.

Park A, Gagner M, Pomp A. The lateral approach to laparoscopic splenectomy. Am J Surg 1997;173:126–130.

Park A, Marcaccio M, Stembach M, et al. Laparoscopic vs. open splenectomy. Arch Surg 1999:134:1263–1269.

17.1. Laparoscopic Ultrasonography: Patient Positioning and Operating Room Setup

Maurice E. Arregui, M.D., F.A.C.S.
Matthew S. French, M.D.

A. Introduction

There are indications and applications for laparoscopic ultrasound during numerous laparoscopic procedures. These situations include evaluation of the biliary tree during laparoscopic cholecystectomy, evaluation of the pancreas and surrounding vasculature during staging of pancreatic cancer, and evaluation of the liver for diagnosis and the ablative treatment of malignant lesions. Other indications include characterization of adrenal tumors, localizing colorectal tumors and retroperitoneal masses, and finding pancreatic islet cell tumors. With increasing experience, the indications for laparoscopic ultrasound continue to expand. This section discusses patient positioning and operating room (OR) setup requirements in patients undergoing laparoscopic ultrasound evaluation.

B. Positioning Patient on the Operating Room Table

Generally, laparoscopic ultrasound is performed in addition to other procedures and therefore positioning the patient is specific to the primary surgical procedure. For this reason, patient positioning is rarely a major issue. With articulating probes, little difficulty is encountered even when the patient must be positioned in the lateral decubitus position for laparoscopic adrenalectomy or splenectomy. The ultrasound equipment can be adapted accordingly. Port placement is more important to successful completion of the examination and is discussed in the next chapter.

C. Equipment

High-quality, up-to-date equipment is essential for performing precise laparoscopic ultrasound evaluations. Numerous companies are now producing equipment dedicated to intraoperative open and laparoscopic use. Most ultrasound units are large with a monitor at eye level for viewing, a keyboard and control panel for manipulating the image, recording equipment for VHS, SVHS, or digital recording, and a printer for making hard copies of an image. Most also have the ability for storing images in the hard drive of the computer for later viewing. Although they are portable, the machines were designed for use in dedicated radiology suites rather than operating rooms. The limited space in the operating room and the relative immobility of most ultrasound units makes them awkward to position. The controls are also designed for manipulation in a radiology suite or office setting, and modifications for use in a sterile environment are lacking. Some of the newer ultrasound units are more compact, and attempts have been made to develop remote hand controls for use by the surgeon under sterile conditions. Currently, for the operating surgeon to control the unit a transparent sterile plastic drape must be placed on top of the controls. This method works reasonably well, but I have found it difficult to position the ultrasound probe and manipulate the controls at the same time. It is more efficient to have the circulating nurse manage the ultrasound unit under the surgeon's direction.

The transducers themselves have been designed for intraoperative open and laparoscopic uses. Most transducers can be sterilized; however, some cannot and must be placed in plastic covers to be used in the operating field. Laparoscopic transducers, in general, are specific to each unit or to the line of units made by each company and thus they are not interchangeable. They are typically made to fit through a 10-mm trocar and are either rigid or made with articulating tips. The tip may articulate in two directions, although newer designs will articulate in four directions. The transducer generally provides a linear ultrasound array at a frequency of 5–10 MHz. This is a higher frequency than that used for transabdominal ultrasound (3.5–5.0 MHz) and results in a more detailed image. The higher frequency is possible due to the close approximation of the probe tip to the structures being evaluated. Guides to assist with biopsy under ultrasound are not easy to find and in general are not helpful. Freehand technique is therefore used for biopsies and placement of radiofrequency probes.

D. Room Setup

Proper positioning of equipment in the operating room is crucial to successful performance of laparoscopic ultrasound. The average OR becomes cluttered during these procedures. The ultrasound machine itself is large and must be positioned in addition to the anesthesia cart, laparoscopic tower, and scrub table. It must also be close enough to allow good visualization. The most effective arrangement is shown in Figure 17.1.1.

There are various options for the room setup. This choice depends on the procedure, positioning of the patient, and additional equipment that may be necessary such as a fluoroscopic unit in the case of laparoscopic common bile duct exploration or for performing radiofrequency tumor ablation. For laparoscopic ultrasound during laparoscopic cholecystectomy, our preferred setup is to have the laparoscopic monitor at the head of the bed (if a flat screen monitor is available) or off the right shoulder of the patient (Figure 17.1.2). The ultrasound unit is located on the right side of the patient adjacent to the armboard. When it is

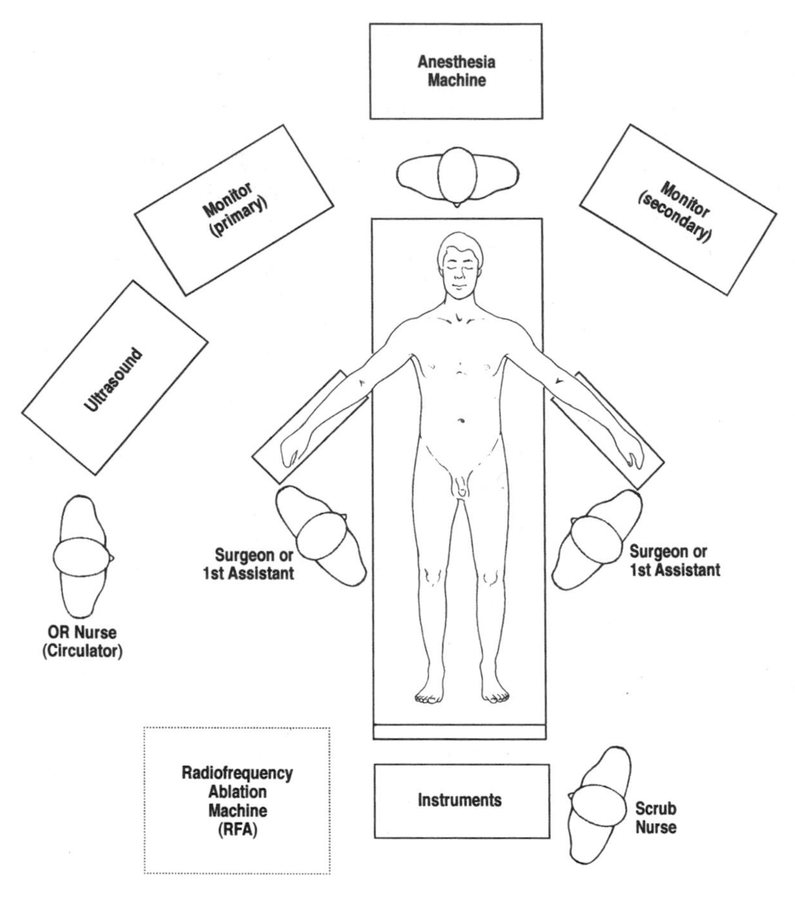

Figure 17.1.1. Operating room setup for laparoscopic ultrasound of upper abdomen (liver, bile ducts, pancreas, stomach, etc.). If a standard CRT monitor is to be used, then it is placed off the patient's right shoulder; if a flat screen monitor or a boom is available, then it is ideally placed at the head of the bed. The ultrasound machine is positioned on the patient's right side. The surgeon stands on the patient's right side and operates the camera and ultrasound probe. This room setup can also be used for radiofrequency ablation (RFA); in this case, the RFA machine is best positioned on the patient's right side.

time to perform the ultrasound, the surgeon goes to the right side of the patient. The surgeon then directs the circulating nurse to adjust the settings in the ultrasound unit. Although this is somewhat cumbersome for the surgeon, we have found that it is easiest for the surgeon to direct the nurse or resident with the ultrasound unit in proximity so that they can more easily show where the correct knobs are located. If the unit is on the other side of the table, the surgeon can more easily see the monitor in a more comfortable manner but has more difficulty seeing the ultrasound console to direct the circulating nurse for the proper adjustments.

We have also tried using picture-in-picture on the monitor at the head of the bed. The image quality is degraded and the same difficulty applies to directing the nurse with the ultrasound console. The same setup, as seen in Figure 17.1.1, is used for laparoscopic staging of pancreatic cancer and for evaluation of the liver during radiofrequency tumor ablation. In thc latter procedure, during placement of the radiofrequency needle, the surgeon stands on the patient's left side while the assistant surgeon holds the ultrasound probe in position to monitor the placement of the radiofrequency needle. The room lights should be turned down

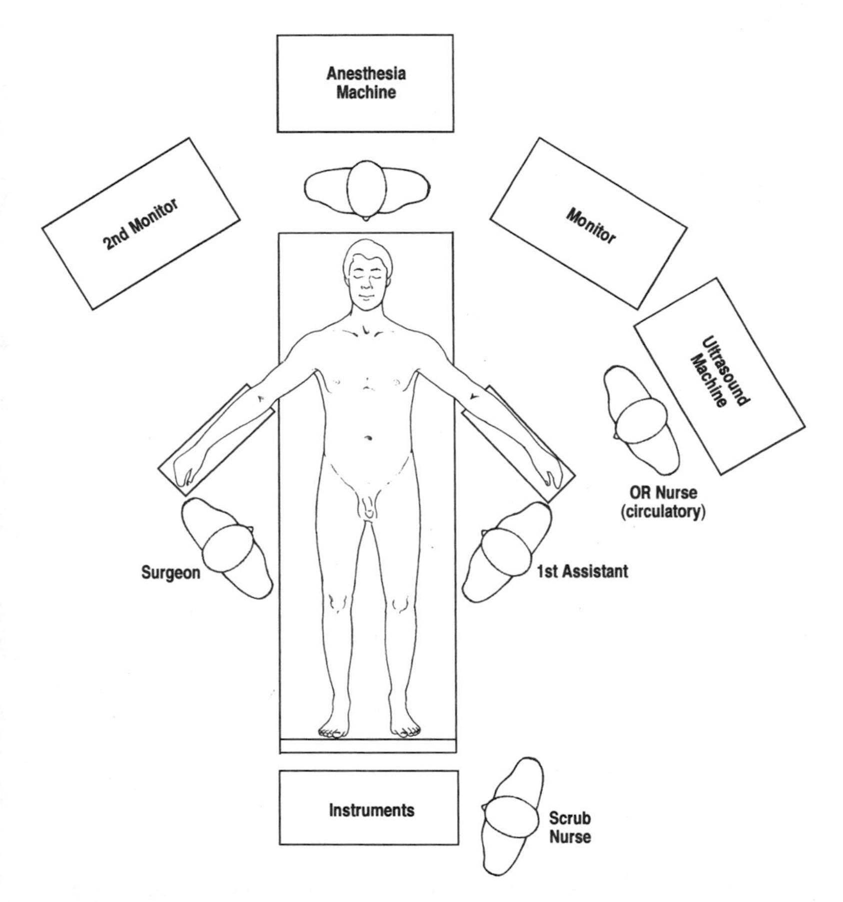

Figure 17.1.2. Alternate OR set up for laparoscopic cholecystectomy or other upper abdominal ultrasound examinations.

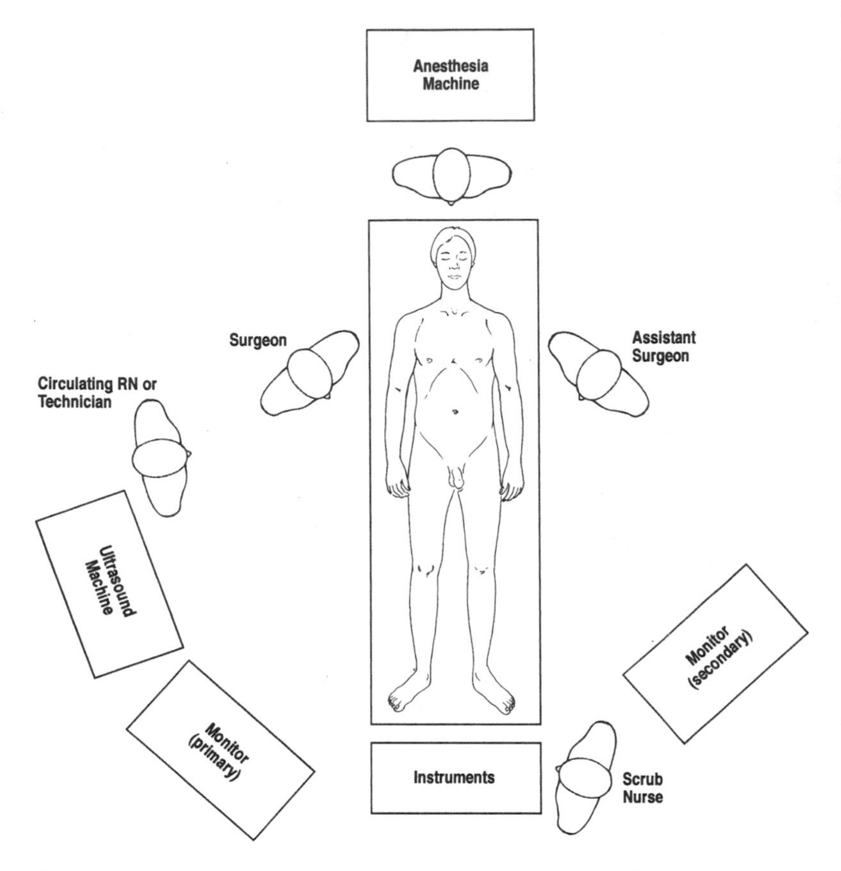

Figure 17.1.3. Operating room setup for use of ultrasound in the pelvis (legs can also be placed in modified lithotomy position).

or off for accurate viewing and the screen turned toward the surgeon. OR staff trained in the operation of the ultrasound console are invaluable but rare.

The recommended OR setup for the performance of pelvic ultrasonography is shown in Figure 17.1.3. Finally, the room setup for ultrasonography with the patient in the left lateral decubitus position is shown in Figure 17.1.4.

E. Discussion

Laparoscopic ultrasound has become very useful during surgery and its indications are increasing. Currently, we use this modality for evaluation of the biliary tree for choledocholithiasis and to confirm normal anatomy before

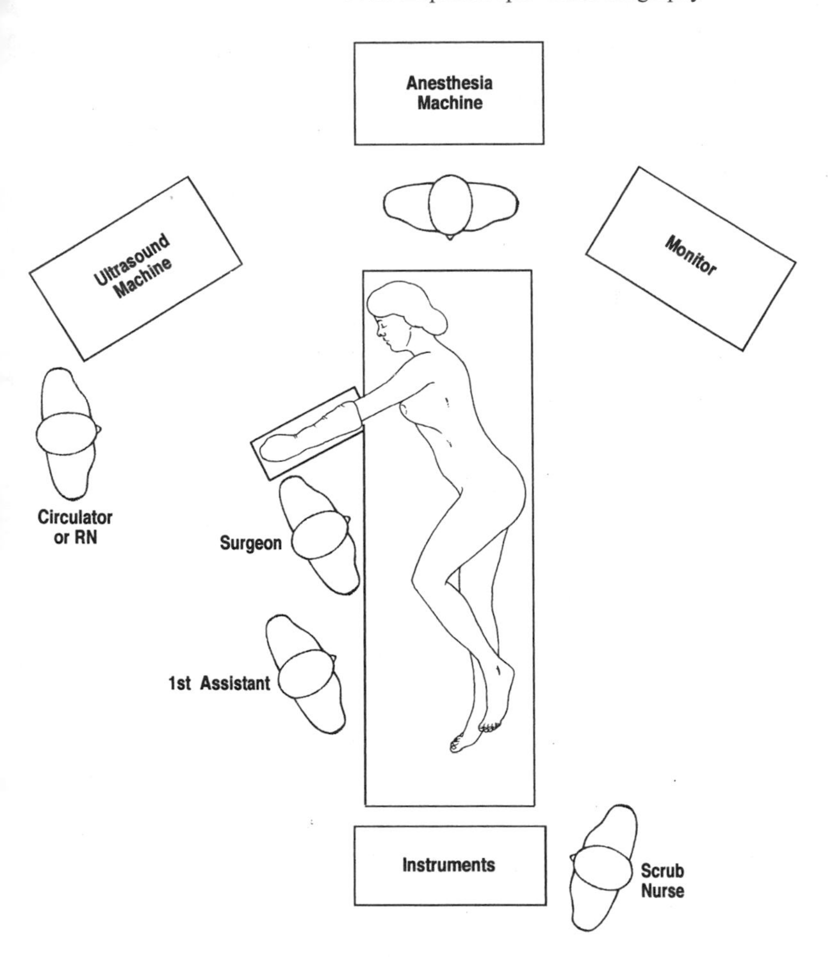

Figure 17.1.4. Operating room setup for use of ultrasound with patient in right lateral patient position (example, left adrenalectomy).

transection of the cystic duct. Anatomic information of the surrounding structures, including the vascular structures, can be very useful when operating on inflamed gallbladders. In our hands, this has effectively replaced intraoperative digital fluorocholangiography. Ultrasound also adds important staging information for intraabdominal malignancies, especially in pancreatic cancer. With the recent interest and increasing use of radiofrequency tumor ablation of hepatic lesions, ultrasound is a requirement. Currently, intraoperative ultrasound has the highest sensitivity for identifying and characterizing hepatic malignancies. It is more sensitive than computerized tomography (CT) scans and magnetic resonance imaging (MRI) scans. We often find many additional lesions intraoperatively when performing radiofrequency tumor ablation. Because of this, intraoperative ultrasound offers the patient the best hope for identification and eradication of all hepatic lesions. The success of radiofrequency ablation, cryosurgery, or resective surgery depends on high-quality ultrasound imaging.

F. Selected References

Bezzi M, Silecchia G, De Leo A, Carbone I, Pepino D, Rossi P. Laparoscopic and intraoperative ultrasound. Eur J Radiol 1998;27(suppl 2):207–214.

Catheline JM, Champault G. Laparoscopic ultrasound in abdominal surgery. Acta Chir Belg 1998;98(2):55–61.

Falcone RA Jr, Fegelman EJ, Nussbaum MS, et al. A prospective comparison of laparoscopic ultrasound vs. intraoperative cholangiogram during laparoscopic cholecystectomy. Surg Endosc 1999;13:784–788.

Jakimowicz JJ. Review: Intraoperative ultrasonography during minimal access surgery. JR Coll Surg Edinb 1993;38:231–238.

Kelly SB, Remedios D, Lau WY, Li AKC. Laparoscopic ultrasonography during laparoscopic cholecystectomy. Surg Endosc 1997;11:67–70.

Lucas SW, Spitz JD, Arregui ME. The use of intra-operative ultrasound in laparoscopic adrenal surgery: The St. Vincent Experience. Surg Endosc 1999;13(11):1093–1098.

Machi J, Schwartz JH, Zaren HA, Noritomi T, Sigel B. Technique of laparoscopic ultrasound examination of the liver. Surg Endosc 1996;10:684–689.

Olsen AK, Bjerkeset OA. Laparoscopic ultrasound (LUS) in gastrointestinal surgery. Eur J Ultrasound 1999;10:159–170.

Thompson DM, Arregui ME, Tetik C, Madden MT, Wegener M. A comparison of laparoscopic ultrasound with digital fluorocholangiography for detecting choledocholithiasis during laparoscopic cholecystectomy. Surg Endosc 1998;12:929–932.

17.2. Laparoscopic Ultrasonography: Port Placement Arrangements

Maurice E. Arregui, M.D., F.A.C.S.
Matthew S. French, M.D.

A. Introduction

Appropriate port placement greatly facilitates the evaluation of intraabdominal structures with laparoscopic ultrasound. Thorough preoperative planning is essential to ensuring a smooth and efficient examination. Two main factors must be considered before selecting trocar sites. First, of course, is the procedure to be performed and organs to be examined, and the second is the type of equipment available.

B. Procedures

As surgeons have become aware of the benefits of laparoscopic ultrasound, the procedure has become increasingly popular. Many articles have been written in the past 5 years describing the use of ultrasound during a variety of general surgical, gynecologic, and urologic procedures. In addition, laparoscopic ultrasound may be the primary procedure to be carried out during staging laparoscopy for pancreatic or other malignancies. Obviously, the location of the organ or organs to be examined will dictate the most appropriate locations for the trocars. Frequently, when ultrasound is performed in conjunction with other procedures, the trocar sites selected for the primary procedure will suffice for the ultrasound examination.

C. Equipment

In general, three types of laparoscopic ultrasound probes exist: rigid, two-direction articulating (up/down), and four-direction articulating (up/down, side/side). These probes are used in conjunction with a free-standing ultrasound module similar to those found in radiology departments, which consist of a monitor, keypad, and recording device or devices. The operating room setup for laparoscopic ultrasound is detailed in the preceding chapter.

D. Port Positioning

During procedures done solely for the purpose of performing laparoscopic ultrasound, the port arrangements shown in Figures 17.2.1, 17.2.2, and 17.2.3 permit laparoscopic examination of the commonly examined upper abdominal structures (liver, bile ducts, pancreas, stomach, etc.). The use of 10-mm ports allows the ultrasound-guided (USG) probe to be inserted via any of the ports, which should facilitate a thorough examination.

In the authors' opinion, the best arrangement for diagnostic ultrasound is that depicted in Figure 17.2.1. Using this port scheme, the ultrasound probe is best placed through the umbilical port while the laparoscope is inserted through the right upper quadrant port. The surgeon can easily control both camera and probe while standing on the patient's right side. If a four-direction articulating probe is used, the entire evaluation can be performed through the periumbilical port. If, however, a rigid probe or two-direction articulating probe is used, then a third port may be needed to complete the examination. When evaluating the liver and bile ducts, the epigastrium just to the right of the midline is the best additional location (see Figure 17.2.2). This position will allow transverse imaging whereas the umbilical position permits only sagittal imaging. The higher location of the epigastric port also allows better access to the dome of the liver. For examination of the pancreas and stomach, the left upper quadrant is probably the best location for a third port (see Figure 17.2.3). This location will facilitate transverse imaging of these structures.

Some surgeons routinely place the ultrasound probe in the right upper quadrant for evaluation of the biliary structures (e.g., Kelly et al.). This technique can result in difficulty evaluating the lower edge of the liver due to its close proximity.

The dome and posterior portions of the liver can be very difficult to evaluate from any port position if a rigid probe is all that is available. Keeping good surface contact under these circumstances is not possible. In this situation, instillation of saline over the dome of the liver will often provide an acceptable window for standoff imaging.

Lower abdominal imaging of the retroperitoneum or colon can almost always be accomplished via the umbilical port with an articulating probe. For pelvic imaging, trocar sites are selected that allow the probe to be positioned adjacent to the structures of interest. The umbilicus is usually a suitable location; however, some patients may require trocars placed in the lower quadrants. Once again additional ports will be required if the surgeon wishes to obtain images in a second plane and does not have access to an articulating ultrasound probe.

E. Conclusion

Optimal port site locations for laparoscopic ultrasound vary with respect to the patient, the procedure performed, and the equipment available to the surgeon. Currently, optimal equipment is not readily available in most operating suites

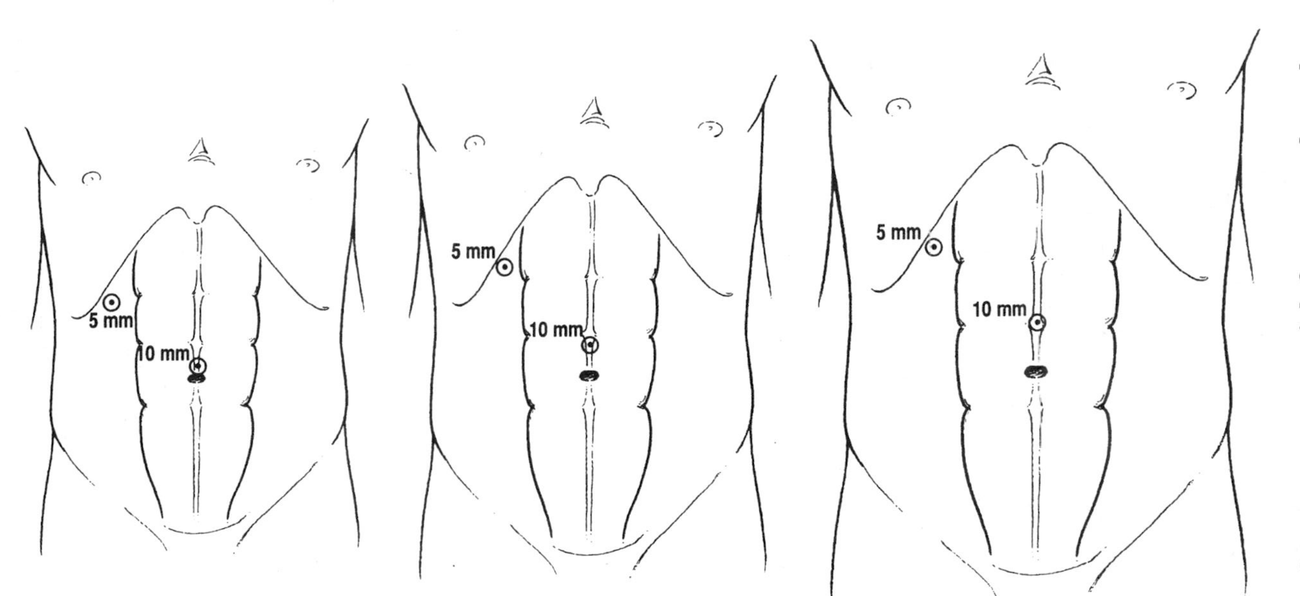

Figure 17.2.1. Trocar placement for laparoscopic ultrasound of the liver, gallbladder, bile ducts, and pancreas. The ultrasound probe is placed through the umbilical port, and a 5-mm scope is placed through the right upper quadrant port.

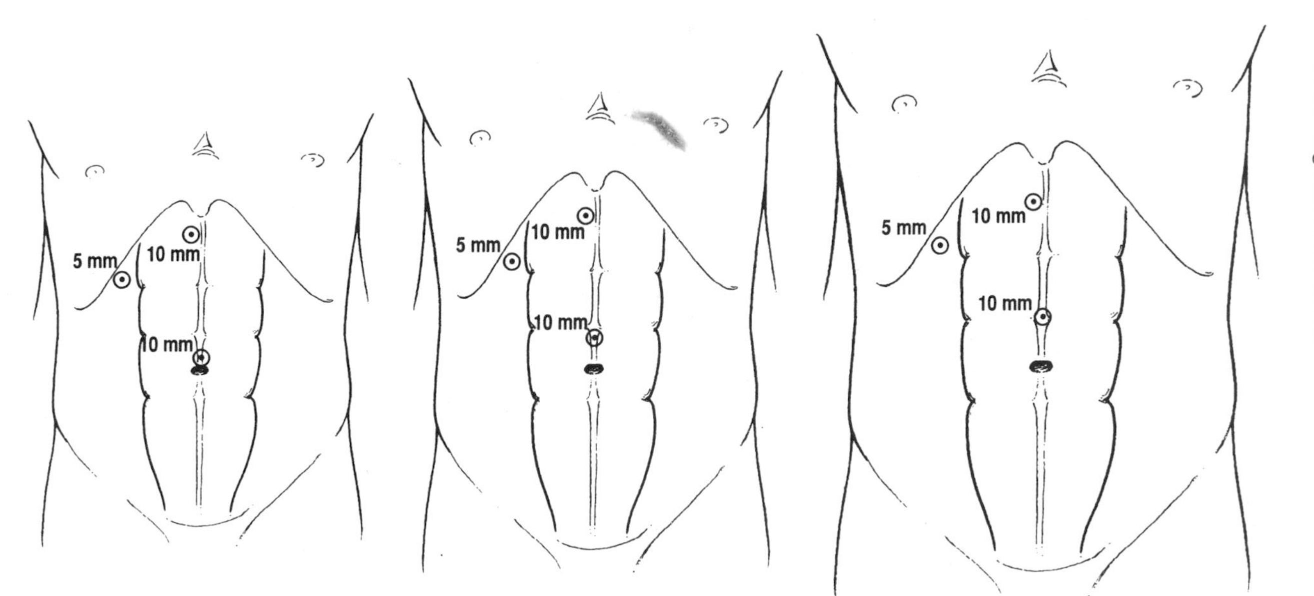

Figure 17.2.2 Alternate trocar arrangement that is useful when using a rigid ultrasound probe. The probe is placed through the umbilical port for sagittal imaging and through the epigastric port for longitudinal transverse imaging.

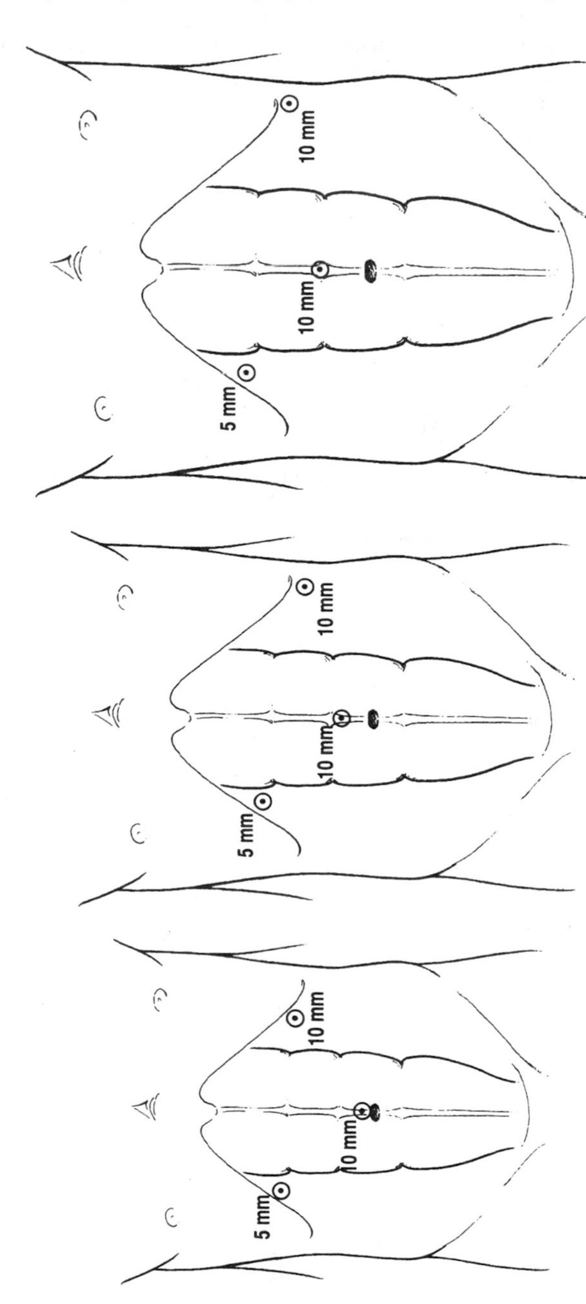

Figure 17.2.3. Trocar placement in the left upper quadrant for evaluation of the pancreas and stomach.

and thus the procedures can be difficult and time consuming. As more surgeons begin to utilize laparoscopic ultrasound, hospital administrators may realize the benefit in obtaining the appropriate ultrasound units and probes.

F. Selected References

Bezzi M, Silecchia G, De Leo A, Carbone I, Pepino D, Rossi P. Laparoscopic and intraoperative ultrasound. Eur J Radiol 1998;27(suppl 2):207–214.

Catheline JM, Champault G. Laparoscopic ultrasound in abdominal surgery. Acta Chir Belg 1998;98(2):55–61.

Falcone RA Jr, Fegelman EJ, Nussbaum MS, et al. A prospective comparison of laparoscopic ultrasound vs. intraoperative cholangiogram during laparoscopic cholecystectomy. Surg Endosc 1999;13:784–788.

Kelly SB, Remedios D, Lau WY, Li AKC. Laparoscopic ultrasonography during laparoscopic cholecystectomy. Surg Endosc 1997;11:67–70.

Machi J, Schwartz JH, Zaren HA, Noritomi T, Sigel B. Technique of laparoscopic ultrasound examination of the liver. Surg Endosc 1996;10:684–689.

Olsen AK, Bjerkeset OA. Laparoscopic ultrasound (LUS) in gastrointestinal surgery. Eur J Ultrasound 1999;10:159–170.

Thompson DM, Arregui ME, Tetik C, Madden MT, Wegener M. A comparison of laparoscopic ultrasound with digital fluorocholangiography for detecting choledocholithiasis during laparoscopic cholecystectomy. Surg Endosc 1998;12:929–932.

18. Intraoperative Upper and Lower Endoscopy Considerations

Keith P. Meslin, M.D.
John M. Cosgrove, M.D.

A. Introduction

There is a growing list of reasonable indications for intraoperative endoscopy. Although this modality may be required for both open and minimally invasive procedures, it will be utilized more often in the laparoscopic setting, excepting hand-assisted procedures, due to the inability to palpate the bowel. In either case, the endoscope can provide information that is not otherwise available to the surgeon which may impact the choice of surgical procedure. Present indications include (1) nonpalpable and nonlocalizable intestinal neoplasms, (2) polypectomy site localization, (3) nonlocalized upper and lower gastrointestinal (GI) bleeding site(s), (4) assessment of the status of the intestinal mucosal lining (for ischemia, colitis, or inflammation) or the bowel lumen (looking for strictures), and (5) searching for other intestinal pathology. Endoscopy may also be used as a technical aid to facilitate the successful completion of a chosen operation. Examples of this type of indication include (1) during low anterior resection to check for an anastomotic leak or bleeding, (2) during gastric bypass surgery, (3) during fundoplication to assess the diameter of the esophageal lumen, and (4) during laparoscopic cholecystectomy with positive cholangiogram to retrieve stones or perform sphincterotomy via intraoperative endoscopic retrograde cholangiopancreatography (ERCP).

When booking and planning an intestinal operation, the surgeon should consider whether intraoperative endoscopy may be required or useful. If there is even a reasonable chance that an intraoperative endoscopic examination may be necessary, the required endoscopy equipment should be specifically requested when the operation is booked, to provide the operating room with ample time to gather the appropriate scope and other equipment. A well-equipped endoscopic cart is required (a single cart can be used for both upper and lower endoscopy). It should have a full array of equipment including biopsy forceps, snare, and some means of coagulation (bipolar cautery, heater probe, or laser). Endoscopic sclerotherapy catheters should also be available.

When intraoperative endoscopy is anticipated, the surgeon should choose the body and table positions that best facilitate the examination and operation. Because unanticipated situations and indications do arise, the operating room should have one or several fully equipped endoscopy carts ready for use as well as clean upper and lower endoscopes.

B. Lower Gastrointestinal Endoscopy

This category includes anoscopy, rigid proctoscopy, flexible sigmoidoscopy, and colonoscopy. Each is discussed separately.

1. **Anoscopy**
   a. Anoscopy permits evaluation of the anorectal sphincter and the distal portion of the rectum.
   b. Outside the setting of an anorectal or perineal procedure, anoscopy should be done preoperatively. The indications for intra-operative anoscopy include:
      1. To rule out neoplasms
      2. To evaluate the anal canal or the distal rectum
   c. Patient position that will permit anoscopy (Figure 18.1)
      1. Modified lithotomy (Figure 18.1A)
      2. Prone (transverse buttock roll and chest rolls are often used) (Figure 18.1B)
      3. Lateral decubitus (Figure 18.1C)
   d. Equipment
      1. Beveled anoscope with obturator (either disposable or reusable)

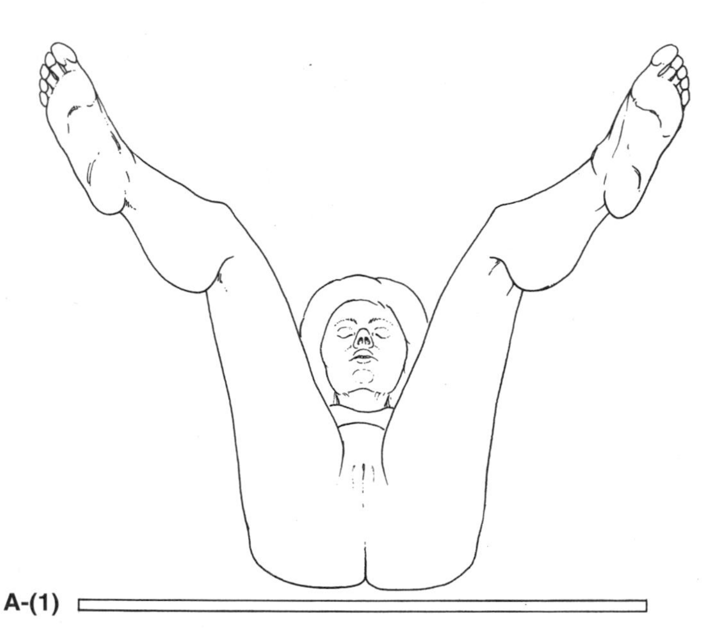

Figure 18.1. (A) Modified lithotomy position (side view and front from foot of bed). (B) Prone position (will roll under pelvis). (C) Sim's position (modified left lateral).

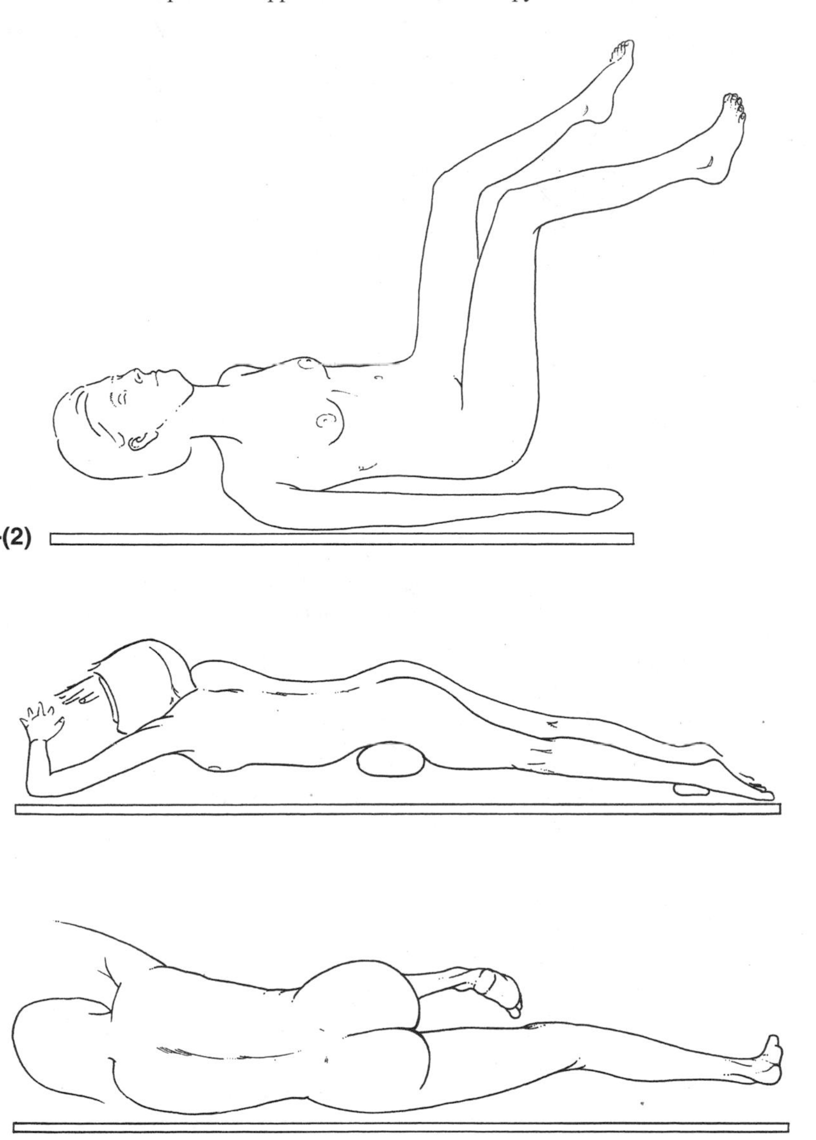

Figure 18.1. *Continued*

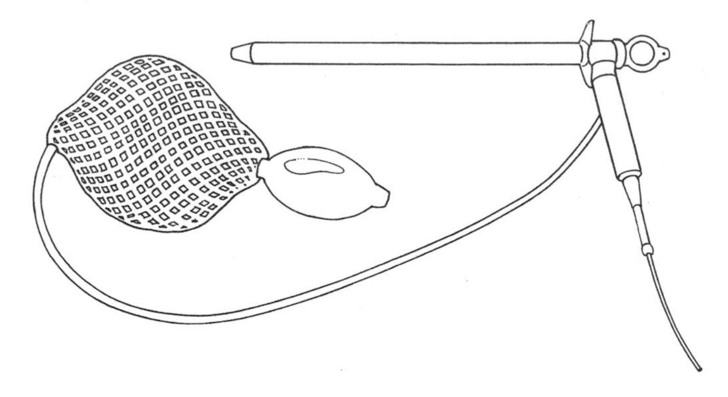

Figure 18.2. Rigid proctoscopy: reusable metal scope.

2. Light source
    a. Some anoscopes have attached light sources
    b. Headlight or other directed light source otherwise needed

2. **Rigid proctoscopy** (Figure 18.2)
    a. Indications
        1. To localize a rectal polyp, polypectomy site, cancer, or other lesion
        2. To check for anastomotic integrity or bleeding
        3. To assess for proctitis, inflammation, etc.
        4. Measurement of the distance between the dentate line (or anal verge) and a neoplasm or anastomosis
    b. Patient position
        1. Modified lithotomy
        2. Prone
        3. Lateral decubitus
    c. Equipment
        1. Length
            a. 25 cm
            b. 15 cm
        2. Scope diameters range from 1.1 to 2.7 cm
        3. Types of scopes
            a. Disposable
            b. Metal, reusable
            c. Plastic, reusable (operating anoscopes)
        4. A working light source with power source in close proximity to table (setting up a rectal cart with all the necessary equipment is advised)
        5. Proper instrumentation includes a proximal magnifying lens and an attachment for the insufflation of air

3. Colonoscopy and sigmoidoscopy (Figure 18.3A,B)

Intraoperative colonoscopy and flexible sigmoidoscopy in both the emergency and the elective situation provide much useful information that is otherwise difficult to obtain.

a. Indications: as per the introduction
b. Equipment
    1. A flexible endoscopy cart with light source, processor, image printer, and monitor (the latter three for videoscopes). An irrigation and air insufflation device (usually part of the light source) and water bottle (with connecting cable) are also needed.
        a. The video monitor may be fixed to the top of the cart (this necessitates that the endoscopist look toward the cart to view the endoscopic image)
        b. The monitor may be kept on a separate mobile stand that can be placed in the ideal position, which is often opposite the endoscopy cart

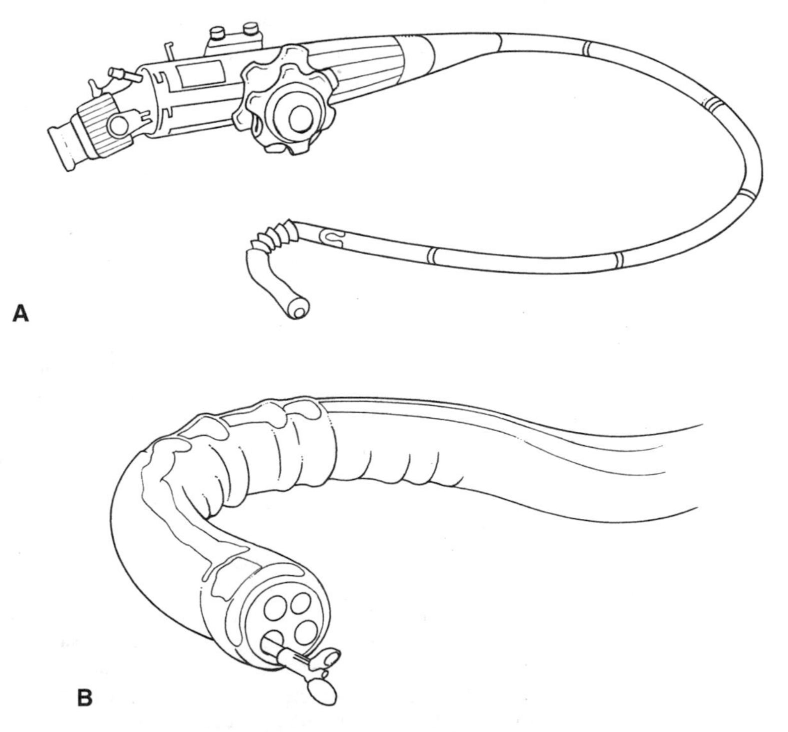

Figure 18.3. (A) Flexible endoscope. (B) Close-up of scope tip showing biopsy forceps from the instrument channel of the scope.

2. The cart should also be stocked with biopsy forceps, snares, sclerotherapy catheters, cleaning brushes, and suction tubing.
3. An appropriate flexible scope (sigmoidoscope or colonoscope) with all the needed detachable components.
   a. Suction and irrigation/insufflation buttons (with appropriate washers)
   b. Instrument channel fenestrated caps (through which biopsy forceps or snare is passed)
4. A dedicated high-volume pump for irrigation is advised for the evaluation of GI bleeders and those patients with incomplete colonic preparations.
5. The flexible endoscopy cart is usually placed at the level of the feet on the patient's right or left if the modified lithotomy position is used. If the patient is left supine with the right mid- and lower leg elevated on one or several pillows, then the endoscopist stands on the patient's right side and the video monitor is placed on the patient's left side.
6. Equipment hookup: It is important that the endoscopist be well acquainted with the operating room (OR) endoscopic equipment to allow rapidly resolving problems that arise. The following steps must be followed before the examination:
   a. Turn on all electronic equipment
   b. Connect the umbilical cable of the endoscope to the light source
   c. Connect the cable/hose of the three-fourths-filled water bottle to the umbilical cable
   d. Connect the suction to the appropriate site on the umbilical cable
   e. Test the insufflation, irrigation, and suction before commencing the procedure
   f. Turn on the light source (ignition)
   g. Check the scopes flexion controls before insertion
   h. Check that the cables from the image processor to the video monitor are connected (for video exams)

C. Patient Position

1. Modified lithotomy position. This is the best position for laparoscopic-assisted colectomy because it facilitates both the colonoscopy and the performance of the colectomy. The endoscopist can either stand or sit on a stool. The patient's thighs should be parallel to the surface of the abdomen if a laparoscopic procedure is planned, because if the thighs are flexed (angled toward the ceiling) they will limit the use of the lower abdominal ports when working in the cephalad direction.
2. Modified supine position: The left leg is elevated by placing several pillows under the lower extremity from just above the knee to the foot.

At the time of the colonoscopy, an additional drape is placed between the legs and the abdomen so as to create a nonsterile working space for the endoscopist. The endoscopist stands on the patient's right side and inserts the scope into the anus from underneath the elevated right upper leg. This can be done from either a sitting or a standing position.

3. Modified left lateral position
   a. Particularly useful for office exams and inspection in the emergency room
   b. Positioning of the legs
      i. The thighs and knees both flexed
      ii. The left leg is kept straight and the right leg is flexed at both the hip and knee
   c. Position particularly suited to the pregnant patient, patients with severe chronic obstructive pulmonary disease (COPD), and patients with severe neurologic impairments
   d. The endoscopist usually stands for the examination

D. Surgeon's Responsibilities (Remains Scrubbed at the Operative Field During the Endoscopy)

1. Must place noncrushing clamp on the terminal ileum to prevent insufflation of the small bowel.
2. Must mark the site of the lesion once it is located with suture, clip, or other means.
3. During laparoscopic case, may be necessary to desufflate abdomen to limit loop formation and to permit application of external pressure to facilitate scope insertion.
4. If intraoperative colonoscopy done with abdomen open, then the surgeon can stent the bowel and facilitate insertion (Figure 18.4). Also, the surgeon and assistant should limit loop size by manually applying pressure to the loops as they form; otherwise, they can enlarge unchecked.

E. Esophagogastroduodenoscopy (EGD)

1. Indications:
   a. Massive suspected upper GI hemorrhage that requires surgery. All upper GI bleeds should undergo endsocopy before surgery; however, if definitive localization was not possible on the preoperative examination(s), then an intraoperative exam for localization may be needed.
   b. Foreign-body removal when the OR is the chosen site for the examination.

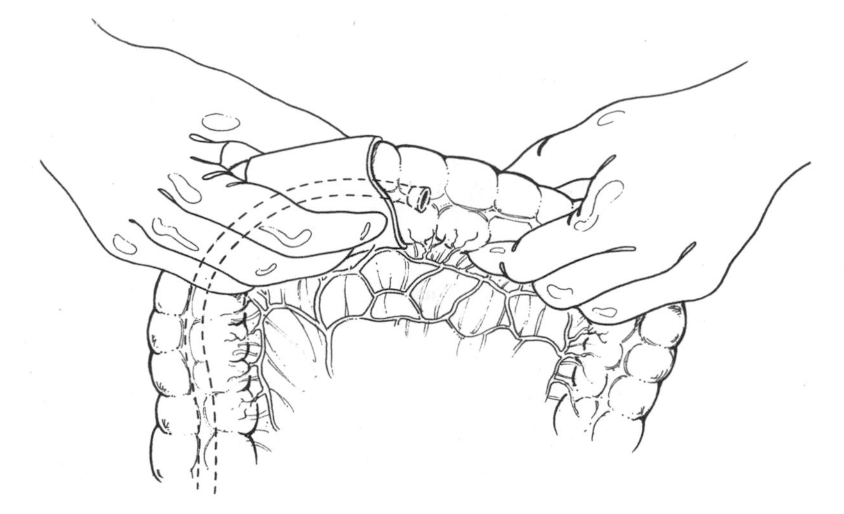

Figure 18.4. Intraoperative colonoscopy during open procedure: manual stenting of the colon to facilitate exam.

   c. During gastric bypass.
   d. During fundoplication to assess the diameter of the esophageal lumen.
   e. To localize a small lesion or ulcer and to inspect the stomach or duodenum for other reasons.
2. Equipment:
   a. As stated in the introduction.
   b. Flexible upper endoscope.
3. Positioning
   a. The patient is usually lying supine with an endotracheal tube in place. This differs from the most commonly used elective position (left lateral decubitis) for examinations performed outside the OR setting.
   b. The endoscopist usually stands on the left side of the patient's head. The video monitor can be positioned close to the head of the table on either the right or left side.
   c. Despite the fact that the patient is under general anesthesia, it is advised that a bite block be used to protect the scope and to facilitate insertion.
4. Surgeon's (at the operative field) responsibilities
      i. The placement of a noncrushing clamp on the proximal jejunum will prevent insufflation of the more distal small bowel.
      ii. If the endoscopy is being done for the purposes of identifying the location of a lesion or of a bleeding site, then the surgeon must mark the site with a suture or clip

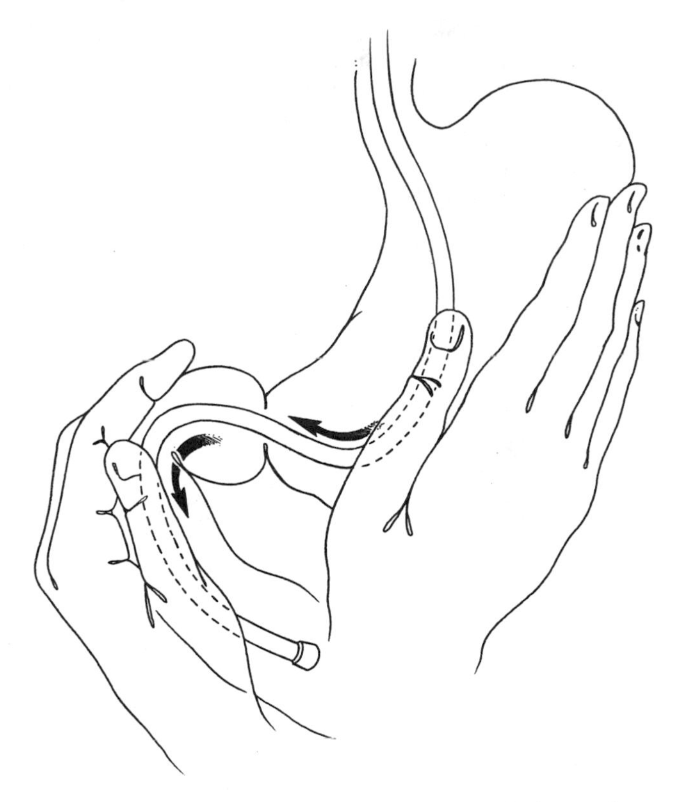

Figure 18.5. Intraoperative endoscopy during open surgical procedure: manual stenting of greater curvature of the stomach and the duodenal "C" loop to facilitate small bowel intubation.

once the site is identified via transillumination or via palpation of the scope tip with an instrument.

iii. If the intraoperative upper endoscopy is being done with the abdomen open, then the surgeon can facilitate the exam and limit loop formation by eternally supporting the greater curve of the stomach and the "C" loop of the duodenum manually (Figure 18.5).

F. Percutaneous Endoscopic Gastrostomy

1. The majority of percutaneous endoscopic gastrostomies (PEGs) are performed in the endoscopy suite; a PEG can also be placed in the intensive care unit, provided the necessary equipment and support are

available. The OR may be chosen as the setting for PEG placement in high-risk patients with multiple medical problems to enlist the assistance of an anesthesiologist. In the majority of patients in whom the PEG insertion is the only procedure to be carried out, intravenous sedation and local anesthesia under the anesthesiologist's guidance and monitoring, so-called monitored anesthesia care (MAC), will suffice. In rare cases, general anesthesia may be required. Uncommonly, PEG insertion may be called for during a lower abdominal operation being carried out under general anesthesia. Rather than extend the lower incision or make a separate upper abdominal incision, a PEG can be placed.

2. The patient should be positioned supine with the head slightly elevated to prevent aspiration. If necessary, in situations where MAC is being given, the left lateral position can be used to intubate the esophagus, after which the patient is rolled to the supine position.
3. Well-functioning suction should be available for oropharyngeal secretions.
4. Please refer to the EGD section above (E, 3) in regard to intubating the esophagus in patients in whom general anesthesia is being used.
5. As for EGD, the endoscopist stands on the patient's left with the video cart on the patient's right.
6. The assistant may stand on either side of the patient depending upon the endoscopist's preference and the patient's body habitus.
7. Once the stomach is intubated and a thorough examination completed, the endoscope is used to transilluminate the anterior abdominal wall and a suitable site for tube insertion chosen.
8. The surgeon then administers the local anesthesia and makes a small skin incision. With the stomach fully insufflated, a long needle is inserted through the abdominal wall toward the light. Once the endoscopist verifies that the needle is in the stomach, a long wire is passed through it from the outside. The endoscopist grasps the wire with a snare and then removes the scope, thus pulling the wire out through the mouth.
9. At this point either the pull or push PEG insertion technique may be used to position the tube. (Please see a standard endoscopy text for details of the procedure.)
10. If a PEG is to be placed in conjunction with a laparoscopic procedure, it will be necessary to desufflate the abdomen completely (after occluding the proximal small bowel) to transilluminate the abdominal wall and choose the best site for the PEG.
11. Standard OR "minor" tray instruments may be used to make the skin incision at the site chosen for the PEG and for the suturing of the tube. Alternately, almost all PEG tubes come in kits that provide adequate disposable instruments for the tube placement.

G. Enteroscopy

Endoscopy of the small bowel is especially useful in the evaluation and treatment of patients with obscure bleeding where prior diagnostic procedures, including upper and lower endoscopy, have failed to determine the bleeding site. Enteroscopy can also be used to locate a small bowel neoplasm, or a lesion, or to investigate a radiologic abnormality. There are four different ways to endoscopically evaluate the small bowel: (1) push enteroscopy, (2) sonde enteroscopy, (3) capsule enteroscopy, and (4) intraoperative enteroscopy. Enteroscopy done during an open abdominal operation allows the surgeon to guide the endoscope through the small bowel as well as to mark the site of important endoscopic findings.

1. Either a pediatric or adult colonoscope should be used because a standard upper scope is not long enough to permit a thorough small bowel examination. The pediatric colonoscope is needed, at times, because it can be difficult to traverse the cricopharynx with a standard diameter colonoscope. However, if the anesthesiologist deflates the endotracheal cuff, passage of the adult scope is usually possible.
2. The endoscopist usually stands to the left of the patient's head above the sterile drapes. The video cart is usually placed on the left side near or above the head.
3. If possible, the endoscopic procedure should be initiated before making the skin incision to facilitate passage of the scope to the level of the proximal jejunum. The intact abdominal wall limits the size of the intragastric loop that forms during insertion through the stomach. If the endoscope is inserted after the abdomen is open, the surgeon can limit the gastric loop by grasping and anchoring the duodenal bulb with one hand while compressing the greater curvature of the stomach with the other hand (Figure 18.5).
4. Concomitant passage of a nasogastric tube is recommended to decrease inflation of the stomach and to limit the development of mucosal lacerations.
5. It is not recommended that the endoscope be passed into the small bowel via an enterotomy because of the increased risk of intraabdominal or wound infections.
6. The surgeon assists the endoscopist in inserting and examining as much of the small intestine as possible.
7. It is not always possible to examine the entire small bowel via an upper approach.
8. Retrograde enteroscopic examination of the terminal ileum and, often, the middle portion of the ileum can be accomplished using a transanally placed colonoscope via the ileocecal valve. In this situation, the upper enteroscopy would be performed first followed by colonoscopy and retrograde distal enteroscopy.

H. Endoscopic Retrograde Cholangiopancreatography

In patients suspected of having common bile duct stones in whom a cholecystectomy is indicated, it is the author's experience that intraoperative ERCP can be quite helpful. During laparoscopic cholecystectomy, an intraoperative cholangiogram is often performed. If the cholangiogram is positive or suggestive of common bile duct stones, an ERCP can be carried out in the OR during the same procedure. This allows the patient to have both procedures under the same anesthesia. Further, if in the midst of intraoperative ERCP large stones (>15 mm) are encountered that cannot be removed by ERCP, the surgeon can next carry out a surgical common bile duct exploration. This approach has not only decreased the percentage of negative ERCPs, it has also decreased the overall length of stay by obviating the need for preoperative or postoperative ERCP and the attendant logistic problems associated with scheduling multiple procedures during a single admission. The method used for intraoperative ERCP is very similar to that used when the procedure is performed in the endoscopy or radiology suite.

1. Patients are placed on a table that permits fluoroscopy in the supine position under general anesthesia.
2. The laparoscopic cholecystectomy is completed, the abdomen desufflated, and all port sites closed and dressed.
3. The endoscopist stands to the left of the patient.
4. The video cart is placed to the right of the patient.
5. The OR needs to be prepared for fluoroscopy. In addition to having the patient on a fluoroscopy capable table, a fluoroscopy machine with a C-arm, a monitor, and a radiology technician must be available. The operating room requirements are similar to those required for operative placement of a long-term central venous access line.
6. A standard ERCP endoscope is required. The scope is connected to the video cart as for other endoscopic procedures.
7. A variety of different endoscopic catheters are used to cannulate the ampulla.
8. Standard ERCP methods are used to carry out the procedure (please consult an endoscopy text for the details).
9. Sphincterotomes, stone retrieval baskets, and balloon catheters are used to facilitate removal of common bile duct (CBD) stones.

I. Selected References

Asao T, Nagamachi Y. Intraoperative colonoscopy during laparoscopic bowel resection. Lancet 1995;345(8957):1123.

Bowden TA. Intraoperative endoscopy of the gastrointestinal tract. In: Dent TL (ed) Surgical Endoscopy. Chicago: Year Book Medical, 1985.

Bowden TA. Intraoperative gastrointestinal endoscopy. GastroEndoscopy 1986;32(6):427.

Cave DR, Cooley JS. Intraoperative enteroscopy. Indications and techniques. Gastro Endosc Clin N Am 1996;6(4):793–802.

Geenen JE. Techniques in Therapeutic Endoscopy. New York: Gower, 1992.

Kalimi R, Cosgrove JM, Marini C, et al. Combined intraoperative laparoscopic cholecystectomy and endoscopic retrograde cholangiopancreatography: lessons from 29 cases. Surg Endosc 2000;14(3):232–234.

Keighley MR. Surgery of the Anus, Rectum and Colon. London: Saunders, 1999.

Kim SH, Milsom JW, Church JM, et al. Perioperative tumor localization for laparoscopic colorectal surgery. Surg Endosc 1997;11(10):1013–1016.

Kuramoto S, Ihara O, Sakai S, et al. Intraoperative colonoscopy in the detection of nonpalpable colonic lesions: how to identify the affected bowel segment. Surg Endosc 1988;2(2):76–80.

Martinez SA, Hellinger MD, Martini M, et al. Intraoperative endoscopy during colorectal surgery. Surg Laparosc Endosc 1998;8(2):123–126.

Ponsky JL, Dunkin BJ. Percutaneous endoscopic gastrostomy. In: Yamada T (ed) Textbook of Gastroenterology. Philadelphia: Lippincott, 1999.

Sakanoue Y, Nakao K, Shoji Y, et al. Intraoperative colonoscopy. Surg Endosc 1993; 7(2):84–87.

Soderman C, Uribe A. Enteroscopy as a tool for diagnosing gastrointestinal bleeding requiring blood transfusion. Surg Laparosc Endosc 2001;11(2):97–102.

Stellato TA. Flexible endoscopy as an adjunct to laparoscopic surgery. Surg Clin N Am 1996;76(3):595–602.

Thorson AG, Blatchford GJ. Operative and anesthetic techniques. In: Beck DE (ed) Fundamentals of Anorectal Surgery. Philadelphia: Saunders, 1998.

Tytgat GN. Upper gastrointestinal endoscopy. In: Yamada T (ed) Textbook of Gastroenterology. Philadelphia: Lippincott, 1999.

Vamosi-Nagy I, Koves I, Szanto I, et al. Intraoperative colonoscopy. Eur J Surg Oncol 1993;19(6):615–618.

19. Choice of Laparoscopic Exposure Method

Christopher A. Jacobi, M.D., Ph.D.
C. Braumann, M.D.

A. Pneumoperitoneum with Insufflation of Gases

Influence of the Type of Gas on Cardiopulmonary and Liver Function

Presently, with few exceptions, carbon dioxide is the gas used for laparoscopic procedures in humans. CO_2 is colorless, noncombustible, odorless, and inexpensive, and, because of its high solubility, is the least dangerous gas should a gas embolism occur during a laparoscopic procedure. Interestingly, several of the major drawbacks associated with the use of CO_2 gas, namely, hypercarbia, acidosis, and other physiologic alterations [8, 27, 37], are also related to the high solubility of CO_2. Deleterious hemodynamic and pulmonary alterations have also been noted to occur in some patients [22]; these changes are related to hypercarbia and acidosis as well as to the elevated intraabdominal pressure. Because hypercarbia stimulates the sympathetic nervous system [21], insufflation of CO_2 may increase blood pressure, heart rate, and the risk of arrhythmia. Furthermore, CO_2 has also been reported to stimulate the growth of malignant tumor cells in vitro [19]. In vivo, CO_2 pneumoperitoneum also has been shown to stimulate tumor growth in a local (i.e., paraabdominal) fashion in small animal models [19, 25, 48]. To avoid the deleterious effects of CO_2, the use of alternative gases and abdominal wall lifting devices have been investigated in animal and in in vitro studies. Helium is the most commonly studied and utilized alternative gas for insufflation. Several studies that assessed helium pneumoperitoneum demonstrated that the negative pulmonary function alterations noted with CO_2 were avoided and that only minor hemodynamic changes occurred [22, 30, 43]. It has also been reported that helium does not stimulate local tumor growth in vivo in recent experimental studies [19, 25, 48]. Furthermore, helium and CO_2 have been compared in several clinical studies [11, 12, 30, 33].

Fernández-Cruz et al. assessed the efficacy of both helium and carbon dioxide pneumoperitoneum in a nonrandomized study of 22 patients with pheochromocytoma who underwent laparoscopic adrenalectomy [11]. There were no conversions to open surgery. Helium insufflation did not cause respiratory acidosis or hypercarbia and provided greater hemodynamic stability during the operation. The authors concluded that helium may be the agent of choice for abdominal insufflation in patients undergoing laparoscopic adrenalectomy for pheochromocytoma because it eliminates the adverse hemodynamic and respiratory changes associated with CO_2 insufflation. Fleming et al. used helium insufflation in 13 patients undergoing different laparoscopic procedures such as colonic resection, lymph node biopsy, or cholecystectomy [12]. A variety of cardiopulmonary parameters were measured in all patients before and after anesthetic induction and every 30 min during the operations, which were carried out via a 10 to 15 mmHg helium pneumoperitoneum. Again, minimal cardiac and pulmonary aberrations were observed; helium seemed to be safe for abdominal insufflation in laparoscopic surgery. They concluded that helium might be the agent of choice for insufflation in patients with significant cardiopulmonary diseases. Neuberger et al. analyzed cardiopulmonary parameters during carbon dioxide and then during helium insufflation in the same patients undergoing laparoscopic cholecystectomy [33]. Although they found significant changes during the period of carbon dioxide insufflation, all values returned to baseline levels under helium pneumoperitoneum. Again, the authors pointed out that carbon dioxide may be harmful in patients with cardiopulmonary disorders and that helium might be a real alternative in these cases. McMahon et al. performed a nonrandomized prospective trial comparing helium and carbon dioxide insufflation during laparoscopic cholecystectomy in 60 patients [30]. They confirmed that helium does not result in significant changes in ventilation requirements whereas carbon dioxide causes an increased ventilatory requirement due to systemic absorption of carbon dioxide.

Horvath et al. analyzed cardiopulmonary changes in pigs undergoing laparoscopic colectomy using carbon dioxide (10 mmHg), helium (10 mmHg), or a gasless procedure [16]. CO_2 pneumoperitoneum caused a significant increase in pulmonary vascular resistance (PVR) as well as hypercarbia and acidosis when compared to the other groups. The elevated intraabdominal pressure in both pneumoperitoneum groups led to a significant decrease of the urine output (UO). The abdominal wall lifting device caused only minor cardiopulmonary changes and had no metabolic and hemodynamic effects in this study. These findings were confirmed in pigs undergoing gasless laparoscopy or carbon dioxide insufflation by Chiu et al. [6]. Both authors suggested that patients with compromised pulmonary function, hemodynamic instability, or preexisting renal insufficiency might benefit from the use of helium or an abdominal wall lifting device. Rademaker et al. studied hemodynamics and gas exchange during insufflation with CO_2 or helium in pigs at different intraabdominal pressures (10, 15, and 20 mmHg) [37]. Although heart rate did not change significantly with either gas, arterial blood pressure was significantly increased with carbon dioxide but not with helium. Cardiac output, mixed venous oxygen saturation, and oxygen consumption did not change, whereas central venous filling pressures increased in both groups. Insufflation with carbon dioxide caused a mild increase of arterial, central venous, and end-expiratory CO_2. The authors suggested that pneumoperitoneum with helium will not be associated with profound circulatory depression, oxygen transport abnormalities, or acid-base disturbances in humans.

Nevertheless, helium insufflation has also been reported to have negative side effects when compared directly to carbon dioxide pneumoperitoneum. Sala-Blanch et al. investigated the effects of peritoneal insufflation with helium and carbon dioxide on hepatic blood flow in a porcine model [39]. Twelve pigs were anesthetized and mechanically ventilated with a fixed tidal volume after the stabilization period. The peritoneal cavity was insufflated with either CO_2 (n = 6) or He (n = 6) to a maximum intraabdominal pressure of 15 mmHg in these animals. Hepatic blood flow, hemodynamic parameters, gas exchange, and oxygen content were studied at baseline, 30 min, 90 min, and 150 min after pneumoperitoneum as well as 30 min after desufflation. Although a similar decrease in cardiac output was observed during insufflation with both gases, hepatic vein oxygen content significantly decreased with respect to the baseline only during helium pneumoperitoneum. Hepatic blood flow was significantly reduced in both the He and CO_2 pneumoperitoneum at 90 min following insufflation. Caution was advised in selecting helium for insufflation during laparoscopic surgery in patients with a limited hepatic reserve or preexisting hepatic dysfunction. Naude et al. investigated stress hormone changes during helium (n = 8) and carbon dioxide (n = 8) laparoscopic cholecystectomy and found significantly higher systemic epinephrine levels in patients undergoing helium insufflation [32]. No significant differences in the other parameters assessed were noted when the results of the two groups were considered.

Furthermore, because of the low solubility of helium in blood, in theory, a fatal gas embolism may occur in the setting of venous injury. Jacobi et al. investigated the cardiopulmonary effects of laceration of the inferior vena cava during laparoscopy with CO_2 or helium in pigs [17]. Twenty pigs underwent laparoscopy (insufflation pressure 15 mmHg) with either CO_2 (n = 10) or helium (n = 10) during which a standardized laceration (1 cm) of the vena cava inferior was intentionally made. After 30 seconds the vena cava was clamped, the laceration closed endoscopically via running suture, and the clamp removed. During the procedure the cardiac output (CO), heart rate (HR), mean arterial pressure (MAP), central venous pressure (CVP), pulmonary artery pressure (PAP), pulmonary artery wedge pressure (PAWP), end-tidal CO_2 pressure ($PETCO_2$), and arterial blood gas analyses (pH, PO_2, and PCO_2) were followed and assessed. MAP and CO decreased after laceration of the vena cava in both groups, with complete hemodynamic compensation noted after the laceration was clamped before the suturing. $PETCO_2$ increased significantly after CO_2 insufflation whereas no significant changes in $PETCO_2$ were noted in the helium group animals. Laceration of the vena cava caused no significant changes in $PETCO_2$ in both groups. Significant acidosis and increase in pCO_2 were only found in the CO_2 group. The authors concluded that the incidence of gas embolism during laparoscopy and accidental vessel injury seems to be very low and that, except for the acidosis and increase of $PETCO_2$ associated with CO_2 insufflation, there were no differences in cardiopulmonary function between CO_2 and helium insufflation.

An interesting study was performed by Schöb et al. who analyzed the influence of different gases (N_2O, CO_2, and helium) during laparoscopy on intracranial pressure and cardiopulmonary functions in pigs [41]. This study was conducted because diagnostic laparoscopy is often performed in trauma patients with intraabdominal injuries in whom concomitant head injury might well be present. Significantly higher intracranial pressures were noted in the CO_2 group; helium and N_2O were associated with significantly lesser increases in the intracranial pressure when compared to the CO_2 group results. As expected, the animals in the CO_2 group showed a significant increase in $PaCO_2$ and $ETCO_2$, as well as acidosis. Thus, helium and N_2O might be an alternative means of establishing pneumoperitoneum in trauma patients. Nevertheless, because N_2O supports combustion, it can only be used in laparoscopic procedures carried out in the absence of diathermy [38].

In summary, carbon dioxide is widely used for the establishment of pneumoperitoneum and the exposure of the operative field with good results. In patients with cardiopulmonary disorders, as well as trauma patients with associated head injury, helium might be an acceptable alternative gas for the establishment of the pneumoperitoneum. The results of both clinical and experimental studies support this position. Unfortunately, helium is more expensive than CO_2. A helium recycling device capable of capturing, filtering, and then reinsufflating the helium gas would be quite useful and would decrease the cost associated with helium use. N_2O cannot be recommended, in general, for the establishment of pneumoperitoneum and the exposure of the operative field because of combustion problems.

Different Gases in Laparoscopic Resections of Malignant Tumors

The most important factor influencing tumor cell spread and growth as well as immunologic suppression during laparoscopic resection of malignant tumors seems to be the surgeon himself. Thus, precise laparoscopic techniques and strict adherence to oncologic surgical principles can minimize the incidence of intra- and extraperitoneal metastases. Reports of large numbers of patients undergoing laparoscopic colon cancer resections have shown that the incidence of port site metastases is similar or even lower in comparison to conventional open resections [13, 24, 26, 46]. Furthermore, the means by which patients are selected for the laparoscopic approach certainly may influence the results and the outcome of laparoscopic cancer surgery. Because of technical limitations, resection of advanced tumors should not be attempted using laparoscopic methods. Although the surgeon probably is the most important variable in the development of port site metastases, other factors have been identified that may certainly influence tumor growth during laparoscopy.

Carbon dioxide, the gas that is most commonly used for the establishment of pneumoperitoneum, has been demonstrated to promote tumor growth and to cause the development of port site metastases. Several different experimental studies about the oncologic effects of different insufflation gases have been carried out; the results are conflicting. Jacobi et al. could demonstrate that incubation of colon cancer cells with carbon dioxide caused a significant increase in tumor cell growth in vitro and ex vivo [19]. Furthermore, these results have been confirmed in vivo in other independent studies with different tumor cell lines [4, 9, 20, 48]. Nevertheless, Neuhaus et al. found no significant difference in tumor growth after carbon dioxide insufflation in comparison to a control group [34]. These differences might be partly explained by the variety of tumor cell lines used in these studies, the varying size of the intraperitoneal tumor cell inoculations, and tumor cell biology. Helium has been investigated as an alternative gas in experimental tumor models and has been demonstrated to be associated with either inhibitory effects or no effect on tumor growth [19, 34]. Helium, therefore, might be useful for laparoscopic cancer surgery. Because of the documented detrimental cardiopulmonary effects and the tumor stimulatory impact associated with CO_2 use [17], the author believes helium should be evaluated in clinical studies.

Increased intraperitoneal pressure has also been correlated with promotion of subcutaneous and intraperitoneal tumor growth in vivo while elevated pressure during in vitro incubation of colonic cancer cells caused suppression of tumor cell growth [18]. These conflicting results might be explained by perioperative immunosuppression caused by higher intraperitoneal pressures.

In summary, helium might be useful for the establishment of the pneumoperitoneum in patients undergoing laparoscopic resection of a malignant tumor. Nevertheless, the stimulating effect of carbon dioxide, found in experimental studies, seems to be marginal in the clinical setting, as confirmed by different prospective studies evaluating laparoscopic and open resection of colonic cancer. Moreover, port site recurrences have also been found after thoracoscopy [2, 5, 7, 10, 14, 40, 47] and thoracotomy [49], where CO_2 is not used for expanding the thoracic wall during the operation. Thus, CO_2 cannot be blamed for the occurrence of port site recurrences observed in these patients.

B. Laparoscopy Using Gasless Procedures

Influence of Gasless Surgery on Cardiopulmonary Function

The first prospective randomized trial comparing gasless laparoscopy and carbon dioxide pneumoperitoneum in advanced surgical procedures, such as colonic resections, was performed by Schulze et al. [42]. Besides cardiovascular and respiratory changes, the authors also investigated the postoperative outcome and immunologic differences in the perioperative course in all patients (gasless: $n = 9$, carbon dioxide: $n = 8$). For gasless surgery, the Laparolift-System (Oregon Medical Systems, San Jose, CA, USA) was used. There were no differences in the duration of surgery or blood loss between the two groups. Central venous pressure, $PaCO_2$ inspiration pressure, and end tidal CO_2 levels were significantly higher in the carbon dioxide group whereas postoperative pain was significantly lower in this group. No other important differences were observed in hemodynamic factors, postoperative convalescence, immunocompetence, or pulmonary function. Thus, laparoscopic colonic resection utilizing a lifting approach seems to be feasible and comparable to laparoscopic resection using a carbon dioxide pneumoperitoneum. These findings were confirmed in an experimental study by Horvath et al. in pigs undergoing either laparoscopic colon resection [gasless ($n = 6$), helium ($n = 6$), carbon dioxide ($n = 6$)] or open resection [16]. No differences were found between the two laparoscopic groups concerning the time of operation, the length of the colonic specimen, or the number of lymph nodes harvested in each group. Laparoscopic treatment of hepatic hydatid disease has also been reported to be feasible using the gasless laparoscopic approach. Berberoğlu et al. compared 31 patients with hydatid disease undergoing laparoscopic surgery using carbon dioxide insufflation to 51 patients undergoing a gasless procedure in a nonrandomized trial [1]. The gasless procedure was shown to be significantly faster while other parameters did not differ between the two methods.

Several studies have been published comparing the gasless and CO_2 pneumoperitoneum exposure methods for laparoscopic cholecystectomy [23, 31, 44]. In a nonrandomized trial, Nanashima et al. assessed immunologic and cardiopulmonary parameters in 16 CO_2 pneumoperitoneum and 11 gasless cholecystectomy patients [31]. Although the length of operation was slightly longer in the gasless group, no significant differences between groups were noted for the other parameters assessed. The authors concluded that both methods of exposure are appropriate for patients with symptomatic cholelithiasis. Koivusalo et al. were able to demonstrate several significant differences in favor of the gasless method of exposure in their cholecystectomy study [23]. Hemodynamic and pulmonary function parameters were reported to be more stable and urine output was higher in the gasless group. Thus, it seems that gasless surgery might be advantageous for routine (i.e., not advanced) procedures in patients with cardiopulmonary or renal disorders.

A third cholecystectomy study yielded conflicting results. Vezakis et al. randomized 36 patients to either low-pressure (carbon dioxide, 8 mmHg) or gasless laparoscopic cholecystectomy using a subcutaneous lifting system (Laparotenser) [44]. Although the procedure was completed in all patients in the low-pressure CO_2 group, 2 patients in the gasless group had to be converted to CO_2 pneumoperitoneum to complete the case. Furthermore, the length of operation was significantly longer in the gasless group. Although there were no significant differences in overall postoperative pain and analgesic consumption, the gasless procedure was associated with shoulder pain more frequently. Despite this, the authors concluded that gasless and low-pressure laparoscopic cholecystectomy were similar with respect to postoperative pain and recovery. Nevertheless, gasless technique provided inferior exposure and the operation took significantly longer. These results suggest that the gasless method might be appropriate in high-risk patients with cardiorespiratory diseases but not for routine cases.

Several studies comparing gasless and CO_2 pneumoperitoneum exposure methods for gynecologic procedures have been carried out. Ogihara et al., in a randomized prospective study, evaluated 12 patients undergoing laparoscopic resection of ovarian tumors and found the gasless method superior to CO_2 pneumoperitoneum [36]. Gasless surgery was associated with normal acid-base balance, a less severe hormonal stress response, and a normal urine output; further, gasless patients avoided derangements of pulmonary mechanics noted in the CO_2 pneumoperitoneum patients. In a porcine study that assessed the utility of the two methods for urologic procedures, Chiu et al. reported similar results [6]. In two other animal studies, Rademaker et al. [37] and McDermott et al. [29] confirmed the advantages of gasless laparoscopy when compared to CO_2 pneumoperitoneum in regard to perioperative cardiopulmonary function. In contrast to the results of these studies, gasless laparoscopic gynecologic surgery was found to be more difficult and time consuming than laparoscopic surgery carried out under a CO_2 pneumoperitoneum in a second prospective and randomized human study.

Goldberg et al. performed a prospective study that involved 57 patients undergoing different gynecologic laparoscopic procedures [15]. Pneumoperitoneum with the use of carbon dioxide ($n = 29$) was compared to a gasless procedure ($n = 28$) using the Laparolift-System. The time to obtain exposure as well as the time of incision closure was significantly longer in the gasless group. Six of the gasless group patients had to be converted to CO_2 pneumoperitoneum because of inadequate exposure. No differences in postoperative pain, morbidity, or length of hospital stay were noted between the two groups. The authors conclude that the gasless system that they utilized was not well suited for infertility procedures and was not associated with any discernible benefits when compared to CO_2 pneumoperitoneum.

In summary, excellent exposure of the operating field can be obtained via CO_2 insufflation. In patients with significant cardiopulmonary disorders, helium may be an acceptable alternative to carbon dioxide. Gasless methods have also been used for different laparoscopic operations including advanced procedures with results comparable to those obtained using CO_2 pneumoperitoneum. Nevertheless, for the majority, the side effects of insufflation are minor and can usually be compensated for by the anesthesiologist during the operation. Reports of technical problems with various abdominal wall lifting systems demonstrate the limits of lifting methods, especially when used for advanced procedures. Thus, we believe that pneumoperitoneum is superior to gasless surgery for the majority of patients so far. Nevertheless, in the future technical innovations and increased experience with abdominal wall lifting may lead to improved gasless methods that provide better exposure.

Gasless Laparoscopy in Resections of Malignant Tumors

To avoid elevated pressure and insufflation of gases, gasless laparoscopy has been used in different tumor models [3, 4, 28, 45]. Tumor growth was significantly lower after gasless procedures than after carbon dioxide insufflation in all experimental models. However, gasless surgery in rodents can hardly be compared to the clinical situation in humans. The abdominal wall of the rat can easily be lifted without causing any tissue trauma or local ischemia of the abdominal wall and almost all operations are feasible with this technique in rodents. In humans the abdominal wall is much heavier, higher pressures are required to obtain exposure; pressure-related tissue ischemia and trauma to the abdominal wall may result. Lifting related abdominal wall injury may account for the findings of a study of laparoscopic cholecystectomy patients by Ninomiya et al. [35]. Systemic interleukin (IL)-6 levels were found to be significantly higher in the gasless surgery patients when compared to results after carbon dioxide pneumoperitoneum. The significance of this finding is uncertain; it is possible that this difference may be associated with impaired postoperative immune function, which in turn may be associated with untoward oncologic effects in cancer patients.

It has also been demonstrated that the exposure obtained with gasless systems is often inferior to that provided by pneumoperitoneum. With suboptimal exposure it may be more difficult or impossible to complete some procedures. Presently, for this and other reasons, gasless surgery has not yet found its way into daily clinical use. Perhaps the gasless methods will prove suitable for some operations restricted to the lower abdomen or pelvis, for example, certain gynecologic procedures. Tissue trauma caused by the retractor itself has also to be considered and might lead to enhanced systemic immune reaction.

In summary, gasless surgery in patients with malignant diseases is presently not advocated by most authorities for advanced procedures because of limited exposure of the operating field and technical problems relating to the lifting devices themselves. In patients with malignancies, tumor manipulation and tumor cell spillage may be more likely to occur because of these problems. Further development might lead to better systems that would then need to be critically evaluated in the clinical setting.

C. References

1. Berberoğlu M, Taner S, Dilek ON, Demir A, Sari S. Gasless vs. gaseous laparoscopy in the treatment of hepatic hydatid disease. Surg Endosc 1999;13:1195–1198.
2. Boutin C, Rey F. Thoracoscopy in pleural malignant mesothelioma: a prospective study of 188 consecutive patients. Part 1: Diagnosis. Cancer 1993;72:389–393.
3. Bouvy ND, Giuffrida MC, Tseng LN, et al. Effects of carbon dioxide pneumoperitoneum, air pneumoperitoneum, and gasless laparoscopy on body weight and tumor growth. Arch Surg 1998;133:652–656.
4. Bouvy ND, Marquet RL, Jeekel H, Bonjer HJ. Impact of gas(less) laparoscopy and laparotomy on peritoneal tumor growth and abdominal wall metastases. Ann Surg 1996;224:694–701.
5. Buhr J, Hurtgen M, Kelm C, Schemmle K. Tumor dissemination after thoracoscopic resection for lung cancer. J Thorac Cardiovasc Surg 1995;110:855–856.
6. Chiu AW, Chang LS, Birkett DH, Babayan RK. The impact of pneumoperitoneum, pneumoretroperitoneum, and gasless laparoscopy on the systemic and renal hemodynamics. J Am Coll Surg 1995;181:397–406.
7. Collard JM, Reymond MA. Video-assisted thoracic surgery (V.A.T.S.) for cancer: risk of parietal seeding and of early local recurrence. Int Surg 1996;81:343–346.
8. Davidson BS, Cromeens DM, Feig BW. Alternative methods of exposure minimize cardiopulmonary risk in experimental animals during minimally invasive surgery. Surg Endosc 1996;10:301–304.
9. Dorrance HR, Oien K, O'Dwyer PJ. Effect of laparoscopy on intraperitoneal tumor growth and distant metastases in an animal model. Surgery 1999;126:35–40.
10. Downey RJ, McCormack P, Lo Cicero J III. Dissemination of malignancies following video-assisted thoracic surgery. J Cardiovasc Surg 1996;111:954–960.
11. Fernandez-Cruz L, Sáenz A, Sabater L, Astudillo E, Fontanals J. Helium and carbon dioxide in patients with pheochromocytoma undergoing laparoscopic adrenalectomy. World J Surg 1998;22:1250–1255.

12. Fleming RYD, Dougherty TB, Feig BW. The safety of helium for abdominal insufflation. Surg Endosc 1997;11:230–234.
13. Fleshman JW, Nelson H, Peters WR, et al. Early results of laparoscopic surgery for colorectal cancer: retrospective analysis of 372 patients treated by Clinical Outcomes of Surgical Therapy (COST) study group. Dis Colon Rectum 1996;39:53–58.
14. Fry WA, Sidiqqui A, Pensler JM. Thoracoscopic implantation of cancer with a fatal outcome. Ann Thorac Surg 1995;59:42–45.
15. Goldberg JM, Maurer W. A randomized comparison of gasless laparoscopy and CO_2 pneumoperitoneum. Obstet Gynecol 1997;90:416–420.
16. Horvath KD, Whelan RL, Lier B, et al. The effects of elevated intraabdominal pressure, hypercarbia, and positioning on the hemodynamic responses to laparoscopic colectomy in pigs. Surg Endosc 1998;12:107–114.
17. Jacobi CA, Junghans T, Peter F, Naundorf D, Ordemann J, Müller JM. Gas embolism during laparoscopy with CO_2 or helium. Surg Endosc 1999;13:45–50.
18. Jacobi CA, Wenger FA, Ordemann J, Gutt CA, Sabat R, Müller JM. Experimental study of the effect of intraabdominal pressure during laparoscopy on tumour growth and port site metastasis. Br J Surg 1998;85:1419–1422.
19. Jacobi CA, Sabat R, Böhm B, Zieren HU, Volk HD, Müller JM. Pneumoperitoneum with CO_2 stimulates malignant colonic cells. Surgery 1997;121:72–78.
20. Jones DB, Guo LW, Reinhard MK, et al. Impact of pneumoperitoneum on trocar site implantation of colon cancer in hamster model. Dis Colon Rectum 1995;38: 1182–1188.
21. Joris JL, Noirot DP, Legrand MJ, Jaquet NJ, Lamy ML. Hemodynamic changes during laparoscopic cholecystectomy. Anesth Analg 1993;76:1067–1071.
22. Junghans T, Böhm B, Gründel K, Schwenk W. Effects of pneumoperitoneum with carbon dioxide, argon, or helium on hemodynamic and respiratory function. Arch Surg 1997;132:272–278.
23. Koivusalo AM, Kellokumpu I, Scheinin M, Tikkanen I, Makisalo H, Lindgren L. A comparison of gasless mechanical and conventional carbon dioxide pneumoperitoneum methods for laparoscopic cholecystectomy. Anesth Analg 1998;86:153–158.
24. Lacy AM, Delgado S, Garcia-Valdecasas JC, et al. Port site metastases and recurrence after laparoscopic colectomy. A randomized trial. Surg Endosc 1998;12:1039–1042.
25. Le Moine MC, Navarro F, Burgel JS, et al. Experimental assessment of the risk of tumor recurrence after laparoscopic surgery. Surgery 1998;123:427–431.
26. Leather AJM, Kocjan G, Savage F, et al. Detection of free malignant cells in the peritoneal cavity before and after resection of colorectal cancer. Dis Colon Rectum 1994;37:814–819.
27. Leighton TA, Liu S, Bongard FS. Comparative cardiopulmonary effects of carbon dioxide versus helium pneumoperitoneum. Surgery 1993;113:527–531.
28. Mathew G, Watson DI, Ellis T, De-Young N. The effect of laparoscopy on the movement of tumor cells and metastasis to surgical wounds. Surg Endosc 1997;11: 1163–1166.
29. McDermott JP, Regan MC, Page R, et al. Cardiorespiratory effects of laparoscopy with and without gas insufflation. Arch Surg 1995;130:984–988.

30. McMahon AJ, Baxter JN, Murray W, Imrie CW, Kenny J, O′Dwyer PJ. Helium pneumoperitoneum for laparoscopic cholecystectomy: ventilatory and blood gas changes. Br J Surg 1994;81:1033–1036.
31. Nanashima A, Yamaguchi H, Tsuji T, et al. Physiologic stress responses to laparoscopic cholecystectomy. Surg Endosc 1998;12:1381–1385.
32. Naude GP, Ryan MK, Pianim NA, Klein SR, Lippmann M, Bongard FS. Comparative stress hormone changes during helium versus carbon dioxide laparoscopic cholecystectomy. J Laparoendosc Surg 1996;6:93–98.
33. Neuberger TJ, Andrus CH, Wittgen CM, Wade TP, Kaminski DL. Prospective comparison of helium versus carbon dioxide pneumoperitoneum. Gastrointest Endosc 1996;43:38–41.
34. Neuhaus SJ, Watson DI, Ellis T. Wound metastasis after laparoscopy with different insufflation gases. Surgery 1998;123:579–583.
35. Ninomiya K, Kitano S, Yoshida T, Bandoh T, Baatar D, Matsumoto T. Comparison of pneumoperitoneum and abdominal wall lifting as to hemodynamics and surgical stress response during laparoscopic cholecystectomy. Surg Endosc 1998;12:124–128.
36. Ogihara Y, Isshiki A, Kindscher JD, Goto H. Abdominal wall lift versus carbon dioxide insufflation for laparoscopic resection of ovarian tumors. J Clin Anesth 1999;11: 406–412.
37. Rademaker BM, Bannenberg JJ, Kalkmann CJ, Meyer DW. Effects of pneumoperitoneum with helium on hemodynamics and oxygen transport: a comparison with carbon dioxide. J Laparoendosc Surg 1995;5:15–20.
38. Robinson JS, Thomson JM, Wood AW. Laparoscopy explosion hazards with nitrous oxide. Br Med J 1995;iii:764–765.
39. Sala-Blanch X, Fontanals J, Martínez-Palli G, et al. Effects of carbon dioxide vs helium pneumoperitoneum on hepatic blood flow. Surg Endosc 1998;12:1121–1125.
40. Sartorelli KH, Partrick D, Meagher DP Jr. Port-site recurrence after thoracoscopic resection of pulmonary metastasis owing to osteogenic sarcoma. J Pediatr Surg 1996; 31:1443–1444.
41. Schöb OM, Allen DC, Benzel E, et al. A comparison of the pathophysiologic effects of carbon dioxide, nitrous oxide, and helium pneumoperitoneum on intracranial pressure. Am J Surg 1996;172:248–253.
42. Schulze S, Lyng KM, Bugge K, et al. Cardiovascular and respiratory changes and convalescence in laparoscopic colonic surgery. Arch Surg 1999;134:1112–1118.
43. Shuto K, Kitano S, Yoshido T, Bandoh T, Mitarai Y, Kobayashi M. Hemodynamic and arterial blood gas changes during carbon dioxide and helium pneumoperitoneum in pigs. Surg Endosc 1995;9:1173–1178.
44. Vezakis A, Davides D, Gibson JS, et al. Randomized comparison between low-pressure laparoscopic cholecystectomy and gasless laparoscopic cholecystectomy. Surg Endosc 1999;13:890–893.
45. Watson DI, Mathew G, Ellis T. Gasless laparoscopy may reduce the risk of port-site metastases following laparoscopic tumor surgery. Arch Surg 1997;132:166–168.
46. Wexner SD, Latulippe J-F. Laparoscopic colorectal surgery and cancer. Swiss Surg 1997;3:266–273.

47. Wille GA, Gregory R, Guernsey JM. Tumor implantation at port-site of video-assisted thoracoscopic resection of pulmonary metastasis. West J Med 1997;166:65–66.
48. Wu JS, Brasfield EB, Guo LW, et al. Implantation of colon cancer at trocar sites is increased by low pressure pneumoperitoneum. Surgery 1997;122:1–7.
49. Yokoi K, Miyazawa N, Imura G. Isolated incisional recurrence after curative resection for primary lung cancer. Ann Thorac Surg 1996;61:1236–1237.

20. Anchoring Laparoscopic Ports

John I. Lew, M.D.
Richard L. Whelan, M.D.

A. Introduction

The majority of laparoscopic ports are not threaded and are of uniform diameter. Unanchored, they are held in place by the abdominal wall, which surrounds or grips the port and provides resistance to outward forces applied to the port. These ports tend to stay in place for short procedures that are carried out in one abdominal quadrant. However, during lengthy procedures that require working in several quadrants, the abdominal wall's hold on the port may weaken and the port may be dislodged altogether, usually at the time of instrument removal. How is the abdominal wall's grip on the port weakened? During any laparoscopic procedure, varying amounts of torque are applied to each port to accomplish the task at hand. Depending on the degree and direction of the torque and the number of times the port is torqued, the port wound at the peritoneal level may enlarge. The fascial wound may also be stretched and enlarged. Each time an instrument is withdrawn from a port, an outward force is applied to the port. When the abdominal wall's grip on the port is sufficiently weak, the port is likely to dislodge. If the port inadvertently comes out of the abdomen, the procedure is disrupted and the pneumoperitoneum is lost. Further, replacing the port back into the abdomen can be difficult and may further enlarge the port wound, which will increase the chances of the port being dislodged again. In the setting of cancer, in theory, the rapid desufflation that occurs when a port is dislodged may serve to transport tumor-laden fluid droplets to the abdominal wound, which may put the patient at risk for a port wound tumor recurrence.

Anchoring ports to the abdominal wall, therefore, is advised for advanced procedures, especially those that require working in multiple quadrants. Well-secured ports will facilitate the timely completion of the case at hand. There are numerous methods of anchoring laparoscopic ports. Some involve modification of the port itself (addition of spiral threads) or of the method of port placement (i.e., bladed trocar versus dilating method) while other methods require the use of a separate device, usually cone shaped, through which the port is placed before insertion. Last, skin sutures can be used to create a tether that will prevent dislodgement. What follows is a brief explanation of these methods.

B. Port Anchoring Methods

1. **Hassan-type devices:** Cone-shaped obturator through which the port is passed before port placement. The original Hassan device was not threaded although threaded versions have since been developed. The original Hassan devices were reusable; there are now several disposable versions. The Hassan is used when the first port is placed via open cutdown. These wounds are usually a bit larger than the port to be placed; the cone-shaped Hassan essentially plugs the wound and prevents loss of gas around the port. The Hassan device is held in place by a fascial suture(s) that is placed at the time of the cutdown and subsequently pulled tight and wrapped around two flanges that extend out from the most external surface of the device.

2. Several companies make threaded disposable **cone-shaped anchoring devices** that are designed for use with ports placed via bladed trocars. The device grips the port tightly once the port has been passed through it. Once the port has been successfully inserted into the abdomen, the trocar is removed and the port is advanced until the innermost edge of the threaded port grip engages the wound edge. Next, the port and the anchor are together screwed into the abdominal wall until at least the first thread of the anchoring device can be seen inside the abdomen via the laparoscope. To loosen the grip of the device on the port, either to push the port further into the abdomen or to withdraw it, the surgeon must pinch together two spring-loaded plastic flanges that extend from the externalmost part of the device. When pinched together, it is possible to slide the port within the sheath. Once the desired position has been obtained, the flanges are released, after which they return to their original position and the port is once again firmly held within the anchor.

3. **Skin suture tether (alone):** A tether can be created with a skin suture that will prevent the port from coming out beyond a certain point. First, the suture is placed through the skin and then tied down loosely just above the skin level. If the port fits snugly in the skin wound then this suture is placed adjacent to the port site. If the port skin incision is too large, the suture can be placed so as to partially close the port wound when tied down; this will serve to limit port slippage and to prevent or minimize the leakage of gas around the port. After the skin suture is placed and tied, several "air knots" are thrown such that a tether of the appropriate length is created. After additional knots are placed at that level, one end of the suture is wrapped around the insufflation arm that extends outward from the port and then is either tied or clamped to the other end of the suture. Ideally, the tether should be long enough so as to permit the port to be withdrawn to within a centimeter or so of the parietal peritoneum. The tether will not prevent the port from moving further into the abdomen. This type of tether should prevent port dislodgement but it does not secure the port in a single position; the port can freely move back and forth for a certain distance.

4. **Skin suture in conjunction with other port-anchoring device:** The addition of a skin suture tether when using other anchoring systems ensures that the port will not become dislodged should the primary anchor fail. Some surgeons believe that this precaution is warranted for cancer cases and in patients with thin abdominal walls and poor tissue integrity. A skin suture is placed close

to the port base and tied loosely at the skin level. One end of the suture is next wrapped several times around the insufflation arm and then pulled down toward the abdominal surface. The other end of the suture is pulled upward, after which the two strands are clamped together. Should the primary anchor fail, this suture will prevent the port from coming out. To reposition the port further in or out of the abdomen, the suture tether must be first released. When the desired position is attained, the suture tether is again wrapped around the insufflation arm and secured with a clamp as described above.

5. **Full-thickness abdominal wall tether:** This type of suture is utilized when trying to limit the expansion of the abdominal wall in the setting of subcutaneous emphysema, usually during a lengthy case. This must be done in conjunction with another anchoring device (for example, a threaded port or a threaded port grip). A large-diameter (#1 or #2) monofilament suture is passed into the abdominal cavity under direct visualization via a retention suture-type needle that has been straightened. Once in the abdomen, the needle is grasped with a laparoscopic instrument and then pulled fully into the abdomen. Next, the needle is carefully turned around and then passed back out of the abdomen close to the port in question. One end of the suture is then wrapped several times around the insufflation arm of the port and then pulled down toward the abdominal surface while the other end is pulled toward the ceiling. The two strands are then clamped together. The primary anchor prevents the port from sliding into the abdomen. The transabdominal wall suture compresses the abdominal wall. This type of suture will also prevent port dislodgement, although it is not primarily used for this purpose.

6. The self-anchoring reusable **Endoscopic Threaded Imaging Port (Endotip)** was developed to prevent the injuries that bladed trocars may incur. The Endotip port uses the principle of Archimedes to lift the abdominal wall tissues along an inclined spiral on the external surface of the port cannula after engaging the most superficial layer with a blunt notched tip. This trocar-less device is literally "screwed" into the abdomen; the blunt tip and the rounded edges of the spiral threads deflect rather than lacerate the vessels and surrounding tissues within the abdominal wall. The external threads also serve to hold the port in place under most circumstances, even during lengthy procedures. Some surgeons use a skin suture anchor, described above, in conjunction with the ENDOTIP port as insurance against the rare port dislodgement event that may otherwise occur. The port position can be altered by screwing the port either inward or outward. The laparoscope can be placed inside the Endotip port before screwing in the initial port after the abdomen has been insufflated via a Veress needle. The scope in the port permits the surgeon to observe the progress of the port as it is advanced into and through the abdominal wall. Secondary ports are inserted under direct laparoscopic vision using the primary port. These reusable cannulas have also been found to be equally safe and effective for use in the bariatric population. At the end of the procedure, the secondary ports are removed under direct laparoscopic vision by rotating them in a counterclockwise direction. For the remaining camera port, the laparoscope is retracted 2 cm into the port cannula and locked into position. The laparoscope is held perpendicular to the patient's abdomen while the port cannula is rotated counterclockwise with the surgeon's dominant hand. This permits visualization of the port wound as the port is removed.

7. **VersaStep-type port:** This bladeless trocar system makes use of an expandable sheath that is passed through the abdominal wall over a Veress-type needle after the abdomen has been insufflated. The synthetic sheath has diamond-shaped skeletal elements embedded in it that serve to neutralize and convert axial force to a purely radial vector. Once the sheath is in position, the needle is removed, after which a blunt obturator, which carries the port, is inserted into the expandable sheath. As the cone-shaped blunt obturator is pushed into the abdomen, the sheath's position is secured with the surgeon's nondominant hand. The wound is dilated by the obturator such that it will accept the port. The port and obturator must be passed far enough into the abdomen such that the port tip extends beyond the inner edge of the expandable sheath. Once in position, the obturator is removed. This device is self-anchoring, and deflects rather than lacerates abdominal wall vessels and structures. When the port and the sheath are removed at the end of the case, a relatively small wound remains because the stretched but uncut abdominal wall tissues return to their original position.

C. Discussion

It is recommended that some type of port anchor be used for advanced laparoscopic cases. Each of the methods described above should suffice; however, each has its benefits and drawbacks. There has been a general trend away from bladed trocars in recent years to avoid sharp trocar-related injuries and to minimize the abdominal wall trauma. Port systems that make use of threaded trocar-less ports as well as those that utilize blunt dilatation are more attractive. After removal of such devices, the remaining defects are reported to be one-half the size of wounds left behind by conventional trocars and therefore are not routinely closed. Although there are studies reporting no cases of port site hernia formation after use of such devices, closure of all fascial defects greater than 10 mm is recommended. Although most hernias are associated with 10-mm ports or larger, there have been many reports of port site hernias occurring through 5-mm ports as well. The reported incidence of port site hernias in the general population after minimal access surgery is approximately 0.2%–3%; however, the true incidence may be actually higher.

Regardless of the anchoring method used, given a long enough case or an abdominal wall with poor integrity, the anchor may fail. In such cases, the surgeon should not hesitate to utilize a suture tether in conjunction with another primary anchor.

D. Selected References

Bhoyrul S, Morui T, Way W. Radially expanding dilatation. A superior method of laparoscopic trocar access. Surg Endosc 1996;10:775–778.

Patterson M, Alters D, Browder W. Postoperative bowel obstruction following laparoscopic surgery. Am Surg 1993;59:656–657.

Plaus WJ. Laparoscopic trocar site hernias. J Laparoendosc Surg 1993;3(6):567–570.

Reardon PR, Preciado A, Scarborough T, et al. Hernia at 5-mm laparoscopic port site presenting as early postoperative small bowel obstruction. J Laparoendosc Adv Surg Tech A 1999;9(6):523–525.

Romagnolo C, Minelli L. Small-bowel occlusion after operative laparoscopy: our experience and review of the literature. Endoscopy 2001;33(1):88–90.

Ternamian AM, Deitel M. Endoscopic threaded imaging port (ENDOTIP) for laparosopy: experience with different body weights. Obes Surg 1999;9(1):44–7.

21. Trocar- and Port-Related Bleeding

Daniel J. Deziel, M.D.

A. Clinical Significance

Some abdominal wall bleeding from trocar or port sites is common during laparoscopic operations. This type of bleeding, while irritating to the surgeon, is usually not a serious problem. However, bleeding from the abdominal wall is a significant complication for 1%–2% of patients undergoing therapeutic laparoscopic procedures in general surgery. In addition, port site hemorrhage accounts for 10%–15% of intraoperative bleeding complications and for more than one-half of postoperative bleeding events. The clinical consequences range in severity from local hematoma formation, obliteration of the operative field, or prolongation of the operation to life-threatening hemorrhage requiring blood replacement and reoperation. In general, bleeding is one of the most frequent complications of laparoscopic surgery and is potentially fatal when a great vessel is involved. Port site hemorrhage is also potentially one of the most preventable complications. Its occurrence can be minimized by recognition of abdominal wall anatomy and patient-specific risk factors and by attention to appropriate technical details during port placement. Adverse consequences of abdominal wall bleeding can be muted by timely recognition and control.

B. Relevant Anatomy

1. **Anatomy of abdominal wall blood vessels**. The vasculature of the anterior and anterolateral abdominal wall consists of superficial subcutaneous vessels, deep subfascial vessels, and vessels to the muscles (Figures 21.1, 21.2).
   a. Superficial vessels
      i. Above the umbilicus, the skin and subcutaneous tissue are supplied by arterial branches from various sources including the superior epigastric artery, musculophrenic artery, and lower intercostal arteries. These anastomosing branches perforate the abdominal wall muscles to reach the subcutaneous tissue. The corresponding superficial veins drain to the superior vena cava via the internal mammary, long thoracic and intercostal veins, and their branches.
      ii. Below the umbilicus, the superficial abdominal wall is supplied by three branches of the femoral artery: superficial epigastric artery (anterior), the superficial circumflex iliac

artery (lateral), and the superficial external pudendal artery (medial groin). The corresponding veins drain to the femoral vein at the saphenous opening and thus to the inferior vena cava.

iii. The superficial veins from the supra- and infraumbilical regions communicate with each other through the thoracoepigastric vein, which ascends from the groin toward the axilla. This vein may be particularly prominent when there is obstruction of the inferior vena cava. The superficial systemic veins of the abdominal wall also communicate indirectly with the portal venous system via the paraumbilical veins and the umbilical vein in the falciform ligament. In cases of portal hypertension, the superficial veins near the umbilicus may become varicose in appearance ("caput medusae").

b. Deep vessels

i. The rectus abdominis muscle receives its blood supply from the superior and inferior epigastric arteries. The superior epigastric artery originates from the internal mammary artery and courses through the costoxiphoid opening at the diaphragm to the posterior surface of the rectus muscle. The inferior epigastric artery branches from the external iliac artery just above the inguinal ligament. It ascends obliquely and medially toward the umbilicus, pierces the transversalis

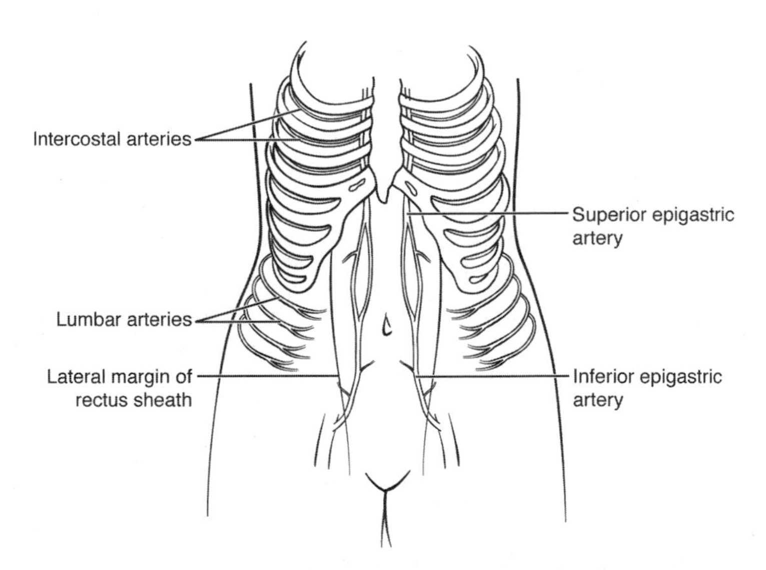

Figure 21.1. Segmental innervations (left) and arterial supply (right) to the abdominal wall.

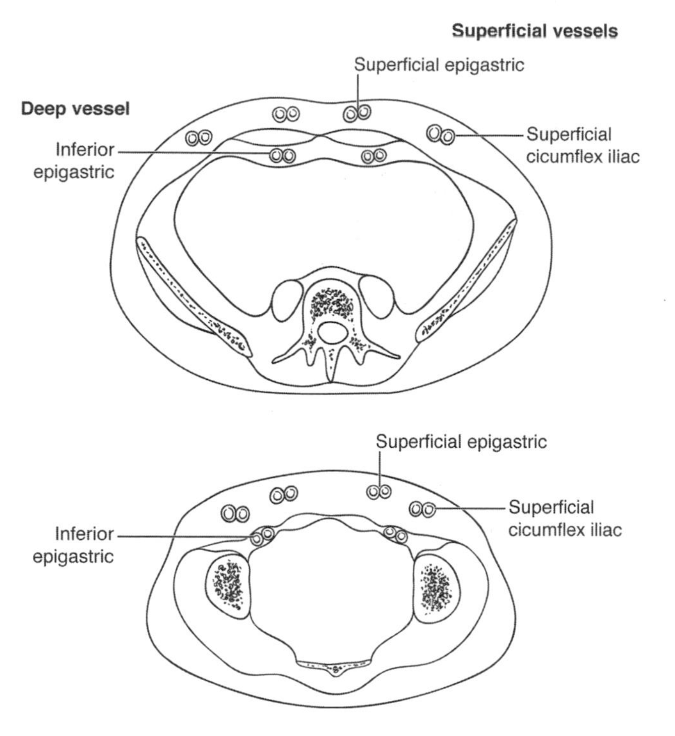

Figure 21.2. Axial view of anterior abdominal wall at (A) 1 cm below umbilicus and (B) 3 cm above symphysis pubis. Soft tissue layers indicated by gray; bone indicated by patterned areas. Vessel locations shown as mean ± SD. Vessel locations without SDs are extrapolated locations.

fascia, and enters the rectus sheath anterior to the arcuate line (the linea semicircularis or semilunar fold of Douglas). The superior and inferior epigastric vessels anastomose with each other at about the umbilical level.

ii. The lower lateral abdominal wall is supplied by the deep circumflex iliac artery, which arises from the external iliac artery lateral to the inferior epigastric artery. It is situated laterally in the iliac fossa between the transversus abdominis and internal oblique muscles. Near the anterosuperior iliac spine, the deep circumflex artery gives off a large ascending branch that can be injured by trocars placed in the low flank. The deep circumflex artery anastomoses with the lumbar and inferior epigastric arteries.

iii. The lateral abdominal wall and flank are supplied by the last six posterior intercostal arteries (from the descending thoracic aorta) and by the four lumbar arteries (from the abdominal aorta). These vessels course between the transversus abdominis and internal oblique muscles. Their branches enter the lateral aspect of the rectus sheath and anastomose with the superior and inferior epigastrics.

C. Surgical Implications of the Vascular Anatomy

The varied and plentiful blood supply of the truncal wall obviously puts many vessels at risk during placement of laparoscopic trocars in the abdomen or flank. The superficial epigastric and circumflex iliac vessels and the deeper inferior and superior epigastrics are probably the most frequently injured. Transillumination of the abdominal wall may identify the superficial vessels in nonobese patients. However, transillumination does not visualize the deeper vessels in the muscular compartments. In the inguinal region, the inferior epigastric vessels can be seen laparoscopically just superficial to the parietal peritoneum and lateral to the medial umbilical ligament (which contains the remnant of the umbilical artery). They are not generally visible at the level of the umbilicus, and they otherwise have no reliable laparoscopic landmarks. The location of the superficial epigastric vessels only roughly correlates with the location of the inferior epigastric vessels. Both occupy a more lateral position in the suprapubic region and become more medial as they rise toward the umbilicus. In overweight individuals, the inferior epigastric artery tends to be slightly more lateral. The lateral border of the rectus abdominis muscle is the least likely area to contain major vessels. Based on the sparse normative data available, it has been recommended that lateral trocars be placed at least 5 cm above the symphysis pubis and approximately 8 cm from the midline (rectus margins) to avoid vessel injury (Figure 21.3).

D. Risk Factors for Trocar- and Port-Related Bleeding

Prevention of trocar and port site bleeding is founded on recognition of risk factors and implementation of measures to reduce risk. A thorough history and physical may reveal conditions or findings that may increase the chances of a port wound bleeding event. Examples of patient-related risk factors follow:

1. Patients with coagulation disorders or thrombocytopenia.
2. Patients with liver disease or portal hypertension.
3. Conditions that alter the configuration of the abdominal wall such as distension, masses, or organomegaly, surgical incisions, or obesity may be associated with variations in the location of abdominal wall vessels.

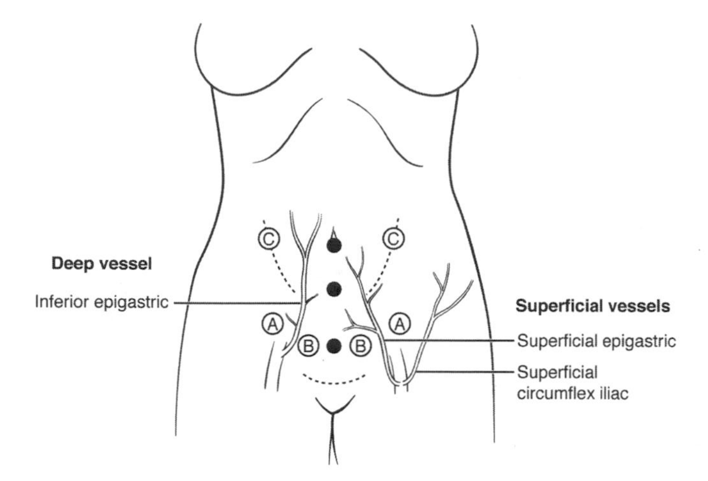

Figure 21.3. Location of deep and superficial vessels of anterior abdominal wall, frontal view. Black vessels with gray shadows indicate mean ± SD for data from computed tomographic scans; vessels without SDs are extrapolated. Dashed lines, relative location of rectus abdominis muscle lateral margin and symphysis pubis; solid circles, standard sites for midline laparoscopic trocar placement; lettered circles, recommended locations for lateral trocar placement: A, ideal location for lateral trocars 5 cm above symphysis, 8 cm from midline; B, alternate location for lateral trocars 3 cm above symphysis, 4 cm from midline; C, location for trocars near level of umbilicus, 8 cm from midline.

E. Trocar Design and Selection of Port Location

1. Trocar design. The type of trocar and port that is utilized impacts on the risk of abdominal wall bleeding.
   a. Larger-diameter trocars cause more injury than smaller trocars, particularly at nonmidline insertion sites. Trocars with a cutting tip are more likely to cause bleeding than are conically tipped, blunt, or radially expanding trocars. Similarly, trocar-less ports that are screwed into and through the abdominal wall via a skin incision are less likely to injure an abdominal wall vessel because these ports push tissue aside and do not actually cut tissue. These are threaded metal reusable ports with an oblique blunt extension from the tip that advances the port through the abdominal wall by applying downward pressure while screwing it into the wall.
   b. Conventional pyramidally tipped nondisposable trocars and cruciate-tipped disposable trocars lacerate tissue as they advance whereas blunt and trocar-less designs split and separate tissue less traumatically.

2. Trocar site. Trocar sites should be selected so as to best avoid major abdominal wall vessels (see preceding section on Anatomy of abdominal wall blood vessels).
   a. Midline sites have a lower risk of bleeding than do more lateral locations.
   b. Transillumination may facilitate identification of superficial vessels in thinner patients.
   c. Nonmidline trocars should be placed lateral to the rectus abdominis muscle, where possible.
   d. In the upper abdomen, the falciform ligament should be avoided.
   e. Secondary ports should be inserted under direct vision.
   f. When the initial port is at a nonmidline position, placement by a direct "cut-down" technique (Hasson) may minimize vessel injury.
   g. In patients at high risk for port wound bleeding and when the situation demands placement of a 10-mm port (or larger) in a high-risk location, it is safest to place the port via the direct cut-down method.

F. Management of Port Site Bleeding

1. **Identification**
   a. Intraoperative bleeding. Port site bleeding is usually manifested intraoperatively by a fairly continuous dripping of blood from around the cannula or as a collection of blood and clot on the surface of the omentum or viscera under the port site. It may also present as external bleeding on the skin surface or as a developing abdominal wall hematoma. It is critical for the surgeon to carefully inspect each port site for bleeding after placement of the port and upon completion of the operation. While this may seem elementary, prospective data demonstrate that the majority (nearly 80%) of abdominal wall bleeding complications are not detected intraoperatively. Because the port itself may tamponade bleeding, each port wound should be observed laparoscopically and externally after the sheath has been removed. Holding a finger *lightly* over the skin as a seal will prevent escape of pneumoperitoneum without tamponading any bleeding vessels. Because the site of the last port removed cannot be viewed laparoscopically, this should be a midline port or one that was initially placed by cut-down under direct visualization.
   b. Postoperative bleeding. A local abdominal wall or port site hematoma is the most often noted sign of abdominal wall bleeding following a laparoscopic operation. Direct bleeding from the port incision may also be noted. Rarely, an abdominal wall or flank ecchymosis may develop if bleeding has been persistent and the blood has tracked along tissue planes. The potentially most dangerous presentation of postoperative port wound bleeding is intraperitoneal hemorrhage. In this circumstance, the patient may

develop abdominal distension and the typical features of hemorrhagic shock (tachycardia, oliguria, cold extremities, hypotension). Obviously, the potential for high-volume blood loss is greater when bleeding into the peritoneal cavity as opposed to bleeding into the abdominal wall itself.

2. **Control of intraoperative bleeding.** Most instances of port site bleeding that are recognized intraoperatively require specific treatment to stop or control the bleeding. A number of techniques may be applicable depending upon the site and extent of the bleeding as well as the size of the patient.
   a. **Compression techniques for intraoperative bleeding**. When bleeding is not severe, several minutes of simple direct pressure or compression may provide adequate hemostasis.
      i. Sharply angling or torquing the port applies direct pressure to one aspect of the abdominal wall adjacent to the wound. While viewing the bleeding port site via the laparoscope, the port is alternately torqued in different directions to determine where the pressure should be applied to stop the bleeding (Figure 21.4). Once the bleeding site is localized, torque pressure should be maintained for several minutes. External pressure can be added by pressing down on the abdominal wall with one or several fingers directly over the site. In this way, the bleeding site is compressed from opposing directions.
      ii. The abdominal wall can also be compressed manually by inserting the second finger into the empty port wound and then applying upward pressure against the opposing thumb, which is pushing downward on the abdominal wall.
      iii. Additional pressure can also be brought to bear on the site by sharply torquing an adjacent port (either alone or with an instrument inserted).
      iv. Alternatively, the wound can be packed with gauze. Another option is to insert a Foley catheter (preferably with a 30-mL balloon) into the abdomen through the wound, inflate it, and then apply direct pressure to the port area by pulling upward on the Foley for several minutes.
   b. **Coagulation methods.** Electrocoagulation can be applied either transcutaneously or transperitoneally with laparoscopic instruments. Ultrasonic instruments, bipolar devices, and other coagulation methods can be similarly used for this purpose. This approach may be effective when the bleeding point is near the skin or peritoneal surface but is not likely to be successful when the source is located more deeply.
   c. **Suture control of bleeding vessels.** Suture ligature is the surest method of hemostasis. Sutures should be used whenever the bleeding is brisk or when injury to a larger artery is suspected or when other methods fail.
      i. Bleeding from larger abdominal wall arteries is probably best managed by extending the incision at the port site to expose the vessel and control it by direct suture ligature.

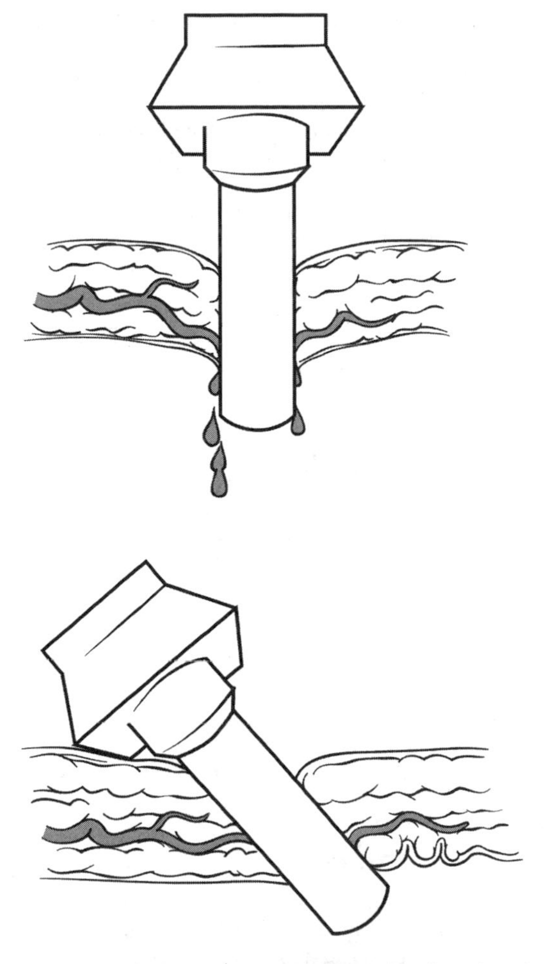

Figure 21.4. (A) Bleeding from a trocar site. (B) Cantilevering the sheath into each quadrant to find a position that causes the bleeding to stop. When the proper quadrant is found, pressure from the portion of the sheath within the abdomen tamponades the bleeding vessel, thus stopping the bleeding. A stitch can then be passed under laparoscopic guidance.

ii. An alternate method that does not require extending the port incision involves the placement of full-thickness abdominal wall horizontal mattress sutures on either side of the bleeding port along the axis of the bleeding vessel. Number one nylon sutures on long curved needles (for placement of retention sutures) are best suited for this purpose. The needle is straightened out before inserting it through the abdominal wall into the abdomen. The needle is then grasped via a laparoscopic needle holder or other grasper and pulled fully into the abdomen. The needle is turned around under direct visualization and then pushed back out through the abdominal wall. These sutures are best tied over a bolster (usually one or several folded-up gauzes) for effective tamponade.

iii. A suture passer can be used to place a suture through the port skin incision (with the port in place) such that the bleeding vessel is encircled. A second suture, placed on the opposite side of the bleeding point, is often needed. These sutures are tied down separately after the port has been removed. The port can then be carefully replaced.

iv. Other local techniques. Packing the trocar tract with hemostatic agents such as gelfoam soaked in thrombin is often effective, particularly when combined with mechanical compression. Injection of epinephrine solution around the port site has also been suggested but is not recommended because it may only provide temporary hemostasis.

3. **Postoperative port wound bleeding.** Local hematomas that develop postoperatively are usually self-limited and can usually be managed conservatively. The rare flank or abdominal wall ecchymoses that result from port wound bleeding are also usually self-limited; however, on occasion, transfusion may be required. Approximately 10% of patients with postoperative abdominal wall bleeding require operative intervention. Most of these patients have had a significant drop in hematocrit and usually have received transfusions. Unless there is an obviously bleeding port site, laparotomy will often be necessary to rule out an intraperitoneal source of hemorrhage in these patients.

G. Selected References

Bhoyrul S, Mori T, Way LW. Radially expanding dilatation: a superior method of laparoscopic trocar access. Surg Endosc 1996;10:775–778.

Deziel DJ, Millikan KW, Economou SG, Doolas A, Ko ST, Airan MC. Complications of laparoscopic cholectectomy: a national survey of 4,292 hospitals and an analysis of 77,604 cases. Am J Surg 1993;165:9–14.

Hurd WW, Bude RO, DeLancey JOL, Newman JS. The location of abdominal wall blood vessels in relationship to abdominal landmarks apparent at laparoscopy. Am J Obstet Gynecol 1994;171:642–646.

Hurd WW, Wang L, Schemmel MT. A comparison of the relative risks of vessel injury with conical versus pyramidal laparoscopic trocars in a rabbit model. Am J Obstet Gynecol 1995;173:1731–1733.

Schäfer M, Lauper M, Krähenbühl L. A nation's experience of bleeding complications during laparoscopy. Am J Surg 2000;80:73–77.

22. Prophylaxis Against Deep Venous Thrombosis

James H. Holmes IV, M.D.
Thomas R. Biehl, M.D.

A. Incidence of Deep Vein Thrombosis

1. Up to 40% of major operations performed by laparotomy are complicated by postoperative deep vein thrombosis (DVT) if no method of prophylaxis is utilized, as determined by screening with the labeled fibrinogen uptake test (FUT). The majority of DVTs are asymptomatic, and the reported incidence of DVT would be less if duplex ultrasound or symptoms were used as the screening modality, given their lower sensitivities relative to FUT.
2. The true incidence of DVT following laparoscopic operations is difficult to determine for a number of reasons:
   a. Clinically evident DVT is an uncommon complication following laparoscopic procedures.
   b. DVT typically presents in a delayed fashion, and symptoms may be disregarded by patients following discharge from the hospital.
   c. No systematic surveillance of venous thromboembolic complications has been carried out and reported in any large laparoscopic series.
   d. The use of DVT prophylaxis has been inconsistently reported.
   e. FUT may lead to infectious complications and, thus, is no longer clinically acceptable as a screening modality for DVT.
   f. The demographics of patients undergoing laparoscopic operations are constantly changing.
3. The reported incidence of DVT following laparoscopic cholecystectomy is approximately 0.03%–0.4%. However, this figure should be viewed as a minimum value given the aforementioned difficulties with establishing an accurate incidence.
4. The true incidence of DVT following other laparoscopic operations is unknown. Minimum estimates may be inferred from the reported incidences of pulmonary embolism listed below.

B. Incidence of Pulmonary Embolism

1. Clinically evident pulmonary embolism (PE) is a complication in ~2% of major open operations when no method of DVT prophylaxis is employed.
2. The true rate of PE following laparoscopic procedures is unknown for reasons similar to those mentioned in the DVT section above.
3. The reported incidences of PE after laparoscopic procedures are as follows:
   a. Cholecystectomy: ~0.02%–0.4%
   b. Antireflux procedures: ~1.8%
   c. Colorectal operations: ~0.7%

C. Risk Factors for DVT/PE

1. Virchow's triad:
   a. Venous stasis
   b. Endothelial injury
   c. Hypercoagulability
2. Surgical risk factors:
   a. Abdominopelvic or lower extremity operations
   b. Operative time >1 hour
   c. General anesthesia
   d. Reverse Trendelenburg position
3. Patient risk factors:
   a. Age >40 years
   b. Prolonged immobility/paralysis
   c. Prior venous thromboembolic event
   d. Malignancy
   e. Obesity
   f. Varicose veins
   g. Congestive heart failure
   h. Myocardial infarction
   i. Inflammatory bowel disease
   j. Nephrotic syndrome
   k. Estrogen use
   l. Hypercoagulable states
4. Most surgical patients have at least two of the risk factors listed above.
5. Laparoscopy-related risk factors:
   a. The reverse Trendelenburg position causes decreased common femoral vein (CFV) flow velocity and increased CFV diameter, promoting venous stasis and potential endothelial injury.
   b. Pneumoperitoneum has been consistently shown to decrease CFV flow velocity and pulsatility while increasing CFV pressure and diameter; these changes promote venous stasis.

D. DVT Prophylaxis for Open, Major Operations

1. Prophylaxis decreases the incidence of DVT by more than 50%. Following is a list of the methods used for prophylaxis for open operations and the incidence of DVT associated with each method.
   a. Low-dose unfractionated heparin (LDUH), usual dose 5000 units via subcutaneous injection q 12 hours: ~8%
   b. Low molecular weight heparin (LMWH): ~7%
   c. Sequential compression devices (SCD)/intermittent pneumatic compression (IPC): ~10%
   d. Graded compression elastic stockings (ES): ~9%
   e. Combining pharmacologic and mechanical modalities of prophylaxis may have additive effects.
2. Prophylaxis with LDUH lowers the rate of *fatal* PE by approximately 50% following open operations for malignant disease.
3. There are few complications of DVT prophylaxis. Low-dose heparin is associated with minor bleeding but no significant increased risk of major hemorrhage. LDUH carries a 3% risk of heparin-induced thrombocytopenia. Mechanical prophylaxis has not been associated with complications.

E. DVT Prophylaxis for Laparoscopic Operations

1. There are no prospective, randomized, clinical trials evaluating DVT prophylaxis for laparoscopic operations.
2. Multiple prospective, randomized studies have analyzed the effect of mechanical DVT prophylaxis modalities on lower extremity venous hemodynamics as a surrogate marker for venous thromboembolism. From the available data, the following may be concluded:
   a. SCD/IPC of any style, either with or without ES, effectively overcomes the lower extremity venous stasis induced by the pneumoperitoneum and reverse Trendelenburg position.
   b. There are conflicting reports regarding the efficacy of ES alone in overcoming lower extremity venous stasis.
3. Recommendations:
   a. Based on the aforementioned data and established recommendations for open operations, all patients undergoing laparoscopic operations should receive DVT prophylaxis in the form of SCD/IPC with or without ES until further data are available.
   b. The substitution/addition of pharmacologic DVT prophylaxis should be at the discretion of the operating surgeon based upon established recommendations and risk assessment for the particular operation to be performed (open data).

F. Selected References

Beebe DS, McNevin MP, Crain JM, et al. Evidence of venous stasis after abdominal insufflation for laparoscopic cholecystectomy. Surg Gynecol Obstet 1993;176:443–447.

Clagett GP, Anderson FA, Geerts W, et al. Prevention of venous thromboembolism. Chest 1998;114:531S–560S.

Ido K, Suzuki T, Kimura K, et al. Lower extremity venous stasis during laparoscopic cholecystectomy as assessed using color Doppler ultrasound. Surg Endosc 1995;9: 310–313.

Jorgensen JO, Lalak NJ, North L, et al. Venous stasis during laparoscopic cholecystectomy. Surg Laparosc Endosc 1994;4:128–133.

Lindberg F, Bergqvist D, Rasmussen I. Incidence of thromboembolic complications after laparoscopic cholecystectomy: review of the literature. Surg Laparosc Endosc 1997;7:324–331.

Millard JA, Hill BB, Cook PS, et al. Intermittent sequential pneumatic compression in prevention of venous stasis associated with pneumoperitoneum during laparoscopic cholecystectomy. Arch Surg 1993;128:914–919.

Moneta GL, Bedford G, Beach K, et al. Duplex ultrasound assessment of venous diameters, peak velocities, and flow patterns. J Vasc Surg 1988;8:286–291.

Nguyen NT, Luketich JD, Friedman DM, et al. Pulmonary embolism following laparoscopic antireflux surgery: a case report and review of the literature. J Soc Laparosc Surg 1999;3:149–153.

SAGES. Global statement on deep venous thrombosis prophylaxis during laparoscopic surgery. Surg Endosc 1999;13:200.

Schwenk W, Bohm B, Fugener A, et al. Intermittent pneumatic sequential compression (ISC) of the lower extremities prevents venous stasis during laparoscopic cholecystectomy. Surg Endosc 1998;12:7–11.

Wilson YG, Allen PE, Skidmore R, et al. Influence of compression stockings on lower-limb venous haemodynamics during laparoscopic cholecystectomy. Br J Surg 1994; 81:841–844.

23. Hypothermia

Catherine Boulay, M.D.

Hypothermia is a known sequela of surgical procedures. It is widely acknowledged that surgical patients with multiple traumatic injuries and those that require massive transfusions are likely to develop hypothermia and, subsequently, the related problems of metabolic acidosis and coagulopathy. However, the prevalence and impact of hypothermia in the standard elective surgical population is largely underestimated. More than half of all surgical patients who receive standard perioperative care experience mild hypothermia, defined as a core temperature less than 36.0°C, while approximately one-third of surgical patients will develop "profound hypothermia," a core temperature of less than 35.0°C [1]. Hypothermia has multiple pathophysiological effects that are briefly discussed.

A. Effects

Hypothermia is associated with measurable cardiovascular alterations. Once core temperature has dropped by 1°C, shivering is induced, which increases the metabolic rate and peripheral oxygen consumption. Perhaps even more importantly, temperature decreases of 0.5°–1.5°C have been associated with an increase in circulating norepinephrine levels, with subsequent systemic vasoconstriction and hypertension [1]. These added stressors are particularly significant in patients with multiple comorbidities. In a study of high-risk vascular patients by Frank et al., there was a significantly higher risk of myocardial infarction during the immediate postoperative period in patients with core temperature less than 35°C [2]. A randomized controlled study of the risk of a cardiac complication [angina, myocardial infarction (MI), or cardiac arrest] in patients at high risk for cardiac disease found hypothermia during surgery to be an independent risk factor for such an event. Patients in the "normothermic" group were maintained at approximately 36.7°C with a forced-air warming blanket whereas the "hypothermic" group reached 35.4°C with standard thermal care [3]. Therefore, prevention of hypothermia during surgery may help decrease the incidence of cardiac complications in surgical patients.

The peripheral vasoconstriction associated with hypothermia is thought to reduce oxygen tension in subcutaneous tissue, which can impair immune defenses against wound infection. Many immune cells such as macrophages and neutrophils are dependent upon oxidative processes and are inhibited by a buildup of nitroso- and oxygen free radicals. Kurz et al. published a prospective randomized double-blind trial comparing colorectal patients who were given standard thermal care versus forced-air warmer and warmed I.V. fluids. Patients with hypothermia reached a mean intraoperative temperature of 34.7°C while the normothermic group had a mean temperature of 36.6°C. The hypothermic patients had a significantly higher incidence of wound infection than the normothermic patients (19% versus 6%). In addition to wound infection, the study found a decreased amount of collagen laid down in the subcutaneous tissue of patients who had been hypothermic. This decrease may be due to diminished hydroxylases for proline and lysine, which in turn would be associated with decreased wound healing [4].

Hypothermia also impairs the function of numerous enzymes that negatively impact coagulation and the degradation of anesthetics. Hypothermia is known to directly affect the enzymes of the clotting cascade and to impair the release of thromboxane A_2, which in turn reduces platelet function and increases the bleeding time [5]. In one study of orthopedic patients, hypothermia of 35.0°C was associated with increased blood loss and increased transfusion requirement [6]. As mentioned above, the pharmacokinetics of many anesthetics are also significantly affected by hypothermia; the enzymes used to metabolize most drugs are sensitive to even small alterations in core temperature [7]. Slower anesthetic recovery leaves patients susceptible to hypoventilation and aspiration, causing longer stays in the recovery room. During the rewarming period in the recovery room, the patient is also susceptible to shivering, which is associated with increased oxygen demand. In patients with significant pulmonary disease, this increased demand can overwhelm oxygen supply, causing a decrease in blood oxygen level. Metabolic derangements such as metabolic acidosis, hypokalemia [8], and negative nitrogen balance [9] have also been associated with hypothermia.

B. Mechanisms

General anesthesia is considered to be the most important contributor to hypothermia in the standard surgical patient. Hypothermia during general anesthesia takes place in three phases. During the first hour of anesthesia, there is a reduction of 1°–1.5°C in core temperature. This is largely caused by the reduction of the thermoregulatory threshold for vasoconstriction, which causes a core-to-periphery redistribution of body heat. The direct vasodilatory effect of many anesthetics and the decreased heat production caused by general anesthesia are much smaller contributors to this phase. The impact of these alterations on obese patients is notably less marked, probably because these patients are normally already in a vasodilated state. During the second phase of anesthesia-induced hypothermia, a slower, linear decrease in core temperature is noted. In addition to the mechanisms listed above, during this phase heat is lost via the following mechanisms: ventilation with cool, nonhumidified gases; third-space fluid losses from the open wound; and the use of unwarmed intravenous fluids. The third phase of intraoperative hypothermia is actually a plateau, where temperature remains constant despite continued surgery-related heat loss. Vasoconstriction, which is triggered at the lower temperature threshold of 34°–35°C, works to reestablish the core-to-periphery heat gradient, which decreases the heat loss from the skin to the atmosphere [7].

C. Preventive Measures

Of the measures used in the operating room to maintain normothermia, the forced-air warming blanket is considered the most effective. In a prospective randomized controlled study, the forced-air warmer maintained patients at a significantly higher core temperature than either cotton sheets or reflective blankets [10]. Other measures to reduce intraoperative hypothermia include the use of warm I.V. fluids as well as warmed and humidified ventilator gases. Although unwarmed I.V. fluids are thought to contribute to hypothermia when administered at rates greater than 2 L/hr, the clinical benefit of warmed ventilator gases remains debatable.

With the advent of laparoscopy, it was thought that minimally invasive methods would be associated with less hypothermia during major abdominal surgery because less heat would be lost via conduction and evaporation as a result of exposure of the peritoneal cavity to the ambient external environment. However, the use of laparoscopic techniques have not been shown to eliminate hypothermia in the surgical patient. Laparoscopy, as practiced by most surgeons, involves insufflation of CO_2 that is cold and dry (approximately 21°C and 0% humidity) [11]. Significant energy is expended by the patient to heat and humidify the gas once it is in the abdomen. Because there is almost always gas leakage from port sites, especially during lengthy advanced laparoscopic procedures, it is necessary to insufflate additional cool dry gas during the case to maintain the pneumoperitoneum. The heating and humidification of intraperitoneal CO_2 is a source of heat loss throughout the case; the extent of these losses is greater in lengthy cases and cases where a high CO_2 insufflation rate is required to maintain an adequate pneumoperitoneum. There is controversy as to what is the net effect on body temperature of laparoscopic methods. Heat is saved because much less of the abdominal cavity is exposed; however, heat is lost due to CO_2 insufflation. Does laparoscopy increase or decrease intraoperative hypothermia? Is it worthwhile to heat and/or humidify the gas itself?

In a case-controlled retrospective study, Berber et al. compared the effect of general anesthesia on body temperature in laparoscopic and open cases of similar duration. In these short cases (<90 min), no warming blankets or warm I.V. fluids were used. Core temperature decreased significantly in both groups, but no significant difference in hypothermia was noted between the two groups [12]. Luck et al. performed a nonrandomized study of open and laparoscopic colorectal surgical patients. Both surgical methods were associated with hypothermia. No significant difference in body temperature was noted between the open and closed groups despite the fact that the laparoscopic cases were significantly longer (180 versus 150 min). Of note, patients in whom a forced-air warming device was utilized were noted to have a significantly higher body temperature at the end of surgery when compared to patients in whom the forced-air device was not used [13]. Danelli et al. carried out a prospective randomized study that assessed hypothermia during laparoscopic and open colorectal surgery. In this study, all patients received both general and epidural anesthesia as well as warmed I.V. fluids and CO_2 gas. Again, no difference was noted in the incidence or the extent of hypothermia between the two groups of patients despite the fact that the laparoscopic cases were significantly longer [14]. In all these studies, the degree of hypothermia is considerable; all groups had an average minimum temperature of less than 36.0°C noted during the case. While several of the mechanisms of heat loss are different during open and closed procedures, both surgical methods appear to result in the same degree of hypothermia.

A number of studies have been carried out that assessed the impact of warm and/or humidified CO_2 during laparoscopy. In a randomized animal study, Bessell et al. compared body temperature after 3 hours of anesthesia alone, after a similar period of pneumoperitoneum with cool dry gas, and following laparoscopy with humidified warmed gas. Warm humid gas resulted in a temperature drop similar to that observed in the anesthetic control animals whereas those animals in whom cool dry gas was utilized manifested a significantly greater drop in temperature [11]. In the clinical setting, the results noted with warm gas have been less impressive. Puttick et al. randomized patients undergoing laparoscopic cases less than 35 minutes long to insufflation with either cool dry or warm dry gas. The mean core temperature of the warm CO_2 group was noted to be 0.18°C higher than the cool gas group; this small difference between the groups was statistically significant [15]. The clinical significance of such a small increase in temperature is unclear. Another randomized prospective study was performed to determine the impact of warm dry versus cool dry CO_2 in laparoscopic cases more than 90 minutes in length. In all patients, cotton blankets, water bath mattresses, and prewarmed I.V. fluids were utilized. Regardless of the type of gas used, the mean temperature of both groups of patients was less than 36.0°C. Similar to the results of Puttick et al., the patients who received warm dry CO_2 had slightly higher temperatures than the cool dry gas patients ($P < 0.05$) [16].

It is possible that humidification of the CO_2 will result in higher core temperatures than the slight benefit noted for warmed CO_2. Thus far, few randomized studies have been performed about the impact of humidified gases in the clinical setting. One such study, by Nguyen et al., assessed temperature in laparoscopic patients who received either cool dry CO_2 or heated and humidified CO_2. The duration of the cases was approximately 90 minutes. Forced-air warming blankets were used on all patients. No difference was seen in core temperature between the two groups [16].

Some surgeons routinely place the legs of patients to undergo laparoscopic colectomy within large plastic bags before placing the legs in the stirrups (modified lithotomy position). The legs can also be wrapped if the patient is to be placed in the supine position. Such a maneuver, in theory, should decrease the heat loss that results from the exposed lower extremities.

D. Summary

Both laparoscopic and open patients are vulnerable to hypothermia during and after surgery. Although some of the mechanisms of heat loss are different for the two surgical methods, the heat loss associated with general anesthesia is similar during both types of procedures. The heat loss from general anesthesia may be more important than the losses attributable to the CO_2 gas. Heating and humidification of the carbon dioxide before insufflation, although logical, to date has not been associated with meaningful increases in core temperature; the small increases in temperature noted with the warmed and/or humidified gas have not been associated with any clinical benefit. Further studies are required. In particular, the impact of humidified CO_2 during longer and more complex laparoscopic cases needs to be better assessed. Currently, the forced-air warmer seems to be the most useful addition to standard thermal care in the operative setting. Efforts to prevent hypothermia are important in all surgical patients, particularly those with comorbid disease, regardless of whether minimally invasive or open techniques are to be employed.

E. References

1. Frank SM, Higgins MS, et al. The catecholamine, cortisol and hemodynamic responses to mild perioperative hypothermia: a randomized trial. Anesthesiology 1995; 82:83–93.
2. Frank SM, Beattie C, et al. Unintentional hypothermia associated with postoperative myocardial ischemia. Anesthesiology 1993;78:468–476.
3. Frank SM, Fleisher LA, et al. Perioperative maintenance of normothermia reduces the incidence of morbid cardiac events: a randomized clinical trial. JAMA 1997;277: 1127–1134.
4. Kurz A, Sessler DI, Lenhardt R. Perioperative normothermia to reduce the incidence of surgical-wound infection and reduce hospitalization. N Engl J Med 1996;334: 1209–1215.
5. Valeri C, Khavvaz K, et al. Effect of skin temperature on platelet function in patients undergoing extracorporeal bypass. J Thorac Cardiovasc Surg 1992;104:108–116.
6. Schmeid H, Kurz A, Sessler DI, Kozek Z, Reiter A. Mild hypothermia increases blood loss and transfusion requirements during total hip arthroplasty. Lancet 1996;347: 289–292.
7. Sessler DI. Perioperative thermoregulation and heat balance. Ann NY Acad Sci 1997; 813:757–777.
8. Laszlo A, Sprung J, et al. Effects of hypothermia and potassium variations on maximum diastolic potential. Anesthesiology 1990;73:3A.
9. Carli FI, Emery PW, Freemantle CAJ. Effects of perioperative normothermia on postoperative protein metabolism in elderly patients undergoing hip arthroplasty. Br J Anaesth 1989;63:76–282.
10. Siew-Fong N, Cheng-Sim O, et al. A comparative study of three warming interventions to determine the most effective in maintaining perioperative normothermia. Anesth Analg 2003;96:171–176.
11. Bessel JR, Ludbrook G, et al. Humidified gas prevents hypothermia induced by laparoscopic insufflation. Surg Endosc 1999;13:101–105.
12. Berber E, String A, et al. Intraoperative thermal regulation in patients undergoing laparoscopic vs. open surgical procedures. Surg Endosc 2001;15:281–285.
13. Luck AJ, Moyes D, Maddern GJ, Hewett PJ. Core temperature changes during open and laparoscopic colorectal surgery. Surg Endosc 1999;13:480–483.

14. Danelli G. Temperature control and recovery of bowel function after laparoscopic or laparotomic colorectal surgery in patients receiving combined epidural/general anesthesia and postoperative epidural analgesia. Anesth Analg 2001;95:467–471.
15. Puttick MI, Scott-Coombes DM, et al. Comparison of immunologic and physiologic effects of CO_2 pneumoperitoneum at room and body temperatures. Surg Endosc 1999; 13:572–575.
16. Nguyen NT, Furdui G, et al. Effect of heated and humidified carbon dioxide gas on core temperature and postoperative pain: a randomized trial. Surg Endosc 2002; 16(7):1050–1054.

24. Implications of Subcutaneous Emphysema and How to Avoid and/or Limit Its Development

Kirk A. Ludwig, M.D.

There are two basic means of providing exposure within the abdominal cavity for laparoscopic procedures: mechanical abdominal wall elevation and pneumoperitoneum. Mechanical lifting devices directly elevate the abdominal wall; however, the exposure obtained is less than ideal. Pneumoperitoneum, which is established via insufflation with some type of gas, currently provides the best exposure for laparoscopic surgery. The ideal gas for insufflation would be nontoxic, nonflammable, colorless, highly soluble in blood, readily available, and cheap. Nitrous oxide, CO_2, helium, air, and argon have all been used to create and maintain pneumoperitoneum. By far the most popular exposure method for laparoscopic procedures is CO_2 gas. The high solubility of CO_2 is an advantage because accidental venous embolism poses far less of a problem than the other less soluble gases used for insufflation; however, it is also a disadvantage because the readily absorbed CO_2 causes hypercarbia, acidosis, and other physiologic alterations. In addition to physiologic side effects, insufflation of gas into the abdomen through the abdominal wall can, on occasion, be associated with other complications such as pneumoperitoneum. Another such complication is subcutaneous emphysema.

Subcutaneous emphysema develops when the gas being insufflated finds its way into the subcutaneous tissues of the abdominal wall. Thankfully, this is generally not a very dangerous complication; however, subcutaneous emphysema at times may threaten the laparoscopic completion of the case. Therefore, it behooves the surgeon to be aware of this complication and to be familiar with methods of dealing with this problem.

A. Incidence of Subcutaneous Emphysema

It is difficult to gather precise data about this complication for several reasons. The extent of the subcutaneous emphysema varies widely from case to case. It may be confined to a small portion of the abdominal wall immediately surrounding a port or extend down into the scrotum and thighs, along the flanks to the back, and up the chest to the neck. Based on the present literature, subcutaneous emphysema has been noted clinically during laparoscopy at a rate between 0.43% and 2.3%. Well-localized subcutaneous emphysema probably occurs more often and goes unnoticed in most cases. Because limited subcutaneous emphysema usually poses no problem clinically, even when detected it may not be noted in the chart. Evidence to this theory is provided by a study reporting that computed tomography (CT) scan of the upper abdomen within 24 hours of laparoscopic cholecystectomy revealed subcutaneous emphysema in 56% of patients. Long operative times (>200 minutes), the use of six or more ports, and extraperitoneal surgery (i.e., adrenal or kidney) may be risks factors for the development of this complication. In rare cases, subcutaneous emphysema may occur in conjunction with pneumothorax or pneumomediastinum.

B. Causes of Subcutaneous Emphysema

When a Veress needle is used to establish the pneumoperitoneum at the start of a case, it is not uncommon to misjudge the position of the needle's tip and to inadvertently insufflate gas into the abdominal wall. This error is usually quickly recognized and corrected. This is probably the most common cause of limited subcutaneous emphysema.

There are numerous other causes or contributing risk factors. In obese patients with a very thick abdominal wall, the port may not reach far enough into the abdominal cavity so that the insufflation hole is actually not in the abdomen. In patients of normal girth, the port may be inadvertently or intentionally pulled back such that the insufflation hole is in the abdominal wall. Torquing of the port in opposing directions during a case may widen the peritoneal defect such that gas more easily tracks into the abdominal wall from the peritoneal cavity. When the "cut-down" method is used for placement of the initial port, an overly large fascial incision encourages desufflation via the port wound, which allows gas to track into the abdominal wall. Repeated dislodgement and reinsertion of the port may enlarge the port wound or result in new tissue paths through the abdominal wall, which makes the development of subcutaneous emphysema more likely. The pneumoperitoneum pressure also plays a role. The higher the pressure setting, the greater the tendency toward the development of subcutaneous emphysema. A faulty pressure gauge on an insufflator may lead to the inadvertent and unwitting use of very high insufflation pressures.

As subcutaneous emphysema develops, the abdominal wall thickness or girth increases as a result of gas dissecting into the subcutaneous tissue planes. This, in turn, shortens the length of the port that extends into the peritoneal cavity beyond the parietal peritoneal level. At a certain point the tip of the port is just barely inside the abdomen; making it more and more difficult to insufflate the peritoneal cavity without also pushing additional gas into the abdominal wall. A "vicious cycle" results wherein the development of the emphysema increases the likelihood that further abdominal wall insufflation will occur. This added insufflation further increases the wall girth, and so on and so on. When this occurs it can become very difficult to complete the operation laparoscopically.

Subcutaneous emphysema can also develop when CO_2 traverses the diaphragm into the mediastinum and results in a pneumomediastinum. From this location the gas can further dissect into the subcutaneous tissue planes of the head, neck, and chest. Barotrauma from high insufflation pressures and positive pressure ventilation can, rarely, cause a pneumoperitoneum that may track into the subcutaneous tissues causing subcutaneous emphysema.

C. Avoiding Subcutaneous Emphysema

1. Veress needle insufflation. Improper technique in inserting the Veress needle can result in extraperitoneal insufflation with resultant subcutaneous emphysema. A summary of the proper technique for insertion and use of the Veress needle in the midline follows:

A. Check the needle for patency by flushing with saline.

B. Occlude the tip of the needle and flush with saline to check for leaks.

C. Push the blunt tip of the needle against a hard surface to be certain that it retracts and springs back into position easily.

D. Pass the needle, grasped by the shaft, via a stab incision, using the dominant hand at a 45°–90° angle to the abdominal wall with the patient in slight Trendelenburg position. Following the initial resistance, there will be two "gives" or "pops" as the needle traverses the linea alba fascia and then the peritoneum. Proper positioning in the peritoneal cavity is confirmed by:

   1) Aspiration to assess for return of blood, urine, or bowel contents.
   2) Instillation of a small amount of saline into the needle to determine if there is free flow into the peritoneal cavity.
   3) Repeated aspiration to be sure that none of the saline is recoverable (saline return indicates that the needle tip is in a hollow organ or other closed space).
   4) Closure of the stopcock on the needle, filling the hub with saline, elevating the abdominal wall, then opening the stopcock to confirm that the saline flows rapidly into the abdominal cavity [the so-called drop test].
   5) Advancement of the needle a short distance further without encountering any resistance.

   Only after confirming proper placement of the needle is insufflation begun. Initial insufflation pressure of greater than 10 mmHg indicates a problem, one of which may be extraperitoneal insufflation. Insufflation is begun at a low flow and increased after 1–2 L CO_2 has been insufflated. If a problem is encountered, stop insufflation, withdraw the needle, and then start over again.

2. Open "cut-down" method. An alternative method for establishing pneumoperitoneum is the "open" technique using a Hasson cannula. A small incision is made at the umbilicus, or an alternate site, and the incision is carried down to the fascia. A small incision is made in the fascia, only large enough to accept an index finger, and the underlying peritoneum is grasped, elevated, and incised. Traction sutures, placed through the peritoneum and fascia, are placed on either side of the fascial incision. Next, the blunt trocar is inserted into the abdominal cavity and its position secured by wrapping each end of the fascial suture around the wings of the cone-shaped tip of the Hasson cannula. The open technique of insufflation is probably safer than the closed technique and, when executed properly, pneumoperitoneum is established just as rapidly, if not more rapidly, than with the closed technique. Development of subcutaneous emphysema with this technique should be a rare occurrence. Keys to avoiding extraperitoneal insufflation are:

A. Keep the skin and fascial incisions small.
B. If possible, place the traction sutures through the peritoneum and the fascia, not just the fascia.
C. Make sure the blunt-tipped trocar is positioned within the peritoneal cavity.
D. Using strong upward pressure on the traction sutures, advance the cone-tipped end of the Hasson cannula into the fascial opening as far and as tight as possible before securing to the wings. High pressures may be noted if insufflation is attempted when the cannula is improperly positioned in the extraperitoneal space.

3. Faulty insufflator. A faulty pressure/flow shutoff mechanism can result in dangerously high intraabdominal pressure and resultant subcutaneous emphysema. The proper function of the insufflator can be checked easily. To assure proper function:

A. Turn the insufflator to high flow (>6 L/min) with the tubing not yet connected to a cannula or Veress needle; the intraabdominal pressure indicator should be 0.
B. Lower the flow to 1 L/min and occlude the tubing. The pressure reading should go to 30 mmHg and the flow indicator should go to 0.

4. Insufflation pressure. For most laparoscopic procedures, the pressure limit should be set at 12–15 mmHg. Intraabdominal pressures higher than this can be problematic and contribute to the formation of subcutaneous emphysema as CO_2 is insufflated under high pressures around cannulas.

5. Number of ports. Subcutaneous emphysema can result from leakage around any port; the more ports that are utilized the greater the incidence. Therefore, the minimum number of ports that will permit safe completion of the case should be placed.

6. Angle of port insertion. The manner in which the cannulas are placed has a bearing on the chances that subcutaneous emphysema may develop. Each cannula should be placed so that its axis is at an appropriate angle for the case at hand. In placing ports, this should be kept in mind, especially in patients with a thick abdominal wall. The cannula should enter the peritoneal cavity at an angle such that there will be minimal movement of the cannula within the abdominal wall during the procedure (generally angled toward the quadrant where the procedure is to be done). If the port is angled toward the head and there is lower abdominal or pelvic dissection to be done, then it will be necessary to torque the port in the opposite direction, which will likely tear and enlarge both the peritoneal defect and the abdominal wall wound.

In patients with a thick abdominal wall in whom the port is placed at an angle, there will be a significant difference between the location of the incision on the skin and the point at which the cannula enters the peritoneum. The surgeon should take this fact into account when choosing the port sites.

7. Port anchoring. Particularly during long cases, port dislodgement or port slippage may occur, which increases the chances of subcutaneous emphysema developing. Therefore, it is advisable to anchor all ports to the abdominal wall to prevent complete dislodgement and to stabilize each port's position in regard to the length of the cannula within the abdominal cavity to prevent slippage.

Threaded ports that are "screwed" into the abdominal wall anchor themselves. Most such ports are reusable. An accessory port anchor or grip of some type is available for most nonthreaded disposable ports. Most such grips are threaded and cone shaped (Christmas tree shaped); the port is inserted through the center of the grip with the narrow end of the grip oriented toward the port tip. Once the proximal end of the port has been inserted into the abdomen, the port anchor is screwed into the abdominal wall. The grip prevents the port from being dislodged and also prevents slippage of the port. The length of the port within the abdomen can be altered, usually by pinching a valve on the grip, which allows movement of the port within the grip.

Regardless of whether a threaded port or port grip is used to anchor the port, it is advisable to further secure the port via a skin stitch placed adjacent to the cannula. A "0"-gauge suture is ideal for this purpose. The suture is loosely tied down to the skin after being placed. One end of the suture is then wrapped around the insufflation arm of the port several times, after which it is pulled down toward the abdominal wall. The opposite end of the suture is then pulled upward and the two lengths of the suture are clamped together. This prevents port dislodgement in the rare instance, usually late in the case, when the port grip or the threaded port fails to anchor the cannula. If this type of anchoring suture is used, it is necessary to unclamp the suture to alter the length of the port in the abdomen. After adjusting the port position, the two ends of the suture are again clamped together after one of them has been wrapped about the insufflation arm.

8. Means of limiting the expansion of the abdominal wall's girth after subcutaneous emphysema has developed. As mentioned, once the problem has been noted, the expanding abdominal wall makes it increasingly difficult to keep the port tip in the abdomen. The following method stabilizes abdominal wall girth near a port and requires only large nylon sutures on "retention suture"-type needles. With the laparoscope observing the port to be anchored, a #2 nylon on the largest available curved needle (which is straightened out before being inserted) is passed through the entire abdominal wall adjacent to the port in question. A laparoscopic needle driver or other grasper is used to grasp the shaft of the needle once it has entered the abdomen. The needle is then carefully pulled into the abdomen and then turned 180° so that the sharp tip is facing the underside of the abdominal wall. As the needle is being pulled into the abdomen, the tip is kept in full view via the laparoscope so that no injuries are made. As the needle is turned around, the heel of the needle is followed rather than the tip, because the heel is now adjacent to the bowel rather than the tip of the needle. The needle is then driven back through the abdominal wall adjacent to the port but some distance away from the entry site. The needle is then pulled back out through the abdominal wall to the outside. In obese patients the needle may not project through the skin, which necessitates careful compression of the abdominal wall to find it. One end of the suture is then wrapped around the insufflation armature three or four times and then pulled down toward the abdominal wall while the opposing end of the suture is pulled upward alongside the port. An assistant then clamps the two strands together, which serves to compress the abdominal wall and drive the port into the abdomen. This method compresses the abdominal wall and keeps the tip of the port within the abdomen. This method is useful in any instance where the port will not stay in the abdomen.

This method works best in conjunction with a port grip but can be used without one if necessary. The grip prevents the external part of the port shaft from being pushed fully into the abdomen by the transabdominal wall nylon suture when it is tightened around the insufflation arm.

D. Recognition of Subcutaneous Emphysema

1. Crepitus. Subcutaneous emphysema can appear early during laparoscopy, but it more typically presents 45–60 minutes after commencement of pneumoperitoneum. When it is limited, it often goes unnoticed until the end of the operation, hidden from the surgeon's view by the drapes as it extends downward into the groin and scrotum or upward into the chest, neck, and head. At that point this complication is usually noted by pushing down on the skin in the affected area, which reveals crepitus. The extent of the crepitus reflects the limits of the subcutaneous emphysema.

2. Insufflation problems. More extensive subcutaneous emphysema may be first noted during the case when maintenance of a sufficient pneumoperitoneum becomes difficult due to an expanding abdominal wall and numerous CO_2 leaks. Examination of the abdominal wall and port sites in this case will reveal crepitus. Placement of the transabdominal full-thickness nylon sutures to compress the abdominal wall and to maximize the length of the port in the peritoneal cavity as described in the above section (Section C.8) usually improves the situation.

3. Hypercarbia and acidosis. CO_2 is readily absorbed from the subcutaneous space; in some cases this absorption will result in notable physiologic changes. When this occurs, the first clinical sign may be a sudden and brisk increase in the end tidal CO_2, which should be detected by the anesthesiologist. At this point, a marked increase in $PaCO_2$ and a systemic acidosis may be noted on blood gas. What determines whether significant physiologic alterations develop is the extent of the subcutaneous emphysema and the ability of the patient to clear the additional CO_2 via the lungs.

4. Pneumoperitoneum-related pneumothorax. In laparoscopic cases where a pneumothorax develops secondary to gas escaping through the diaphragm into the chest, the anesthesiologist may recognize an increase in airway pressure or a decrease in lung compliance. The associated hypercarbia and acidosis can lead to cardiac arrhythmias (particularly ventricular), sinus tachycardia, and hypertension. An examination of the patient for subcutaneous emphysema and auscultation of the chest for breath sounds should be carried out if the pulmonary end-tidal CO_2 increases substantially during a laparoscopic case. A portable chest X-ray will demonstrate a pneumothorax, which can be managed via needle decompression of the hemithorax followed by placement of an anterior chest tube, if needed. Tension pneumothorax, with its attendant hemodynamic effects, is managed directly without a chest X-ray by immediate decompression. The surgeon should also remember that pneumothorax can develop from rupture of a pulmonary bleb and thus, in this case, not be related to the pneumoperitoneum at all.

5. Pneumoperitoneum-related pneumomediastinum. Insufflated CO_2 can also track from the abdominal cavity into the mediastinum and result in a pneumomediastinum. This can occur at congenital weak points or defects in the diaphragm, or it can occur when tissue planes along the vena cava, aorta, or retroperitoneum are disturbed, thus providing a pathway to the mediastinum for the gas. Most cases of pneumomediastinum associated with laparoscopy resolve spontaneously with observation and without major intervention. However, lifethreatening complications can occur if insufflation is continued once the pneumomediastinum has developed. Pneumopericardium in association with pneumomediastinum and subcutaneous emphysema has, very rarely, been reported and may be associated with potentially life-threatening cardiac tamponade.

E. Management of Subcutaneous Emphysema

1. When noted during the case. The patient should be quickly evaluated for the presence of a pneumothorax via auscultation of the lungs and, if necessary, by obtaining a chest radiograph. The patient's pulmonary end-tidal CO_2 and arterial CO_2 levels should be checked and, if high, the minute ventilation and inspiratory pressure adjusted to lower the $PETCO_2$ and $PaCO_2$ to acceptable levels. The anesthesiologist should also discontinue the use of nitrous oxide because it rapidly enters the space containing the CO_2, adding to the gas volume in the subcutaneous tissues. The insufflation pressure should be reduced to as low a level as possible to maintain adequate exposure and the operation completed promptly. If expanding abdominal wall girth and maintenance of an adequate pneumoperitoneum is a problem, then full-thickness nylon sutures should be placed adjacent to the ports and used as described in Section C above to compress the abdominal wall and keep the port tip in the abdomen. Obviously, if it is not possible to sufficiently lower the $PaCO_2$ levels via manipulation of the respirator settings, or it is not possible to maintain adequate laparoscopic exposure, then conversion to an open procedure will be necessary.

2. When noted at the end of the case. The patient should be evaluated for pneumothorax and the $PETCO_2$ and $PaCO_2$ levels assessed as described above. Before extubation, it is crucial that the end-tidal and arterial CO_2 levels be within normal limits. In patients with severe chronic obstructive pulmonary disease or those with ventilatory dysfunction due to medications (opioids or anesthetic medications), mechanical ventilation may need to be continued postoperatively until the CO_2 levels normalize. If the subcutaneous emphysema involves the chest and neck then, before extubation, the upper airway is carefully evaluated to be sure there is no airway compression. It is important to reassure the patient that the subcutaneous emphysema will resolve spontaneously over a relatively short period of time.

F. Selected Refercnces

Abe H, Bandai Y, Ohtomo Y, et al. Extensive subcutaneous emphysema and hypercapnia during laparoscopic cholecystectomy: two case reports. Surg Laparosc Endosc 1995; 5:183–187.

Hasel R, Arora SK, Hickey DR. Intraoperative complications of laparoscopic cholecystectomy. Can J Anaesth 1993;40:459–464.

Holzman M, Sharp K, Richards W. Hypercarbia during carbon dioxide gas insufflation for therapeutic laparoscopy: a note of caution. Surg Laparosc Endosc 1992;2:11–14.

Kent RB. Subcutaneous emphysema and hypercarbia following laparoscopic cholecystectomy. Arch Surg 1991;126:1154–1156.

Klopfenstein CF, Gaggero G, Mamie C, et al. Laparoscopic extraperitoneal inguinal hernia repair complicated by subcutaneous emphysema. Can J Anaesth 1995;42:523–525.

Pearce DJ. Respiratory acidosis and subcutaneous emphysema during laparoscopic cholecystectomy. Can J Anaesth 1994;41:314–316.

Richard HM, Stancato-Pasik A, Salky BA, et al. Pneumothorax and pneumomediastinum after laparoscopic surgery. Clin Imaging 1997;21:337–339.

Rudston-Brown BCD, MacLennan D, Warriner CB, et al. Effect of subcutaneous carbon dioxide insufflation on arterial pCO_2. Am J Surg 1996;171:460–463.

Wahba RWM, Tessler MJ, Kleiman SJ. Acute ventilatory complications during laparoscopic upper abdominal surgery. Can J Anaesth 1996;43:77–83.

Wolf JS, Clayman RV, Monk TG, et al. Carbon dioxide absorption during laparoscopic pelvic operation. J Am Coll Surg 1995;180:555–560.

25. Fluid Management and Renal Function During a Laparoscopic Case Done Under CO_2 Pneumoperitoneum

Gamal Mostafa, M.D.
Frederick L. Greene, M.D.

Minimally invasive surgery aims to attenuate the stress of surgical trauma while achieving the desired therapeutic effect. The pneumoperitoneum and the patient's position required for laparoscopy induce pathophysiologic changes that complicate intraoperative and anesthetic management. In addition, the long operative time of some laparoscopic procedures and the difficulty in evaluating the volume of blood loss are factors that make laparoscopic surgery a potentially high-risk procedure. Carbon dioxide is currently the most commonly used gas for creating pneumoperitoneum. Insufflation of CO_2 into the peritoneal cavity is known to have certain cardiorespiratory and hemodynamic consequences. These changes affect intraoperative renal function and are also closely related to intravascular volume status and intravenous fluid therapy during the procedure. Although the hemodynamic, renal, and fluid management aspects of laparoscopic surgery might not be of obvious concern in a young, healthy individual who is undergoing a brief laparoscopic procedure, this is certainly not the case when a long, complicated procedure is performed on a high-risk patient. An understanding of the physiologic changes of carboperitoneum is essential for formulation of an appropriate intraoperative management plan, which may entail invasive perioperative monitoring to optimize hemodynamic performance. Under optimal conditions, pneumoperitoneum can be tolerated by patients with limited physiologic reserve who can, therefore, benefit from minimally invasive surgery. Because more complicated laparoscopic surgery is now being performed and the application for these procedures is extending to older and perhaps sicker patients who are medically compromised, clear understanding of the physiologic changes in different body systems caused by pneumoperitoneum is essential for both the surgeon and the anesthesiologist.

A. The Intraperitoneal Pressure

The normal mean intraabdominal pressure is zero (equal to atmospheric pressure) or less. Peritoneal insufflation during laparoscopic procedures is one of several important clinical conditions causing elevation of intraabdominal pressure. Pathophysiologically, this is defined as compartment syndrome, a condition in which increased pressure in a confined anatomic space can adversely affect the circulation and function of the tissues therein. Deleterious consequences of elevated intraabdominal pressure appear gradually in a graded response that is related to the level of pressure. Operative laparoscopy is usually performed with a constant pneumoperitoneum at 10–15 mmHg pressure.

B. Renal response to CO_2 Pneumoperitoneum

The main effect of increased intraabdominal pressure associated with CO_2 pneumoperitoneum on renal physiology is decreased renal blood flow and glomerular filtration rate. The decrease in renal blood flow mainly affects the renal cortex. The superficial cortical arteries are particularly sensitive to increased sympathetic activity because of their rich innervation and high blood flow rate compared with other regions of the kidney. Insufflation of the abdomen to 15 mmHg pressure has been shown to cause 60% reduction in renal cortical perfusion. This decrease in renal cortical blood flow translates clinically into a 50% reduction in urine output. Oliguria is a universally observed phenomenon during laparoscopic pneumoperitoneum. It can be profound and is always greater than observed with the same procedure performed through a laparotomy. An increase of intraabdominal pressure to 40 mmHg induces complete anuria. After evacuation of the pneumoperitoneum, renal cortical perfusion returns to normal almost immediately. Oliguria, on the other hand, remains for almost an hour after the procedure.

C. Mechanisms of Carboperitoneum-Induced Oliguria

Peritoneal insufflation triggers two important mechanisms that lead to reduction in urine output; one is pressure mediated and the other is hormonal (Figures 25.1, 25.2).

1. The direct compressive effect of pneumoperitoneum on the renal parenchyma and the renal vein causes decreased renal cortical perfusion and subsequent oliguria.
2. The hormonally mediated reduction in urine output occurs, in part, because of the stimulatory action of pneumoperitoneum on the peritoneal stretch receptors leading to antidiuretic hormone and aldosterone release.
3. Also important is the documented activation of the renin-aldosterone mechanism observed with pneumoperitoneum (see Figure 25.2). This not only causes oliguria but also leads to renal vasoconstriction, further decrease in renal perfusion, and perpetuation of the cycle.
4. The compressive effect of pneumoperitoneum on the renal parenchyma and renal vein is immediately and completely reversed on deflation of the abdomen with return of renal blood flow to baseline.

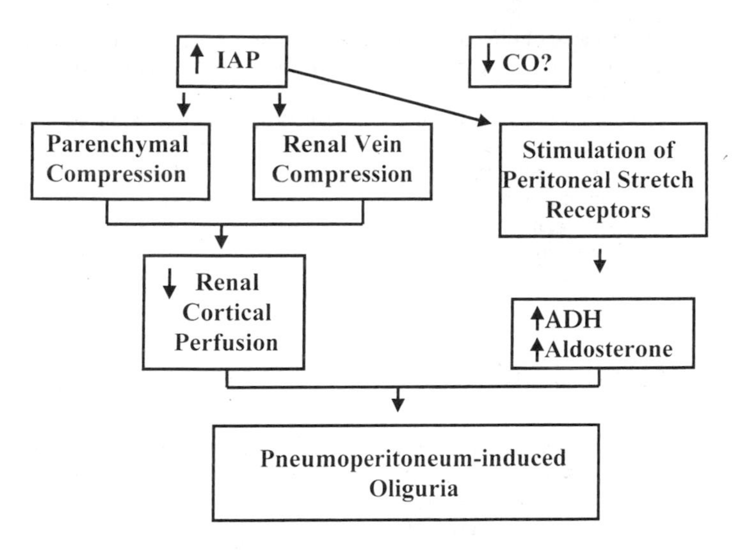

Figure 25.1. Mechanism of oliguria in laparoscopic cases. The role of decreased cardiac output is questionable. IAP, intraabdominal pressure; CO, cardiac output; ADH, antidiuretic hormone.

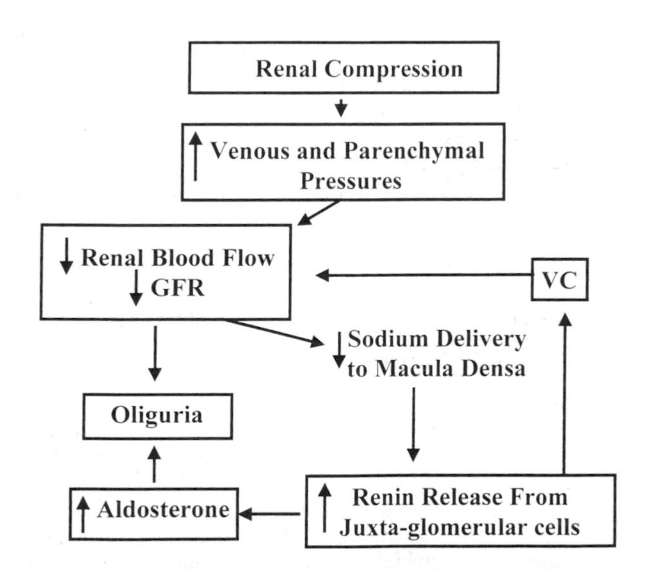

Figure 25.2. The intrinsic hormonally mediated renal mechanism for oliguria in laparoscopic procedures. VC, vasoconstriction; GFR, glomerular filtration rate.

5. Persistence of oliguria after completion of a laparoscopic procedure is hormonally mediated due to high levels of antidiuretic hormone and aldosterone.
6. It is important to remember that pneumoperitoneum-induced oliguria is completely independent of the effect of increased intraabdominal pressure on the cardiac output and is mainly a local renal effect of pneumoperitoneum.
7. In addition, neither bilateral ureteral compression nor decrease in renal artery pressure has a role in the mechanism of oliguria associated with laparoscopy.

D. Clinical Significance of Oliguria

The decreased renal perfusion and the resultant drop in the urine output during and for some time after a laparoscopic procedure should be considered by the surgeon and the anesthesiologist.

1. If possible, the lowest insufflation pressure should be used during gaseous laparoscopy to minimize the potential for significant hemodynamic renal alterations.
2. This is even more prudent when performing a laparoscopic procedure on a patient with borderline renal function. In these instances, it is also important to avoid the concomitant use of any potentially nephrotoxic medication or anesthetic agent as this may have an additive effect on the already compromised renal function.
3. Pulmonary edema from excessive intraoperative fluid administration is a main concern with pneumoperitoneum-induced oliguria. This complication occurs due to vigorous attempts to reverse the oliguria. It is important to remember that the decreased urine output, in this instance, is independent of the cardiac output and cannot be corrected by administering fluids in a futile attempt to achieve a predetermined bias of what intraoperative urine output should be. This will only lead to pulmonary edema.

E. Volume-Dependent Response to CO_2 Pneumoperitoneum

The response of cardiac output to pneumoperitoneum is dependent on two major variables: the increase in intraabdominal pressure and the baseline intravascular volume status of the patient (Figure 25.3). When the intravascular volume is low, increased intraabdominal pressure compresses the inferior vena cava (IVC) and impedes right ventricular filling, causing a decrease in cardiac output. On the other hand, with high intravascular volume, venous return is aided by the pneumoperitoneum, and cardiac output is increased.

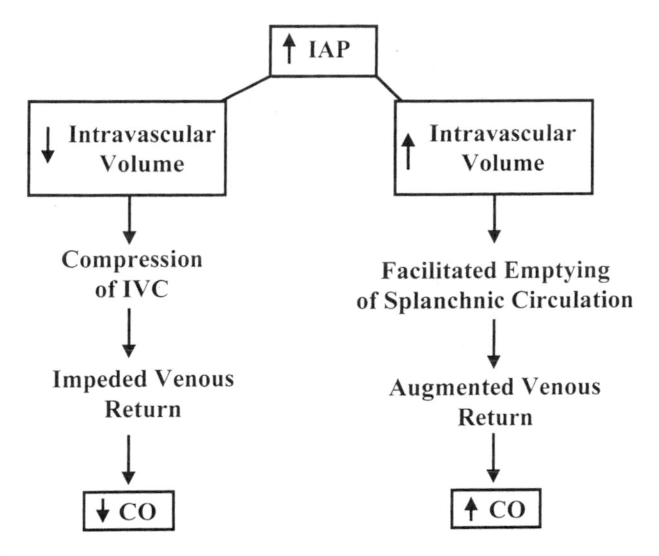

Figure 25.3. The distinctive influence of volume status on the effect of pneumoperitoneum on cardiac output. IAP, intraabdominal pressure; IVC, inferior vena cava; CO, cardiac output.

F. Principles of Intraoperative Fluid Management in Uncomplicated Laparoscopic Surgery

1. Urine output is not an accurate reflection of the intravascular volume status during laparoscopy, as oliguria is the norm. Therefore, intravenous fluid administration during an uncomplicated laparoscopic procedure should not be guided by urine output.
2. Excessive fluid loss that normally takes place in open abdominal surgery is avoided during laparoscopy. Because of this, the need for supplemental fluid is usually eliminated. Intraoperative fluid administration should not exceed a maintenance rate (110 mL/hr for a 70-kg adult) in an uncomplicated procedure on a healthy individual.
3. The appropriate volume of fluid required intraoperatively is given as balanced salt solution. The additional use of colloids or albumin solutions is unnecessary and is potentially harmful.
4. It is important to remember that oliguria will last for about an hour after completion of the procedure due to the hormonal effects of pneumoperitoneum.

5 It is important to remember that patients who have undergone a mechanical bowel preparation are almost always hypovolemic at the start of the case. Ideally, these patients should be given one or several liters of I.V. fluids prior to anesthetic induction in an effort to restore them to the euvolemic state.

G. Laparoscopy in the Compromised and Critically Ill Patient

Certain clinical situations make fluid management during a laparoscopic procedure more complicated. This is essentially because, in these situations, the physiologic response to pneumoperitoneum cannot be considered isolated as it is compounded by coexisting factors that can lead to harmful consequences even with a mild elevation of intraabdominal pressure.

1. Patients with hemorrhagic shock and hypovolemia have aggravated hemodynamic and renal consequences of pneumoperitoneum. This is particularly pertinent in the acutely injured patient in whom diagnostic laparoscopy may be used. If the volume status of the patient is not corrected before the procedure, diagnostic laparoscopy may amplify the hemodynamic instability.
2. Critically ill patients may require diagnostic laparoscopy for the diagnosis of sepsis. It is important to consider that these patients are frequently hypovolemic and are receiving mechanical ventilation with high positive end-expiratory pressure (PEEP). These two factors can compound the effect of pneumoperitoneum leading to acute circulatory compromise if adequate intravenous fluids are not administered.
3. The high-risk cardiac patient requires accurate fluid management. Invasive monitoring with a pulmonary artery catheter and intraoperative assessment of mixed venous saturation are useful in evaluating and correcting intraoperative events of decreased tissue perfusion as indicated by decrease in mixed venous saturation. Volume loading can be used to reverse these events.
4. Prophylactic volume expansion, in euvolic patients, is recommended in instances when the anticipated period of pneumoperitoneum is longer than 4 hours. This practice has been shown to have a protective effect on renal hemodynamics. This concern can be important in certain procedures such as laparoscopic donor nephrectomy.

H. Selected References

Andrus CH, Wittgen CM, Naunheim KS. Anesthetic and physiological changes during laparoscopy and thoracoscopy: the surgeon's view. Semin Laparosc Surg 1994;1: 228–240.

Chiu AW, Chang LS, Birkett DH, Babayan RK. The impact of pneumoperitoneum, pneumoretroperitoneum, and gasless laparoscopy on the systemic and renal hemodynamics. J Am Coll Surg 1995;181:397–406.

Doty JM, Saggi BH, Sugerman HJ, et al. Effect of increased renal venous pressure on renal function. J Trauma 1999;47:1000–1003.

Harman PK, Kron IL, McLachlan HD, Freedlender AE, Nolan SP. Elevated intra-abdominal pressure and the renal function. Ann Surg 1982;196:594–597.

London ET, Ho HS, Neuhaus AMC, Wolfe BM, Rudich SM, Perez RV. Effect of intravascular volume expansion on renal function during prolonged CO_2 pneumoperitoneum. Ann Surg 2000;231:195–201.

Safran DB, Orlando R. Physiologic effects of pneumoperitoneum. Am J Surg 1994; 167:281–286.

Safran D, Sgambati S, Orlando R. Laparoscopy in high-risk cardiac patients. Surg Gynecol Obstet 1993;176:548–554.

Schein M, Wittmann DH, Aprahamian CC, Condon RE. The abdominal compartment syndrome: the physiological and clinical consequences of elevated intra-abdominal pressure. J Am Coll Surg 1995;180:745–753.

26. Port Site Closure Methods and Hernia Prevention

Chandrakanth Are, M.D.
Mark A. Talamini, M.D.

Laparoscopic port site hernias have been frequently reported (incidence of 0.02%–5% with an average of 1%) since the first case was documented in 1968 by Fear et al. Larger port size and increasing numbers of ports required to perform more complex laparoscopic procedures are likely to increase the incidence of port site hernias (PSH). PSH tend to develop more frequently at umbilical and midline port sites due to the thinness of the umbilical skin and weaknesses in the linea alba. The presence of an undetected umbilical hernia when the port site is near the umbilicus can also increase the incidence of a PSH in that location if both the port site and the preexisting umbilical hernia are not closed with a formal herniorrhaphy. About one-quarter of PSH are umbilical. Overlapping muscle and fascial layers explains the reduced incidence of PSH at lateral port locations. Closure of the fascial defect does not completely prevent the development of PSH, although the incidence is higher if a fascial closure is not attempted. PSH have been reported through port sites of all sizes (including 5 mm). However, more than 90% of PSH occur through trocar sites 10 mm or larger.

Patients usually present within 2 weeks of surgery, although some cases have been reported years after the initial surgery. The development of unremitting pain, fever, or other gastrointestinal complaint after laparoscopic surgery requires immediate investigation. The contents of these hernias are usually small bowel or omentum or, on rare occasions, large bowel. The spectrum of symptoms range from no symptoms to pain due to omental infarction or small bowel obstruction. Richter's hernia is very common among PSHs due to the small size of the fascial defect. The insidious nature of Richter's hernia can lead to significant morbidity. PSH should be suspected in all patients with bowel obstruction up to 1 year after laparoscopic surgery. A computed tomography (CT) scan can be helpful in making the diagnosis. Comorbid conditions that can increase the incidence of PSH include diabetes mellitus, wound infection, and obesity.

Laparotomy or repeat laparoscopic surgery is required to repair the PSH. Adhesiolysis and bowel resection are also necessary in up to 10% of the patients. The associated morbidity of these iatrogenic hernias underscores the importance of preventing the condition. Every attempt should be made to keep the incidence less than the expected 1% by closing the fascia *and* the peritoneum. Trocars used for laparoscopic surgery usually range between 5 and 15 mm. Port sites (PS) 10 mm or greater should be closed if at all possible. Current consensus is not uniform about the management of PS less than 10 mm. In this chapter, we detail the indications, various methods, and techniques to ensure proper port site closure to minimize the occurrence of PSH.

A. Methods

The ideal method of closure should be quick, easy to perform without enlarging the skin incision, safe, inexpensive, and provide adequate closure of fascia and peritoneum. Several methods and instruments are available to help close the trocar sites. The more commonly used techniques are described below. The ideal method for each patient depends on the incision characteristics, the body habitus, and the surgeon's preference.

Standard Closure (Via Skin Wound)

This method entails direct visualization of the defect through the skin wound once the pneumoperitoneum has been released and the port removed. Usually, the fascial edges are grasped with a Kocher or Allis clamp and the various layers are sutured together with a simple or figure-of-eight suture. This can be difficult in obese patients with a large breadth of subcutaneous fat. Every attempt should be made to include all fascial layers and the peritoneum in the closure. It can be very difficult to include the peritoneum when dealing with patients of moderate to high body mass index (BMI). In some cases, the skin incision may have to be enlarged to permit adequate closure; in this case, the morbidity of an incisional hernia outweighs the benefit of a small skin incision. Although this method is a reasonable alternative, in the author's opinion, one of the laparoscopically visualized methods of suture placement is preferred.

Laparoscopic Direct Visualization Fascial Closure Methods

There are a number of fascial and peritoneal closure methods that permit accurate placement of sutures under direct laparoscopic visualization. The goal of all these methods is a subcutaneous knot that well approximates the peritoneal and the fascial wound. These methods are carried out with the pneumoperitoneum intact. The sutures can be placed either with the port in place (by working adjacent to the port) or after the port has been removed. In the latter case, the surgeon usually "plugs" the hole with the second or third finger to prevent gas desufflation while carefully inserting the suture passer, needle, or other device through the skin wound adjacent to the finger. The laparoscope is used to visualize the port wound in question and the passage of the suture bearing instrument directly observed. By moving the laparoscope to different ports it is possible to use this method for all ports that require closure. The advantages of this type of method when compared to the standard open method described in the section above include (1) more accurate placement of suture under direct vision, (2) possible decrease in operative time, (3) elimination of the possible need to extend the skin incision, and (4) suture placement may be technically easier. Numerous devices have been designed for this purpose including the Grice method, the Carter-Thomson Needle-Point suture passer, the Maciol suture needle, and the Endoclose suture carrier. These suture placement methods can also be used to control bleeding from abdominal wall vessels injured during port placement or surgery.

Using a Spring-Loaded Needle or Suture Passer Needle

Several of these devices consist of a needle with a plastic or metal oversheath. The needle is notched or has a groove within which the suture is intended to lie. The spring-loaded sheath is retracted to expose the notch or groove. When released, the sheath returns to its neutral position, which covers the notch, thus entrapping the suture. An alternative design is a laparoscopic suture passer that has a spring-closed handle. Commonly, these instruments have a jawed needle tip that has a conical shape. One jaw of the tip has a groove that is meant to hold the suture. To open the device to release or grasp a suture, it is necessary for the surgeon to forcibly spread the hands apart, thus overcoming the spring on the handle. Regardless of which type of device is used, the method is similar (Figure 26.1A–D).

The device is loaded with a suture by retracting the outer plastic sheath or by opening the jaw of the instrument. Once the suture is locked in the suture notch, the plastic sheath is released or the spring-closed handle is released, thus securing the suture. The tip of the needle is directed at a 30°–45° angle through the abdominal wall adjacent to the fascial defect. Once the tip is inside the peritoneal cavity, the suture is released by either opening the instrument jaws or retracting the sheath. A grasper introduced through another port is used to grasp the intraperitoneal end of the suture and thus prevent the suture from being pulled back out of the abdomen when the suture passer is withdrawn. The empty suture passer is inserted through the opposite side of the fascial defect, 180° from the initial insertion site. Once inside the peritoneal cavity, the free intraperitoneal end of the original suture is grasped. Placing mild tension on the suture by pulling on the extraabdominal component of the suture material can facilitate reloading the needle. Next, the suture passer is withdrawn from the abdomen. The two ends of the suture that are now outside the abdominal cavity can either be tied or "tagged" with a clamp and a second interrupted suture placed. Alternatively, the process can be repeated with the same suture to create a figure of eight.

Angiocatheter Technique

This method utilizes a 14-gauge angiocatheter that is universally available and is inexpensive. At the end of the procedure, with the trocar in place, a 14-gauge angiocatheter is inserted into the subcutaneous tissue between the skin

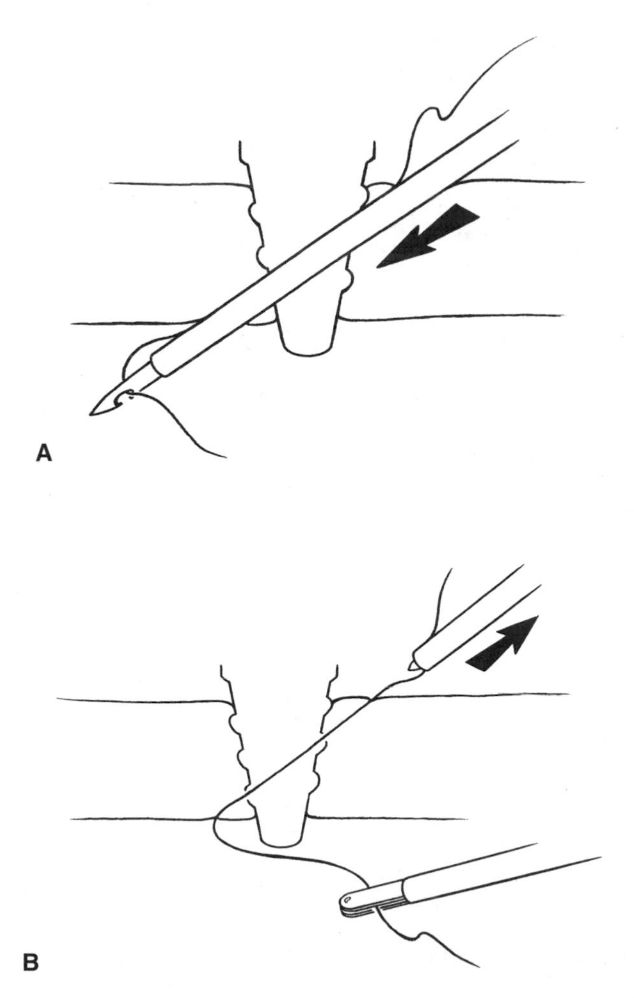

Figure 26.1. (A) Suture containing suture passes is inserted into the abdomen. (B) Intraabdominal instrument grasps suture and suture passer is withdrawn.

edge and trocar. The angiocatheter is inserted at an angle of 30° away from the trocar to capture as much fascia as possible. Under laparoscopic direct visualization, the angiocatheter is inserted completely into the abdominal cavity. A pre-tied loop of suture is inserted through the plastic cannula after removing the metal needle. With the help of a laparoscopic grasper introduced through another port, the loop is drawn further into the abdomen and held in place while the plastic cannula is withdrawn. The angiocatheter is then inserted on the opposite side of the trocar site (180°) in similar fashion. One end of a second long suture

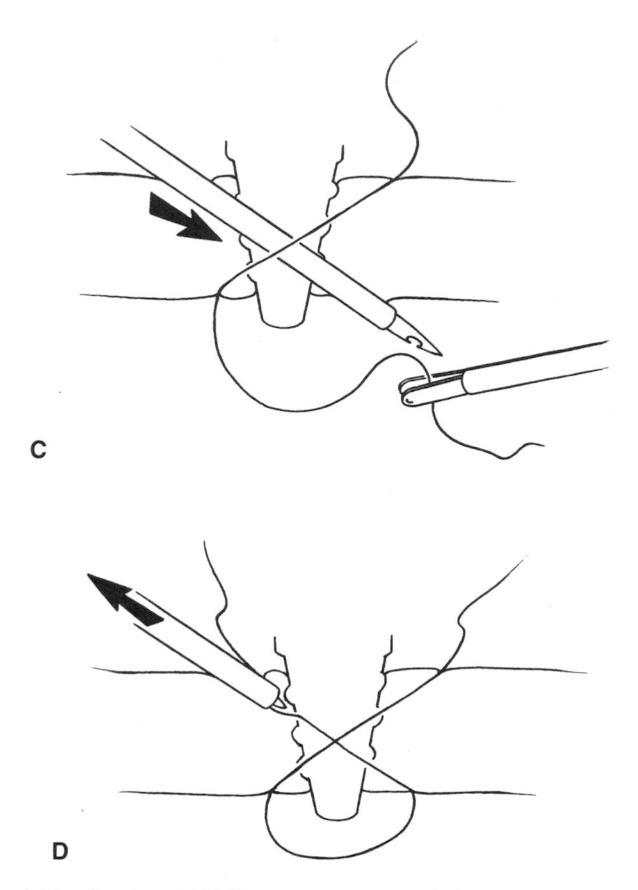

Figure 26.1. *Continued* (C) Empty suture passer is inserted back into abdomen on opposite side. (D) Suture has been passed to the suture passer that is being withdrawn from the abdomen.

is now introduced into the peritoneal cavity via the cannula, after which it is passed and then pulled a good distance through the looped end of the first suture. After removing the plastic cannula, the loop-ended suture is then pulled out of the abdomen, hopefully carrying the other suture with it. The nonlooped second suture that has now been passed into and out of the abdominal wall can then be tied. The knot will lie in the subcutaneous tissue. This method can be used to suture all ports under direct vision and also to control abdominal wall bleeding. While sharing the benefits of the Grice needle, it has the added advantage of being inexpensive (about $3). The only disadvantage of this approach is that the standard angiocatheter may not be long enough for obese patients. In this case, 16- or 18-gauge spinal needles can be used.

Use of a Heavy Spatulated Needle

This method utilizes a 110-mm heavy spatulated suture needle (5/8 circle). The suture is placed under direct vision. With the port in place, the needle is inserted perpendicular to the abdominal wall, about 1–2 cm from the skin edge. The laparoscope is used to directly view the needle as it enters the peritoneal cavity. The needle is pushed through the abdominal wall on the opposite side of the port site, again 1–2 cm from the skin edge. This step can be facilitated by levering or bending the port so that it is almost parallel to the abdominal wall. Once the needle has been passed, the port is removed and both ends of the suture are lifted to make them taut. A nerve hook is then inserted into the subcutaneous tissue and an attempt is made to entrap the suture, after which the hook is removed. The goal of this maneuver is to redirect the suture end out through the subcutaneous fat layer. After retrieving both ends in this manner the suture can be tied; the knot will lie in the subcutaneous fat. By rotating the camera between the different trocars, all port sites can be sutured.

Using a Suture Carrier

This approach uses a hook suture carrier, which is a 24-cm-long modified hook retractor with an eye drilled into its tip. The fascial edge is lifted vertically and the suture carrier is passed into the abdomen via the open wound. Under direct laparoscopic visualization, the end of the hook is then pulled up through the peritoneum and fascia (from the inside out) such that the tip reenters the wound via the subcutaneous fat. The suture is then threaded into the eye and the carrier is withdrawn back into the abdomen pulling the suture with it. With one end of the suture still loaded in the eye, the instrument and the hook's tip are turned to the opposite side of the wound, and then the hook is driven up through the peritoneum and fascia, again from the inside out, into the wound via the subcutaneous tissue once again. This brings the two ends of the suture into the subcutaneous tissue.

Alternatively, after the first pass, the suture is unloaded from the hook, and the carrier without a suture is passed from inside out again on the opposite side of the wound. The external free end of the suture is then passed through the hook tip and the carrier withdrawn into the abdomen. Both ends of the suture now lie in the abdominal cavity. This method is used if the surgeon chooses to bury the knot.

B. Recommendations Regarding Port Wound Closure

Although several approaches have been described here, it should be noted that there are several other methods as well. The choice of method will depend on the individual patient characteristics (such as body habitus, number and size of ports), the surgeon's preference, and available resources. Regardless of the specific approach, the authors recommend that the following principles be adhered to in regard to closure of port wounds. Admittedly, it is not possible to provide supporting published data for each of these recommendations.

1. All ports greater than 10 mm (midline and lateral) should be closed at the fascial level.
2. It is advised that 5-mm ports may need to be closed if the peritoneal and/or fascial defect has enlarged significantly during the procedure as a result of lengthy or extensive manipulation during the procedure. This is more likely to be necessary when the port is located in the midline.
3. Enlarging the incision to allow proper closure should take precedence over obtaining a good cosmetic result.
4. Port closure should include fascia *and* peritoneum.
5. In thin patients, midline port sites can be closed using standard methods via the skin wound.
6. Where possible, it is advised to view the abdominal side of each wound during fascial closure via the laparoscope.

C. Tips to Avoid Port Site Hernia

1. Use the minimum number of ports needed.
2. Use ports of the smallest possible diameter.
3. Avoid violent or severe levering or torquing of the ports as this can enlarge the fascial defect.
4. Attempting to insert the ports in a "Z"-shaped fashion with some subcutaneous travel may help reduce herniation.
5. Desufflate the abdomen carefully when removing ports. If this is not done, escaping CO_2 can draw the bowel or omentum into the port sites (chimney effect) or the wound utilized for specimen removal.
6. After completion of surgery and before closure of ports, shake the abdomen to dislodge any bowel stuck in the port sites.
7. The fascial defects should be closed before the patient wakes up. Coughing and gagging can make closure very difficult.
8. Palpate the abdomen before closure to identify any unrecognized or preexisting hernia defects that may require repair.
9. Presence of incidental paraumbilical or umbilical hernias dictates enlarging the incision and performing a formal umbilical herniorrhaphy. This sometimes may require placement of a mesh patch.
10. Obese patients can pose a problem due to the thickness of the abdominal wall. Long needle carriers may be needed to secure proper closure.

D. Conclusions

In summary, every attempt should be made to ensure the proper closure of port sites. Otherwise, the morbidity associated with a port site hernia will negate the expected benefits of the intended minimally invasive surgery.

E. Selected References

Ammori BJ, Morias JC. A simple method of closure of a laparoscopic trocar site. J R Coll Surg Edinb 1996;41:120–121.

Fear R. Laparoscopy, a valuable aid in gynaecologic diagnosis. Obstet Gynecol 1968;31: 297–309.

Garzotto MG, Newman RC, Cohen MS, Rout R, Grice OD. Closure of laparoscopic trocar sites using a spring-loaded needle. Urology 1995;45:310–312.

Li P, Chung R. Closure of trocar wounds using a suture carrier. Surg Laparosc Endosc 1996;6:469–471.

Nadler RB, McDougall E, Bullock AD, Ludwig MA, Brunt LM. Fascial closure of laparoscopic port sites; a new technique. Urology 1995;45:1046–1048.

27. Decision to Convert to Open Methods

Valerie J. Halpin, M.D.
Nathaniel J. Soper, M.D.

A. Conversion Versus Complication

1. **Definitions**
   a. **Elective conversion** is defined as a laparoscopic case that is opened in the absence of a complication. **Elective conversion should NOT be considered a complication of laparoscopic surgery**.
   b. **Emergent conversion** is defined as a laparoscopic case that must be converted to an open approach because of the development of a complication that cannot be adequately managed using laparoscopic techniques.
   c. Complications are defined as unintentional events occurring intraoperatively that require additional maneuvers to correct and/or increase the risk of a poor outcome.
   d. The reported conversion rates of commonly performed laparoscopic procedures vary greatly (Table 27.1). The right-hand column includes the estimated number of cases in a surgeon's learning curve. If a surgeon is learning under the supervision of another trained laparoscopist, the learning curve is shorter and generally requires fewer cases. Most publications have demonstrated that conversion rates decrease after the initial learning curve to the lower numbers in the conversion rate column. Some authors have found that their conversion rates remain relatively constant due to their selection of straightforward, technically simple cases early on in their experience with a particular procedure. More challenging cases are attempted only after gaining experience.
2. **Effect of conversion on complication rates**
   a. **Laparoscopic cholecystectomy.** Recent data by Thompson comparing laparoscopic to open cholecystectomy have shown that the complication rate is independent of the approach when analyzed on an intention to treat basis in three cohorts of patients (group one, open cholecystectomy; group two, laparoscopic cholecystectomy with 5.8% conversion rate; group three, laparoscopic cholecystectomy with 1.2% conversion rate). This observation remained true even in group three where the conversion rate

Table 27.1. Conversion rates in commonly performed laparoscopic cases.

Procedure	*N*	Conversion rates	Number of cases in learning curve
Cholecystectomy	100	<1%–10%	30–50
Acute cholecystitis	100	5%–40%	
Colorectal operations	50	1%–40%	15–50
Diverticulitis	50	4%–61%	
Crohn's	25	5%–25%	
Cancer	100	4%–25%	
Antireflux surgery	50	0%–10%	15–50
Inguinal hernia repair	100	1%–8%	30–50
Splenectomy	25	1%–18%	20–50
Adrenalectomy	25	0%–20%	10–20
Nephrectomy	50	5%–14%	10–50
Gastric bypass	25	0%–10%	10–50
Appendectomy	100	<1%–23%	20
Peritonitis		0%–25%	

N is the minimum number of patients in series included in analysis of conversion rates.

approached 1%. The severity of complications was comparable in all three groups. Notably, the converted patients in group two did have a higher complication rate than the entire group of open patients but these two groups cannot be considered equivalent in disease severity.

b. **Laparoscopic nephrectomy.** Data by Keeley on laparoscopic nephrectomy have shown that complication rates are more likely related to diagnosis rather than operative approach.
c. **Laparoscopic colectomy.** Converted patients experience longer operating times and longer hospital stays than laparoscopically completed patients. There are insufficient data in the literature to assess the complication rates of laparoscopic and converted colorectal procedures when analyzed on an intention-to-treat basis.
d. Given this information, the surgeon, when faced with a difficult operation, should feel justified in converting to an open approach rather than risk a serious complication such as a bile duct injury with much greater clinical consequences.

B. Preoperative Factors Affecting Conversion to Open Surgery

Ideally, it would be possible to accurately predict which patients are highly likely to require conversion for a given laparoscopic operation. This subgroup, once identified, would be advised to undergo an open procedure. There are many studies concerning a variety of laparoscopic procedures that have addressed this issue.

1. **Laparoscopic cholecystectomy.** Investigators have attempted to identify risk factors associated with a high rate of conversion. The results of these studies have been variable; however, most suggest that preoperative factors are, in general, not reliable predictors of conversion. Many different factors have been analyzed:
   a. The presence of **acute cholecystitis** at the time of the surgery has been associated with higher conversion rates in multiple studies.
   b. A **previous history of cholecystitis,** often elicited in older patients, may be associated with the operative findings of a densely adherent gallbladder and a foreshortened cystic duct. In patients without a clear history of cholecystitis, a history of more than 10 attacks of biliary colic may indicate the presence of unrecognized chronic cholecystitis.
   c. Some studies have found that **male gender** is a predictor of higher conversion rates. The reason(s) for this are unclear; it is possible that males may neglect their symptoms for a longer period of time than females and, therefore, present with more inflammation.
   d. **Age greater than 65–70 years** has not consistently been associated with increased rates of conversion.
   e. **Leukocytosis** has been shown, in some studies, to predict higher conversion rates, particularly in patients with acute cholecystitis.
   f. It was once widely held that it was best to delay surgery for acute cholecystitis once the "golden" 72- to 96-hour window had passed. The literature suggests that this may not be the case.
   g. The impact of **obesity** on conversion has been variable. Some authors have postulated that obesity may increase the operative difficulty early in the experience of the surgeon or when proper instrumentation is not available. Problems associated with obesity include difficult cannula placement, obscured anatomy due to excessive intraperitoneal fat, hepatic steatosis interfering with access to the subhepatic area, or difficulty with instrument manipulation in an excessively thick abdominal wall.
2. **Laparoscopic colorectal procedures.** Similar to the situation for laparoscopic cholecystectomy, there are conflicting reports in the literature concerning risk factors for conversion. The following factors have been analyzed:
   a. **Inflammatory conditions**
      i. Diverticulitis: A recent meta-analysis by Gervaz identified diverticulitis as a risk factor for conversion. Several series have reported higher conversion rates with more complicated diverticular disease. The highest conversion rates for diverticular disease have been in the 50% range. Patient selection may also figure heavily in the determination of conversion rates. Series that report lower conversion rates may have avoided patients with complicated disease (large inflammatory masses, colovesical fistulas, etc). One series

reported a conversion rate of 18% for patients with complicated disease as opposed to a rate of 4.8% for uncomplicated patients.

ii. Crohn's disease: Inflammatory bowel disease was not associated with higher conversion rates in a recent meta-analysis.

b. **Surgeon inexperience** (<50 cases) may be associated with higher conversion rates unless patients are very carefully selected.

c. The effect of patient **age** has not been consistent in all studies. The 55- to 64-year-old age group may be at a higher risk due to a higher incidence of diverticulitis.

d. The impact of **male gender** on conversion is also not clear. Some authors have found increased conversion rates in males and have postulated that this finding may be due to a higher prevalence of anatomic difficulties (narrow, deep pelvis).

e. **Obesity** will make a technically difficult case more challenging, similar to laparoscopic cholecystectomy; however there are conflicting data as to whether conversion rates are higher when obesity is specifically studied.

f. **A diagnosis of malignancy** in some colorectal resection series has been associated with a higher conversion rate. A recent meta-analysis of the literature confirms this finding. Notably, there are widely varying reports of conversion rates in oncologic laparoscopic colorectal procedures ranging from 4% to 25%. These disparate results may be related to case selection. A high conversion rate would be anticipated for patients with large lesions and advanced disease.

g. **Rectal resections.** A review of independent reports demonstrate a fairly broad range of conversion rates in regard to rectal resections. The meta-analysis by Gervaz identified anterior resection of the rectum as a risk factor for conversion. Many surgeons have been reluctant to laparoscopically pursue middle and low rectal cancers when performing a sphincter-saving procedure because it is very difficult to divide the distal rectum transversely with existing linear staples. A few authors suggest either a hand-assisted approach for these lesions or a hybrid laparoscopic and open method. The latter hybrid method includes laparoscopic proximal devascularization, splenic flexure takedown, and initial rectal mobilization followed by a planned limited inferior laparotomy through which the procedure is completed.

h. A logistic regression analysis by Schwander showed probabilities of conversion of 3.3%, 8.2%, 4.0%, and 5.8% in the presence of male gender, age (55–64 years), extreme body-mass index (= 27.5), and diverticular disease, respectively. If all four factors were present the probability of conversion increased to 70%.

i. A simple scoring system has been developed by Schlachta to predict conversion rates in laparoscopic colorectal procedures (Table 27.2). For 0 to 4 points, the conversion rate can be predicted to be 1.1%, 3.3%, 9.8%, 25.4%, and 49.7%, respectively.

Table 27.2. Point system for predicting conversion to open surgery in colorectal procedures.

Factor	Points
Diagnosis	
—Malignancy	1
—Benign disease	0
Patient weight	
—<60 kg	0
—60 to <90 kg	1
—90 kg or more	2
Surgeon experience	
— = 50 cases	1
— > 50 cases	0

3. **Laparoscopic nephrectomy.** Factors that predict a more difficult operation and higher conversion rates include inflammatory conditions such as history of pyonephrosis, previous renal surgery, staghorn calculi, polycystic kidney disease, and xanthogranulomatous pyelonephritis
4. **Laparoscopic adrenalectomy.** The size of the adrenal has been shown to have an impact on the conversion rate. Large adrenals (upper size limit varying from 5 to 15 cm) are associated with a higher conversion rate.
5. **Laparoscopic splenectomy.** Large spleens (length greater than 30 cm and weight greater than 3200 g) and platelet count less than 35,000 have been associated with higher conversion rates.

C. Intraoperative Decision Making: Indications for Conversion

1. **Planned conversion. Failure to progress** should be considered an indication to convert. Not surprisingly, the case may fail to progress in a variety of situations.
   a. Adhesions from prior surgeries or from past or recent inflammatory events are a common reason for conversion. In most patients with a history of prior abdominal surgery, the adhesions, if present, can be lysed and the case completed laparoscopically. However, in a significant percentage, the adhesions will preclude the safe and timely laparoscopic completion of a case. Pelvic and lower abdominal adhesions, in particular, can be a problem. Most recommend placing the first port via an open cutdown well away from the site of the prior operations. If it proves very difficult to find a quadrant where there is adequate space for one or several other ports, then the patient should be converted promptly. Like-

wise, once several ports are placed, if the early adhesiolysis efforts suggest that the adhesions are very dense or extensive, then early conversion is advised. In these cases, it may be possible to at least clear the abdominal wall adhesions beneath the planned incision site so that the open entry into the abdomen will be safe and rapid.

b. Acute and chronic inflammatory changes may make dissection very difficult. Inflammation may result in increased vascularity and/or dense adhesions. The extent of inflammation may preclude laparoscopic completion. In the case of laparoscopic cholecystectomy there may be difficulties due to cirrhosis/portal hypertension, a large stone in the neck, or a tethered gallbladder. It can be difficult to grasp an edematous or gangrenous gallbladder. In regard to diverticulitis or Crohn's disease, a large inflammatory mass or especially dense adhesions to the pelvic sidewall, bladder, or gynecologic structures may make safe dissection very difficult. Radiation-related inflammation or adhesions may also be particularly difficult. There are no precise rules as to how much time to allow before converting. The surgeon should take into account the time of dissection versus the progress made as well as the remaining tasks to be completed.

c. **Exposure** may be poor or inadequate. Obesity may preclude placement of the ports due to an excessively thick abdominal wall. It may also prove difficult to obtain an adequate working space via pneumoperitoneum in obese patients. Last, the weight and size of the abdominal structures in some obese patients may not permit completion of a laparoscopic operation. For example, an omentum 1–2 inches thick cannot be easily lifted or reflected using the laparoscopic instruments that are available today. Minor bleeding, although not life threatening, can certainly prevent adequate visualization. Finally, in lengthy cases, it may prove difficult to maintain the pneumoperitoneum because of gas leaks around and through port incisions.

d. **Altered, aberrant, or unclear anatomy.** In patients who have undergone certain prior operations, the anatomy in a region may be altered such that safe laparoscopic dissection may not be feasible. For example, in a patient with a history of gastrectomy and retrocolic gastrojejunostomy, it may not be possible to carry out a right hemicolectomy or a transverse colectomy, which would require dissection near and around the retrocolic window. Acute inflammation, in the absence of prior surgery, may also distort or alter the anatomy. In acute cholecystitis, the cystic duct may become foreshortened with the gallbladder densely adherent to the common bile duct. The anatomy may also vary considerably for certain structures such as the cystic duct. The surgeon needs to be secure as to the location and junction of the common duct and cystic ducts. In cases of unclear anatomy, avoiding injury to the common bile duct should take precedence over avoiding laparotomy.

e. **Surgeon inexperience** is critical. During a surgeon's initial experience with new laparoscopic procedures, the surgeon should be selective and choose uncomplicated cases. Adequately experienced assistants should be secured. The surgeon's threshold for conversion should be low while gaining experience. Once familiar with a given operation and having done a reasonable number of cases, the surgeon can gradually advance to more complicated cases.
f. When is the surgeon "**in difficulty**?" If the surgeon is unable to obtain adequate exposure or traction or "the instruments won't do their job," he or she should consider themselves in difficulty. In addition, if the surgeon is not sure precisely "where they are" anatomically then they are "in difficulty." When in difficulty, one should convert sooner rather than later.

2. **Emergent conversion. Cases in which complications occur that are** not manageable laparoscopically should be immediately converted to an open procedure. Severe bleeding, which may be from a major mesenteric or retroperitoneal vessel, will most often require rapid conversion. It is important to try and limit the bleeding by carefully applying direct pressure to the vessel or area with a laparoscopic instrument while the laparotomy incision is made. Care must be taken not to make the problem worse by tearing or injuring adjacent structures. Abdominal wall port wound bleeding can often be controlled without conversion (see Chapter 21 on port wound bleeding). Certain bowel injuries or other hollow viscus injury may require conversion. Simple enterotomy or colotomy can be repaired via laparoscopically placed sutures or a linear stapler. If the colotomy is in a segment of bowel to be resected, then a loop tie can be used to close the opening. A lengthy or complex bowel injury would almost always mandate conversion. In the case of laparoscopic cholecystectomy, one should convert if there is a suspected biliary injury that cannot be ruled out by cholangiography or if there is a documented biliary injury.
3. Surgeons need to recognize **disease that is not appropriate for minimally invasive methods,** such as gallbladder cancer or colon cancer that invades an adjacent organ such as the kidney, spleen, or bladder.
4. **Technical problems/instrument malfunction** may on occasion mandate conversion. The surgeon must check that the necessary and appropriate laparoscopic equipment is available and in working order before starting the case, and that backups are available for critical pieces of equipment.
5. **Anesthesia-related issues.** Conversion may also prove necessary if the patient is poorly tolerating the pneumoperitoneum. Pulmonary problems such as hypercarbia, hypoxia, and the need for very high inspiratory pressures (to deliver the desired volume of gas) may mandate conversion. This is most likely to occur in patients who have a history of lung disease. Brief pneumoperitoneum "breaks" during which the abdomen is desufflated may permit completion of the case in patients in whom hypercarbia develops. Patients with marginal cardiac function may also not tolerate a pneumoperitoneum. It is

critical that the surgeon and anesthetist communicate well and often during the operation so that timely conversion can be carried out. Please refer to the chapters concerning the cardiac and pulmonary ramifications of pneumoperitoneum as well as the anesthesia chapters for a full discussion of these issues.

D. Selected References

Fried GM, Barkun JS, Sigman HH, et al. Factors determining conversion to laparotomy in patients undergoing laparoscopic cholecystectomy. Am J Surg 1994;167:35–41.

Gervaz P, Pikarsky A, Utech M, et al. Converted laparoscopic colorectal surgery. A meta-analysis. Surg Endosc 2001;15:827–832.

Higashihara E, Baba S, Nakagawa K, et al. Learning curve and conversion to open surgery in cases of laparoscopic adrenalectomy and nephrectomy. J Urol 1998;159:650–653.

Hutchinson CH, Traverson LW, Lee FT. Laparoscopic cholecystectomy: do preoperative factors predict the need to convert to open? Surg Endosc 1994;8:875–878.

Keeley FX, Tolley DA. A review of our first 100 cases of laparoscopic nephrectomy: defining risk factors for complications. Br J Urol 1998;82:615–618.

Pandya S, Murray JJ, Coller JA, Rusin LC. Laparosopic colectomy: indications for conversion to laparotomy. Arch Surg 1999;134:471–475.

Rutledge D, Jones D, Rege R. Consequences of delay in surgical treatment of biliary disease. Am J Surg 2001;180:466–469.

Schlachta CM, Mamazza J, Seshadri PA, Cadeddu MO, Poulin EC. Predicting conversion to open surgery in laparoscopic colorectal resections. Surg Endosc 2000;14:1114–1117.

Schwandner O, Schiedeck THK, Bruch HP. The role of conversion in laparoscopic colorectal surgery. Do predictive factors exist? Surg Endosc 1999;13:151–156.

Strasberg SM, Hertl M, Soper NJ. An analysis of the problem of biliary injury during laparoscopic cholecystectomy. J Am Coll Surg 1995;180:101–125.

Thompson MH, Benger JR. Cholecystectomy, conversion and complications. HPB Surg 2000;11:373–378.

Part III
Postoperative Management of the Laparoscopic Patient

28. Perioperative Fluid Management

Joseph F. Sucher, M.D.
Bruce V. MacFadyen Jr., M.D.

A. Basic Physiology

1. **Total body water** (TBW) is approximately 50%–60% of adult body weight (Figure 28.1).
   a. **Lean body mass** dictates the amount of TBW for any given person. The higher the fat content in an individual, the lower the TBW. In other words, muscle contains more water than fat. Estimation of TBW in obese individuals should be decreased by approximately 10%.
   b. **Sex** influences TBW. Adult females TBW average 50%; males average 60%.
   c. **Age** is a predictor of TBW. Neonate TBW is 70%–80% of their body weight; this decreases through the first year to more closely resemble that of an adult. The elderly person's TBW averages 40%–50% of body weight, accounting for loss of lean body mass.
2. **Body water is divided into three functional compartments.**
   a. **Intracellular fluid (ICF)** accounts for two-thirds of TBW or 40% of body weight.
   b. **Extracellular fluid (ECF)** accounts for one-third TBW or 20% of body weight. This compartment is further broken down into:
      i. Intravascular (plasma), which accounts for 25% of the ECF volume (5% of body weight).
      ii. Extravascular (interstitial), which accounts for 75% of the ECF volume (15% of body weight).
3. **Fluid physiology** is governed by the dynamics of the semipermeable cellular membrane in relation to the osmotically active plasma and cellular solutes.
   a. **Osmotic pressure**
      i. Activity of **electrolytes** (Figure 28.2) within a compartment depends on:
         a. Number of particles present (mmol/L).
         b. Number of electric charges (mEq/L).
         c. Number of osmotically active particles (mOsm/L).
      ii. Normal osmolality is 290–310 mOsm/L.
      iii. **Plasma proteins** are responsible for "effective" osmotic pressure (colloid osmotic pressure).
      iv. **Sodium (Na^+)** accounts for most of the osmotic pressure of the interstitial fluid.

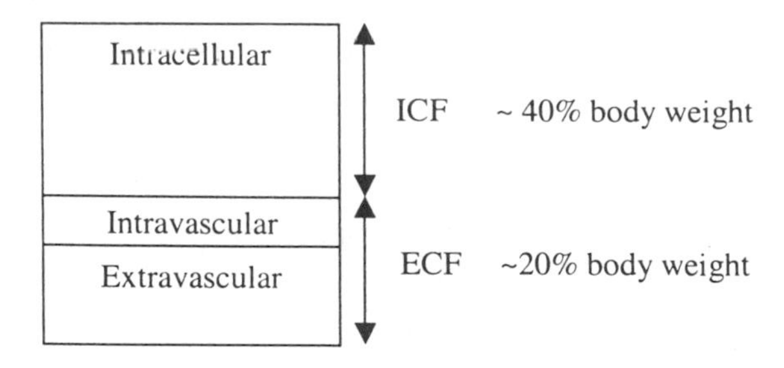

Figure 28.1. Composition of total body weight (TBW) for a typical 70-kg male. ICF, intracellular fluid; ECF, extracellular fluid.

v. **Glucose and blood urea nitrogen (BUN)** increase the osmotic pressure.

b. **Homeostatic control mechanisms**
 i. The **kidney** is the cornerstone of control.
 ii. Extracellular water is controlled largely by **plasma volume** and **serum Na^+**.
 iii. **ADH** and **mineralocorticoids** affect Na^+ and water balance.

4. **Normal exchange of water**
 a. Average consumption is 2000–2500 mL water/day

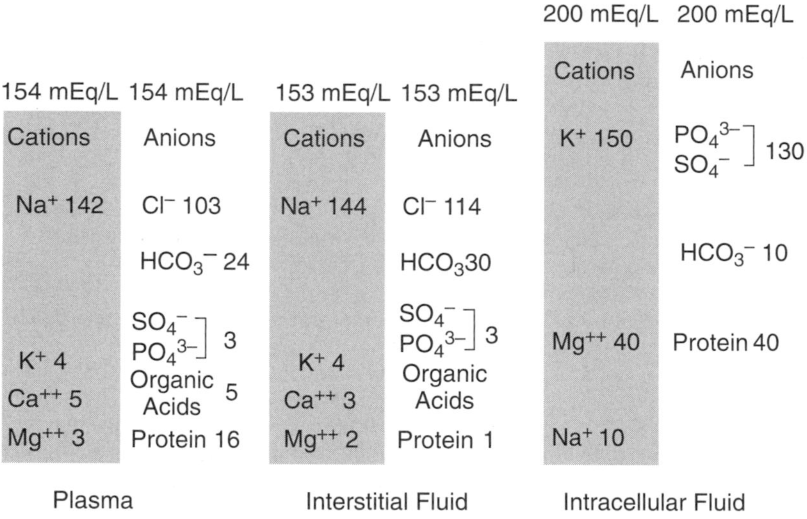

Plasma: Cations (154 mEq/L)	Plasma: Anions (154 mEq/L)	Interstitial Fluid: Cations (153 mEq/L)	Interstitial Fluid: Anions (153 mEq/L)	Intracellular Fluid: Cations (200 mEq/L)	Intracellular Fluid: Anions (200 mEq/L)
Na^+ 142	Cl^- 103	Na^+ 144	Cl^- 114	K^+ 150	PO_4^{3-}, SO_4^- 130
K^+ 4	HCO_3^- 24	K^+ 4	$HCO_3$30	Mg^{++} 40	HCO_3^- 10
Ca^{++} 5	SO_4^-, PO_4^{3-} 3	Ca^{++} 3	SO_4^-, PO_4^{3-} 3	Na^+ 10	Protein 40
Mg^{++} 3	Organic Acids 5	Mg^{++} 2	Organic Acids		
	Protein 16		Protein 1		

Figure 28.2. Electrolyte composition of body fluid compartments.

b. Daily water losses
   i. 250 mL stool
   ii. 800–1500 mL urine
   iii. 600 mL insensible losses
      a. 75% skin
      b. 25% lung
   iv. Minimum excretion is 500–800 mL to excrete products of catabolism.

B. General Principles of Fluid Requirements

1. **Maintenance** requirements. The average 70-kg male requires 2000–2500 mL/day.
2. Underlying **disease process** and **fluid deficit/overload** should be used to make appropriate adjustments in fluid maintenance.
3. **Intraoperative fluid loss**
   a. Blood loss
   b. Extracellular loss (third space)
      i. Edema of the bowel, including luminal sequestration
      ii. Interstitial tissue edema
      iii. Accumulation of fluid in peritoneal cavity
      iv. Wound loss
   c. Evaporative losses (insensible losses)

C. General Principles of Fluid Therapy

1. Approximate **calculation of maintenance** volume for a 24 hour period.
   a. 100 mL/kg for the first 10 kg
   b. 50 mL/kg for the next 10 kg
   c. 25 mL/kg for each 1 kg over 20 kg
2. **Rules of thumb for acute resuscitation**
   a. Replace 3 × volume loss with balanced salt solution [normal saline (NS) or lactated Ringers (LR)].
   b. Large resuscitation volumes with NS can lead to hyperchloremic acidosis.

D. General Consideration in Postoperative Fluid Management

1. Use **NS or LR for the first 24 hours postoperatively.**
   a. Fluid status should be closely monitored to ensure good renal function.

b. With **good renal function** ensured, switch **to D5 $^{1}/_{2}$ NS with 20 mEq/L KCl.**

2. Because of **corticoid release perioperatively**, some patients may develop increased blood glucose, leading to an osmotic diuresis. This hyperglycemia is short lived and usually does not require treatment.

E. Specific Considerations in Perioperative Fluid Management of the Laparoscopic Patient

Most laparoscopic procedures are performed with CO_2 insufflation. CO_2 gas is used in preference to other gases (nitrogen, helium, argon, etc.) because it is inexpensive, easy to handle, noncombustible, and dissolves quickly in plasma (helping to decrease the risk of serious complications due to vascular embolism). However, CO_2 gas, in conjunction with the pressures used to create a surgical pneumoperitoneum, can lead to significant and reproducible hemodynamic changes, as well as reversible acid-base disturbances.

Gaining an understanding of this pathophysiology will aid in the perioperative fluid management of the laparoscopic patient. Three major factors determine the physiologic derangement encountered during typical laparoscopic procedures that utilize CO_2 insufflation to create an optimal operative environment.

1. **Acid-base** changes occur as a direct result of CO_2 diffusion through the peritoneum. This results in a "pseudoventilatory" acidosis, which can be seen by rising end-tidal CO_2 ($ETCO_2$) measurement. This reversible acidosis is significant, but manageable, via increased intraoperative ventilation. An increase in minute ventilation of 25%–35% is typically necessary to prevent significant acidemia. However, even at this rate, $ETCO_2$ concentrations will increase, reaching a plateau at 40 minutes. Thereafter, CO_2 begins to accumulate in the body, the bone being the largest reservoir. This may lead to significant postoperative CO_2 retention and prolonged acidosis. Postoperatively, adequate pulmonary toilet should be ensured to aid in clearing excess CO_2. The mild to moderate degree of acidemia (7.30–7.40) produced during CO_2 insufflation stimulates release of epinephrine from the adrenal medulla, resulting in systemic and pulmonary hypertension, decreased stroke volume, and concomitant tachycardia. If $ETCO_2$ is allowed to rise so much that severe acidemia (<7.30) results, then cardiac dysfunction may ensue, leading to bradycardia, depressed myocardial contractility, and ventricular fibrillation. Of note, increased vagal stimulation as a result of peritoneal stretching has also been implicated as potentially playing a causal role in the development of myocardial dysfunction.
2. **Increased intraabdominal pressures** during routine laparoscopy negatively impact renal blood flow and hepatic portal and arterial blood flow, as well as venous return to the right atrium. These hemodynamic changes create a complex problem in perioperative fluid management. Significant hemodynamic changes occur at pressures above 20 mmHg. With these pressures, there is decreased venous return to the heart

(decreased preload), increased systemic vascular resistance, and increased mean arterial pressure, resulting in decreased stroke volume and, ultimately, depressed cardiac output. This causes an added burden on the already impaired renal and hepatic blood flow, necessitating early intraoperative volume loading. It appears that renal function deteriorates at pressures above 10 mmHg, resulting from decreased renal cortical perfusion. This causes activation of the renin-angiotensin-aldosterone system (Figure 28.3). Therefore, cardiac output, which is depressed during the initiation of the pneumoperitoneum, subsequently increases, likely as a result of surgical stress.

3. **Gas temperature** impacts hemodynamics, as most gas insufflation is not routinely coupled with heating the gas to that of body temperature. During prolonged operations, room temperature gas insufflation is associated with decreased core-body temperature and slower return to normal body temperature than in those patients who undergo warmed gas insufflation. The decreased core-body temperature is associated with decreased cardiac output in addition to decreased renal blood flow.

The goals of **preoperative and intraoperative fluid management** for laparoscopic surgery are based on the same principles that govern traditional open surgical procedure, which are:

a. Optimize adequate oxygen delivery
b. Ensure normal electrolyte concentrations and pH balance
c. Maintain normoglycemia

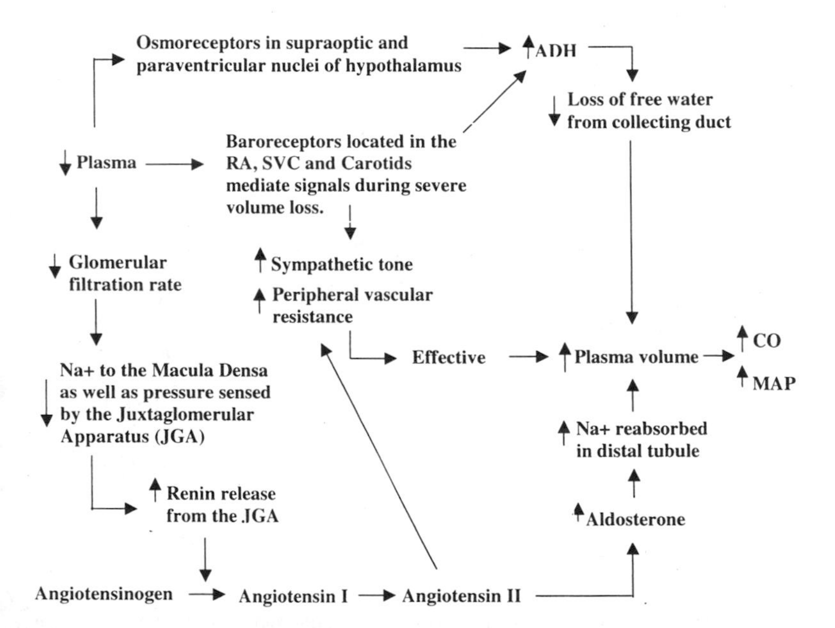

Figure 28.3. The renin-angiotensin-aldosterone system. ADH, antidiuretic hormone; SVC, superior vena cava; MAP, mean arterial pressure.

Contributing factors that together determine the total fluid requirement are

a. The compensatory intravascular volume expansion (CVE) that accompanies anesthesia
b. The preoperative deficit carried into the operation
c. Calculated maintenance fluids
d. Operative losses
e. Fluid redistribution (i.e., third-space losses).

Total fluid requirement = CVE + deficit + maintenance + loss + third space

CVE is that volume needed to compensate for the venodilation and cardiac depression incurred as a result of anesthesia. This is especially important in laparoscopic surgery, as the pneumoperitoneum creates an additional burden, as mentioned above. The fluid deficit is the maintenance volume multiplied by the hours since last intake added to any preoperative external or third space deficits. The losses are any fluid loss (blood, urine, ascites, or evaporative) that occurs during the procedure. During laparoscopic surgery, there is much less evaporative loss compared to that seen during a traditional laparotomy. Third-space losses are difficult to estimate. Traditionally, the anesthesiologist utilizes a variety of vital statistics [mean arterial pressure (MAP), pulse, urine output, etc.] to aid in optimizing the fluid resuscitation.

Typically, the solution of choice intraoperatively is normal saline (NS) or lactated Ringers (LR). In some instances, such as donor nephrectomy, hypertonic saline (7.5%) loading has been suggested to aid in improving renal blood flow. However, this may promote the acidemia caused by the CO_2 gas typically used during these procedures and, thus, should be used with caution.

Postoperative fluid management is directed at preventing further acidemia, as well as ensuring optimal volume loading. LR is a good choice intraoperatively as well as in the early postoperative setting. This balanced salt solution is nearly isotonic and has two important advantages over most other solutions. First, the lactate in this solution directly addresses the acid-base disturbance caused by CO_2 retention. Lactate is readily converted to bicarbonate within the liver, thus improving the acid-base ratio and facilitating return to normal pH. In addition, LR is low in potassium (4 mEq/L). This low level of potassium provides a margin of safety for those patients who may have postoperative impairment of renal function.

Prolonged (>2 hours), complex procedures may lead to extended postoperative myocardial depression owing to the acid-base derangement. During this time, optimal volume loading is key to ensuring adequate cardiac output, and renal perfusion. Urine output (the "poor man's CVP", central venous pressure) should be studiously monitored after these lengthy procedures. As the pH returns to normal, there is a return of cardiac and renal function, which should cause an increase in urine output owing to an improvement in overall hemodynamics.

F. Conclusion

Comprehension of basic physiology is the fundamental cornerstone for the practice of modern medicine. As such, understanding the homeostatic mechanisms for maintaining normal fluid volume, electrolytes, and pH is of critical importance when performing surgery. During laparoscopy, a number of physiologic derangements occur, including decreased plasma pH and reduced effective intravascular volume. In addition, there are direct and indirect alterations in cardiac function, resulting in depressed myocardial contractility with potential for mild to severe cardiac arrhythmias. Continued research into the pathophysiology of laparoscopy is needed to help improve its safety.

G. Selected References

Backlund M, Kellokumpu I, Scheinin T, et al. Effect of temperature of insufflated CO_2 during and after prolonged laparoscopic surgery Surg Endosc 1998;12:1126–1130.

Blobner M, Bogdanski R, Kochs E, et al. Effects of intraabdominally insufflated carbon dioxide and elevated intraabdominal pressure on splanchnic circulation: an experimental study in pigs. Anesthesiology 1998;89(2):475–482.

Dexter SPL, Vucevic M, Gibson J, McMahon MJ. Hemodynamic consequences of high- and low-pressure capnoperitoneum during laparoscopic cholecystectomy. Surg Endosc 1999;13:376–381.

Faber MD, Schmidt RJ, Bear RA, Narins RG. Management of fluid, electrolyte, and acid-base disorders in surgical patients. In: Narins RC, ed. Maxwell & Kleeman's Clinical Disorders of Fluid and Electrolyte Metabolism, 5th edition. New York: McGraw Hill, 1994:1407–1436.

Gunther RA, Wolfe BM. Intraperitoneal carbon dioxide insufflation and cardiopulmonary functions. Laparoscopic cholecystectomy in pigs. Arch Surg 1992;127(8):928–932; discussion 932–933.

Joris JL. Anesthesia for laparoscopic surgery. In: Miller RD, ed. Anesthesia, 5th edition. New York: Churchill Livingstone, 2000:2003–2017.

Junghans T, Bohm B, Grundel K, Schwenk W, Muller JM. Does pneumoperitoneum with different gases, body positions, and intraperitoneal pressures influence renal and hepatic blood flow? Surgery 1997;121(2):206–211.

Kaye AD, Grogono AW. Fluid and electrolyte physiology. In: Miller RD, ed. Anesthesia, 5th edition. New York: Churchill Livingstone, 2000:1601–1606.

Koivvusalo AM, Kellokumpu I, Sheenin M, et al. A comparison of gasless mechanical and conventional carbon dioxide pneumoperitoneum methods for laparoscopic cholecystectomy. Anesth Analg 1998;86:153–158.

Kraut EJ, Anderson JT, Safwat A, et al. Impairment of cardiac performance by laparoscopy in patients receiving positive end-expiratory pressure. Arch Surg 1999;134:76–80.

Saunders CJ, Gunther RA, Wolfe BM. Effector of hemodynamics during laparoscopy: CO_2 absorption or intra-abdominal pressure? J Surg Res 1995;59(4):497–503.

Saunders CJ, Corso FA, Wolfe BM. The effects of CO_2 pneumoperitoneum on hemodynamics in hemorrhaged animals. Surgery 1993;114(2):381–387; discussion 387–388.

29. Ambulation and Early Postoperative Performance Criteria

Frank H. Chae, M.D.
Greg V. Stiegmann, M.D.

A. Postanesthesia Recovery

1. **Goal:** Adequate pain control with prevention of nausea and vomiting. These factors are the keys to success in achieving early postoperative ambulation and discharge from hospital.
2. **Objective evaluation of the recovering patient:** A postanesthetic recovery score is commonly used to evaluate patients recovering from surgery. It includes evaluation of motor activity, respiration, circulation, consciousness, and cutaneous color at timed intervals during the course of recovery. Scores range from 0 to 2 for each category, and a patient must achieve a total score of 10 to be discharged from the recovery room or Post Anesthesia Care Unit (PACU).
3. **Discharge from the PACU:** Discharge from the PACU to a secondary recovery unit (hospital bed or outpatient discharge center) is possible when the following criteria have been met: the acute effects of anesthesia and surgery have resolved, the patient no longer requires continuous monitoring, and the risk of abrupt catastrophes such as airway obstruction or profound hypotension is minimal. The decision to discharge the patient from the PACU usually requires a period of time during which no special intervention is required. For a healthy patient after a minor procedure, this period may be as brief as 20–30 minutes; for a sick patient, a period of several hours may be required. A discharge protocol based on an arbitrary period of observation for all patients is inappropriate.

B. Early Postoperative Performance Criteria

1. **Ambulation:** When the performance criteria (Table 29.1) have been met, the clinical judgment of the health care provider examining the patient becomes the single most important factor in determining the patient's readiness to ambulate.
2. **Steps:** Once the patient's vital signs have been stabilized for at least 30 minutes with pain and nausea well controlled, the oxygen mask is removed. Movement from side to side is encouraged and gradually the

Table 29.1. Early postoperative performance criteria for ambulation.

1. Vital signs satisfactory and stable
2. Ability to recognize time, place, and person
3. Return to preoperative mental state
4. Adequate pain control
5. Adequate treatment of nausea or vomiting
6. Securing all drains, catheters, tubes, and dressings
7. No new symptoms that may threaten a safe recovery
8. Minimal oozing from wound
9. Good circulation in extremities
10. Postoperative orders verified to double-check appropriate restrictions
11. Minimal dizziness or shortness of breath after sitting for 10 minutes

sitting position is achieved. Deep breathing and leg movement are encouraged. While sitting, the patient is allowed time to adjust (10 minutes recommended) and then is carefully helped to their feet. It is critical that all I.V. lines, tubes, catheters, and drains be secured and then prepared for ambulation. A nasogastric tube and all drains attached to wall suction, if present, need to be disconnected from the wall suction and clamped. The urinary drainage bag needs to be attached to the I.V. pole or carried by either the nursing team member or the patient. Next, after establishing that the patient is able to stand, the patient is encouraged to walk with assistance. For outpatient surgery, the patient is urged to take liquid when appropriate and to void an adequate volume. If the patient fails this trial, the entire procedure is repeated from the start with the patient in the supine position with oxygen in place. In this case, the pain or nausea medication may need to be adjusted.

C. Laparoscopic Surgery and Postoperative Pain

1. **Pain after laparoscopy:** Pain after laparoscopy is multifactorial: it results from a combination of inflammation, ischemia, and tissue trauma at the surgical site. Some of the potential sources of pain are unique to laparoscopic procedures whereas others are not.
   - **a. Incision:** Almost all patients have some incisional pain, although usually less than that experienced by patients undergoing the equivalent open procedure.
   - **b. Intraperitoneal insufflation:** Carbon dioxide may cause peritoneal irritation. Subdiaphragmatic free air has been demonstrated as long as 3 days postoperatively in some patients. Gas-induced irritation of the diaphragm and phrenic nerve is the probable cause of shoulder pain after laparoscopy. Ambulation or erect posture tends to exacerbate shoulder pain because intraperi-

toneal gas rises to the diaphragm. Intraabdominal gas should be minimized before closure of the wound.

c. **Intraperitoneal fluid:** Peritoneal fluid accumulation may cause patients to experience pain exacerbation when in the supine position and alleviation of pain when in the sitting or erect position. Blood and other fluids that remain in the peritoneal cavity may irritate the diaphragm and peritoneum while the patient is supine; in the sitting position, irritating fluid accumulates in gravity-dependent areas.

2. **Pain control measures:** In addition to the standard intramuscularly, intravenously, or orally administered pain medications, there are several other strategies that can be employed to limit the pain.
   a. **Local anesthetic:** The use of locally infiltrated 0.25% bupivacaine may aid in postoperative pain management. For optimum benefit, long-acting local anesthetic agents should be injected at the incision sites at the start of the operation.
   b. **Epidural:** Patients undergoing major laparoscopic surgery may benefit from central neuraxial analgesia administered via the epidural route. Epidural morphine or bupivacaine will help control the patient's pain and may decrease the amount of systemic pain medication that is required. A continuous infusion technique alone or in combination with patient-assisted epidural bolus allows greater analgesic titratability than a single epidural bolus injection.
   c. **Patient-controlled analgesia (PCA):** Compared with traditional methods of R.N.-administered on-demand intravenous morphine or meperidine delivery, PCA may provide optimal analgesia with less total drug use, less sedation, less sleep disturbance, and a more rapid return to physical activity. Patients titrate the medication boluses via a programmed pump device. In addition, a baseline continuous infusion can also be given. The amount of drug per bolus and the length of the "lock-out" period can be adjusted. Optimum results depend on the patient's ability to use the device, the dose size, the lock-out interval, and the recognition that a continuous infusion may be indicated.

D. Postoperative Nausea

1. **Risk factors:** Predisposing factors include: young age (peak incidence between the ages of 11–14 years), female gender (three times more common than males), obesity, history of motion sickness, history of postoperative nausea, anxiety, gastric distension from ventilation, nitrous oxide, ketamine, etomidate, neostigmine, and prolonged operation time.
2. **Laparoscopic surgery:** Antiemetic administration is not indicated for all procedures because the side effects of these drugs include sedation to a varying extent. For patients at high risk of postoperative vomit-

ing, prophylactic therapy is justified. Few definitive studies have compared the efficacy of the different antiemetics in use today; therefore, one drug cannot be recommended over another. Because postoperative nausea may have a multifactorial origin, at times a combination of drugs may be required to provide relief.

3. **Opioids:** All opioids may produce nausea and vomiting. Despite these unwanted side effects, it is essential that pain be adequately controlled with opiates because postoperative pain itself may cause nausea. Therefore, control of pain should take precedence over nausea.

E. Venous Thromboembolism

1. **Impedance of venous return:** Several factors in laparoscopic surgery may enhance the risk of venous stasis, deep vein thrombosis (DVT), and subsequent pulmonary embolism. Use of reverse Trendelenburg or modified lithotomy positioning, long operative times, and the elevated intraabdominal pressure all favor pooling of venous blood in the lower extremities.
2. **Prophylactic measures:** Thromboembolic prophylaxis such as pneumatic compression devices and/or subcutaneous low-dose heparin is recommended in the recovery room and on the hospital floor postoperatively until the patient is ambulating adequately. Early ambulation is a key component to DVT prophylaxis.

F. Selected References

Airan M, Appel M, Berci G, et al. Retrospective and prospective multi-institutional laparoscopic cholecystectomy study organized by the Society of American Gastrointestinal Endoscopic Surgeons. Surg Endosc 1992;6:169–176.

Aldrete JA, Kroulik D. A postanesthetic recovery score. Anesth Analg 1970;49:924–934.

Egan KJ, Ready LB. Patient satisfaction with intravenous PCA or epidural morphine. Can J Anaesth 1994;41:6–11.

Hanley ES. Anesthesia for laparoscopic surgery. Surg Clin N Am 1992;72:1013–1019.

Hodgson C, McClelland RMA, Newton JR. Some effects of the peritoneal insufflation of carbon dioxide at laparoscopy. Anaesthesia 1970;25:383–389.

Natof HE. Complications associated with ambulatory surgery. JAMA 1980;244:1116–1118.

Weinmann EE, Salzman EW. Deep vein thrombosis. N Engl J Med 1994;331:1630–1641.

30. Pulmonary Considerations

Desmond H. Birkett, M.D.

The term minimal access has led to the misconception that a laparoscopic operation is a small or minor procedure and as a result is not associated with pulmonary complications. Proponents believe that minimally invasive procedures are associated with fewer postoperative pulmonary complications when compared to results after open operations; however, this has not been definitively proven, thus far. Both open and laparoscopic operations are associated with sizeable decreases in the tidal volume and forced expiratory volume (FEV)-1. It has been demonstrated that, following laparoscopic-assisted colon resection, patients recover their pulmonary function more rapidly than after the same open procedure. This faster recovery may or may not be associated with a lower incidence of actual complications. When considering the possibility of pulmonary complications, after either open or closed procedures, attention must be paid to the magnitude of the operation, the length of the operation, and the expected postoperative course of the patient.

Before undertaking a laparoscopic procedure, as is the case for open operations, the patient's baseline pulmonary function must be considered and assessed. Similarly, postoperative patient management must take the lungs into account and should include measures that will improve postoperative pulmonary function and minimize the chances that a pulmonary complication will develop. Last, all involved in the care of the patient should be "on the lookout" for signs and symptoms of pulmonary complications.

A. Preoperative and Intraoperative Considerations

I. **Preoperative evaluation.** A careful pulmonary history should be taken from every patient undergoing any operation, be it open or laparoscopic. Attention must be given to breathlessness, exercise tolerance, and a smoking history. Enquiries must be made into a history of any prior pulmonary complications that may have occurred with any previous operation. For those patients whose history suggests they may have significant pulmonary compromise, a preoperative assessment with pulmonary function tests may be necessary. Such tests will objectively assess a patient's lung function and will establish their baseline level of function. A formal consultation and evaluation by a pulmonary specialist is advised for patients with severe pulmonary disease and for some patients with moderate disease.

A pulmonologist, where appropriate, will institute a medication regimen that will maximize the patient's function. Furthermore, the pulmonary M.D. will outline a treatment plan for the early postoperative period and can follow the patient after surgery. Rarely, a patient's pulmonary function may be so poor as to preclude the use of laparoscopic methods. Of note on this account, the first decade of advanced laparoscopic procedures has taught us that it is possible to complete laparoscopic procedures in some patients with moderate or even severe pulmonary disease by reducing the maximum insufflation pressures, minimizing the use of Trendelenburg position, and by taking short breaks during which thc abdomen is fully desufflated. It has also been made clear that there is a small group of severely diseased patients who will not tolerate even a low-pressure pneumoperitoneum; early conversion in these cases is necessary and appropriate.

II. **Preoperative dietary instructions.** Probably the most devastating procedure-related pulmonary complication is aspiration at the time of intubation. Although this is primarily an anesthesiology problem, the surgeon can play an important part in its prevention by providing clear and explicit preoperative instructions. The patient groups that are at risk for this problem are those with gastric emptying problems and patients with esophageal abnormalities such as gastroesophageal reflux, achalasia, and esophageal obstruction due to tumor. All patients must be told to stop eating and drinking from midnight on the day of the operation. Patients who have achalasia of the cardia and those with known gastric cmptying problems, such as diabetic gastroparesis, should be placed on liquids for at least 48 hours before the operation in an attempt to empty the esophagus and stomach of residual solid food.

III. **Explanation of operation and anticipated postoperative course.** The need for postoperative pain medications can be reduced if the patient has a clear understanding of the procedure to be carried out, the anticipated postoperative course, and the amount and duration of pain they are likely to experience. Therefore, it behooves the surgeon to spend time with a patient preoperatively going over the planned procedure and these points. The fact that incision-related pain will make deep breathing difficult and that pulmonary complications can develop after surgery should be explained to the patient. The importance of taking adequate pain medication and of using the incentive spirometer, of coughing, and of taking deep breaths postoperatively needs to be stressed. The fact that the patient can lower their chances of developing a pulmonary problem by doing these exercises should be made clear.

IV. **Intraoperative pain management measures.** A patient's postoperative pulmonary management may be significantly improved by the following intraoperative manipulations.

1. Intraoperative infiltration of the port sites with a mixture of short- and long-acting local anesthetics before making the incision and placing the port. Proponents believe that this practice reduces postoperative pain.
2. The intravenous administration of the NSAID (nonsteroidal anti-inflammatory drug) Toradol (15–30 mg) at the end of the opera-

tion can reduce early postoperative pain. It may not be advisable to use Toradol in patients in whom bleeding has been a problem during the laparoscopic operation because of the antiplatelet side effects of this group of drugs. Of note, the bleeding side effects have not been reported with 15 mg Toradol given intravenously. This drug should be avoided in patients with a history of peptic ulcer disease or gastritis.

V. **Prevention of postoperative vomiting.** Vomiting and retching is a major postoperative complication that prolongs the patient's recovery, enhances the postoperative pain, and may result in respiratory complications as a result of aspiration. This complication can be minimized or prevented via the intravenous injection of antiemetics at the end of the operation.

B. Postoperative Management

Careful consideration must be given to the ventilation and oxygenation of a postoperative patient who has just undergone a minimal access procedure. The following must be considered.

I. **Patient monitoring**

1. **Ventilation:** To ensure adequate ventilation in the recovery room, the respiratory rate and the adequacy of ventilatory excursion must be carefully monitored. The ventilatory demands are greater for laparoscopic patients as they recover from the CO_2 pneumoperitoneum when compared to open patients due to the postoperative resorption of residual CO_2 in the abdomen and soft tissues (subcutaneous emphysema), which increases the $PaCO_2$. This excess CO_2 must be "blown off" by increasing the minute ventilation. Signs of inadequate ventilation include restlessness, agitation, and confusion. Pain will also limit ventilation; therefore, an adequate pain management strategy must be in place for these patients immediately after surgery. An arterial blood gas should be obtained if there is doubt about the adequacy of ventilation. At times, reintubation will be necessary.
2. **Oxygenation:** The pulse oximeter presently is the best way to assess oxygenation. The oximeter sensor is placed on the patient's finger or ear. If possible, the oxygenation status of the patient should be followed during transportation to the recovery room. Certainly, in the recovery room continuous pulse oximetry should be employed until the patient is fully recovered. If oxygenation saturation values are not adequate, then oxygen in the form of nasal cannulae or mask should be administered. If, despite these measures, concern remains about the adequacy of oxygenation, then an arterial blood gas analysis should be carried out. A decision can then be made as to whether the patient needs to be reintubated or whether some lesser measures will correct the problem.

3. **Chest X-ray:** There is no reason to perform a routine chest X-ray in the recovery room. However, patients in whom a central venous line was placed in the neck or upper chest during the procedure and those in whom physical examination reveals poor breath sounds in one or the other lung, a chest film is indicated. Also, patients with persistently low oxygen saturation values or who are ventilating poorly merit a chest film. The anesthesiologist may request chest films in laparoscopic patients with severe subcutaneous emphysema that extend up to and include the neck to rule out barotrauma-related pneumomediastinum or pneumothorax. In this setting, provided that physical examination of the lungs is unremarkable and that the patient is well ventilated and oxygenated, chest X-rays are probably not required. An upright X-ray should be taken, if possible, to better demonstrate pneumothorax and pleural effusions.
4. **Electrocardiogram:** Routine EKGs are not necessary for healthy patients whose operation went smoothly and are without signs of cardiac instability. However, an EKG should be obtained in the immediate postoperative period if there are concerns about myocardial ischemia or infarction as well as if there is suspicion of a pulmonary embolus. In regards to the latter, an EKG may reveal right heart strain. Patients with a history of significant coronary artery disease, even if the case went smoothly, should also have an EKG.

II. Postoperative pain management. As already mentioned, pain must be controlled for the patient's comfort and to permit adequate inspiration such that the patient is well ventilated and well oxygenated. Although overmedication with narcotics can suppress respiratory function and must be avoided, it should be noted that it is far more common to undermedicate patients after surgery. In addition to the intraoperative pain measures already mentioned, one or several of the following should be ordered:

1. Patient-controlled analgesia: Usually morphine sulfate or demerol.
2. Intermittent intravenous or intramuscular injections of narcotics.
3. Intravenous or intramuscular Toradol or other appropriate NSAIDs (if not already given at the close of the operation).
4. Epidural analgesia: If an epidural catheter has been placed in the patient, it should be utilized. The anesthesiologist normally manages the use of these lines. This is an excellent way to control pain without suppressing respiratory function.
5. Oral pain medications in appropriate situations:
   a. Narcotic-containing preparations
   b. Nonsteroidal antiinflammatory drugs

III. Pulmonary toilet, chest physical therapy, and pulmonary medications

1. As mentioned, abdominal incisional pain impairs postoperative pulmonary function. An aggressive effort should be made, especially following major procedures, to educate the patient about

the dangers of postoperative atelectasis and infection. The patient and nursing staff should also be instructed as to how they can improve the patient's pulmonary function.

a. Spirometer use for 5 minutes each hour while awake
b. Coughing (after being medicated)
c. Deep breathing
d. Sitting in chair and ambulation
e. Nursing orders to make sure that patient does the above exercises
f. Where necessary, chest physical therapy (PT) should be ordered
    i. Chest clapping combined with the above measures should improve pulmonary function.
    ii. Nasotracheal suctioning helps to clear mucous plugs and to reinflate atelectatic segments.
    iii. Determining vital capacity, FEV-1, and other pulmonary function parameters, at the bedside with a pocket spirometer, can help clarify a patient's problem and also allow their progress to be monitored.

2. In patients with significant pulmonary disease, bronchodilators, aerosolized treatments, and other specific pulmonary medications may be needed. At times, steroids may be needed. Ideally, a pulmonologist would manage or assist with the pulmonary care of these patients. These patients are likely to require continuous oxygen, at least for the first few postoperative days.

C. Pulmonary Complications

I. The type of laparoscopic operation carried out will help determine the chances that a pulmonary complication may develop; some procedures are more likely to be accompanied by pulmonary problems than others. Obviously, a patient's baseline pulmonary function and their general medical condition are also important variables. The physician caring for the patient should be familiar with the patient's history and should carefully review the operative course. The common complications that may be encountered are listed and briefly discussed below.

1. **Atelectasis and consolidation:** Atelectasis is probably the most common pulmonary complication encountered after surgery. These complications are observed more frequently in patients who have undergone long operations or operations in the upper abdomen. Atelectasis can often be avoided with good pain control and aggressive chest physical therapy and pulmonary toilet.
    a. Occasionally, a segment can fully collapse. Careful pulmonary auscultation should alert the physician to this possibility, and a plain chest film should confirm the diagnosis. Nasotracheal suctioning and bronchoscopy are usually required to reinflate the segment in question.

b. An infiltrate or consolidation may develop in an atelectatic area. This is usually heralded by the development of a productive cough or secretions, fever, and an elevated white blood cell count.
   i. If suspected, sputum cultures and Gram stains should be obtained and chest films taken.
   ii. If evidence is found supporting the diagnosis, then an appropriate antibiotic agent should be started.
   iii. An aggressive chest PT program should be initiated, if not already in place.
   iv. At times, in a minority of cases, a bronchoscopy may be indicated.

2. **Pneumothorax:** Postoperative pneumothorax is a rare complication that can occur in patients undergoing an upper abdominal operation during which mediastinal dissection has been necessary. It results most commonly from a pleural injury; direct pulmonary injuries are rare.
   a. The pleural injury permits CO_2 to enter the hemithorax. Because the patient is intubated and receiving positive pressure ventilation, the lung does not collapse. Postoperatively, in most cases, it is not necessary to place a chest tube because CO_2 is rapidly absorbed from the pleural space. The patient must be carefully observed, however, and serial chest films and frequent lung examinations should be carried out.
   b. On the rare occasion when pneumothorax is due to direct pulmonary injury and an air leak develops from the lung, then a true pneumothorax (with air) will develop after surgery. The body is not able to absorb most of the components of air; therefore, a chest tube will be necessary. The surgeon should be alerted to this situation by a deterioration in the pulmonary examination and a worsening of the chest X-ray findings.
   c. Very rarely, intubation or mechanical ventilation-related barotraumas can cause a pneumomediastinum or pneumothorax. A chest X-ray, if it demonstrates the former, will help establish the diagnosis. This diagnosis should be kept in mind especially in patients with significant pulmonary disease who demonstrate poor early postoperative pulmonary function.

3. **Pleural effusion:** A rare complication that can occur in patients who undergo significant mediastinal dissection as well as in those with preexisting significant heart or pulmonary disease. An effusion may also develop in a patient who develops a subphrenic abscess or collection. When suspected clinically, it should be confirmed by X-ray. The cause of the effusion must be carefully considered and then the appropriate treatment initiated. If small and asymptomatic, then observation would most likely be appropriate. Larger effusions, especially in symptomatic patients, may require thoracentesis. Fluid obtained should be sent for the appropriate chemistry tests and for cultures.

4. **Deep venous thrombosis and pulmonary embolus**
   a. **The incidence and prophylactic measures:** Laparoscopic proponents believe that the incidence of deep vein thrombosis (DVT) and pulmonary embolus should be lower after a minimally invasive procedure because patients ambulate sooner and further than after open procedures. However, the argument can be made that the elevated intraabdominal pressure associated with pneumoperitoneum reduces lower extremity venous return, thus increasing the chances of venous stasis and DVT formation. There are not sufficient or adequate data, thus far, to settle this issue. Clearly, these problems do occur, rarely, after minimally invasive procedures. Therefore, the usual preventive measures should be undertaken.
      i. Venous compression boots on the legs applied before the induction of anesthesia have been shown to reduce the incidence of DVT.
      ii. Minidose heparin or similar agents given perioperatively. The first dose should be given well before the incision is made. (Please see the chapter regarding prophylaxis against DVT.)
      iii. Early ambulation.
   b. **Diagnosis:** It is important to consider this diagnosis in patients who develop chest pain (most often pleuritic), dyspnea, tachypnea, apprehension, or hypoxia. It is important to rapidly workup patients suspected of having a pulmonary embolus. The following tests are helpful in this workup.
      i. Arterial blood gases
      ii. Chest films
      iii. Electrocardiogram
      iv. Ventilation/perfusion scan
      v. Pulmonary angiogram
      vi. Pulmonary arterial CT scan
   c. **Treatment**
      i. Supplemental oxygen
      ii. Hemodynamic support
      iii. Intensive care setting
      iv. Intravenous heparin: this should be started before confirmation of the diagnosis in a patient with a high index of clinical suspicion.
      v. Long-term treatment: coumadin therapy
      vi. Placement of an inferior vena cava (IVC) umbrella or filter (if anticoagulation contraindicated)

D. Summary

Although laparoscopic procedures are associated with less pain and more rapid ambulation and mobilization of patients, as well as shorter length of hospital stay, pulmonary complications still pose a threat in the postoperative period. Respiratory function, similar to the situation after open surgery, is temporarily impaired postoperatively. Therefore, surgeons caring for patients who have undergone minimally invasive operations must motivate both patients and staff to make a concerted effort to maximize pulmonary function early after surgery. They must also remain vigilant in regard to the development of pulmonary complications. When a pulmonary problem is suspected, a rapid evaluation and, when indicated, appropriate treatment must be promptly initiated.

E. Selected References

Fitzgerald SD, Andrus CH, Baudendistel LJ, et al. Hypercarbia during carbon dioxide pneumoperitoneum. Am J Surg 1992;163:186–190.

Milsom JW, Bartholomäus B, Hammerhofer KA, Fazio V, Steiger E, Elson P. A prospective randomized trial comparing laparoscopic versus conventional techniques in colorectal cancer surgery: a preliminary report. J Am Coll Surg 1998;187:46–57.

Schauer PR, Luna J, Ghiatas AA, et al. Pulmonary function after laparoscopic cholecystectomy. Surgery 1993;114:389–399.

Schwenk W, Bohm B, Witt C, et al. Pulmonary function following laparoscopic or conventional colorectal resection: a randomized controlled evaluation. Arch Surg 1999;134:6–13.

Wittgen CM, Andrus CH, Fitzgerald SD, et al. Analysis of the hemodynamic and ventilatory effects of laparoscopic cholecystectomy. Arch Surg 1991;126:997–1001.

Wittgen CM, Naunheim KS, Andrus CH, et al. Preoperative pulmonary function evaluation for laparoscopic cholecystectomy. Arch Surg 1993;128:880–886.

31. Resumption of Diet and Recovery of Bowel Function

Robert W. Beart Jr., M.D.
James A. Olson, M.D.

To understand our approach to the resumption of diet and recovery of bowel function, we must first review the physiology and motility of the gastrointestinal tract, focusing on the stomach, small intestine, and colon. Using this framework, a rational algorithm guiding management can be formulated.

A. Physiology and Motility

1. **Stomach:** Anatomically, the stomach is divided into the cardia, fundus, corpus, and antrum. With respect to motility, the stomach is divided into two different regions, the proximal one-third and the distal two-thirds.
   a. The **proximal stomach** has three layers of gastric smooth muscle: an inner oblique layer, a middle circular layer, and an outer longitudinal layer. The proximal stomach has no intrinsic electrical activity, and peristalsis is absent. Muscle contraction in the proximal stomach is tonic and sustained for several minutes, increasing intraluminal pressure. When coupled with distal gastric contraction, this results in a churning action, mixing the food particles and digestive enzymes.
   b. The **distal stomach** is also composed of three muscle layers. The outer longitudinal layer predominates and the inner oblique layer is indistinct. Unlike the proximal stomach, the smooth muscle of the distal stomach has spontaneous electrical activity called pacesetter potentials. These represent partial depolarization of the gastric smooth muscle cells that discharge approximately three times per minute in humans. This intrinsic myoelectric activity originates along the greater curvature of the stomach, which when superimposed by an action potential results in gastric contraction. An action potential is a rapid change in the membrane potential that conducts over a short distance. The peristaltic contraction, once initiated, moves distally toward the pylorus.
   c. Various **neurohumoral agents** stimulate and inhibit gastric smooth muscle contraction (Table 31.1).
   d. **Vagally** mediated reflexes influence gastric contractile activity. Relaxation of the proximal stomach to increasing gastric volume

Table 31.1. Neurohumoral agents that affect gastric motility.

Stimulatory	Inhibitory
Acetylcholine	Vasoactive intestinal polypeptide (VIP)
CCK-8	Secretin
Substance P	Glucagon
Enkephalins	

is termed receptive relaxation. This occurs during ingestion of a meal and allows for gastric accommodation with little increase in intragastric pressure. This reflex is ablated following truncal or proximal vagotomy, resulting in increased gastric pressure following ingestion of a meal. This may also result in accelerated emptying of liquids. However, vagal denervation of the distal stomach may result in delayed emptying of solids greater than liquids.

2. **Small intestine:** The small intestine is composed of three layers: the mucosa, submucosa, and muscularis. The mucosa is responsible for absorption and secretion. The submucosa harbors the blood vessels, lymphatics, and nerves. The muscularis is composed of an inner circular layer and an outer longitudinal layer, which are responsible for intestinal motility. Between these muscle layers lie the Auerbach myenteric plexus and a plexus of ganglia for nonmyelinated nerve fibers.

   Small bowel motility appears to result from a sophisticated harmony between the intrinsic electrical activity in the smooth muscle and the myenteric nerve plexus. The motility of the small bowel promotes contact of enzymes and the ingested material with the mucosa for digestion and absorption, in addition to evacuating harmful material such as bacteria and toxins.

   a. **Intrinsic electrical activity:** Similar to the stomach, the small bowel also has a pacemaker potential; however, it decreases in frequency as one moves distally. It ranges from 11–12 cycles/minute in the duodenum to 8–9 cycles/minute in the ileum. An action potential may be triggered by a food bolus. When an action potential coincides with a slow wave or pacemaker potential, smooth muscle contraction results.
   b. **Myenteric nerve plexus:** The nerves between the muscle layers have efferent, afferent, and intrinsic reflex functions. Each neuron can have multiple dendritic processes that function independently of each other, that is, one inhibitory and one excitatory. This results in a peristaltic reflex with contraction above a site of small bowel distension and relaxation below. The neurotransmitters responsible for inhibition are neither adrenergic nor cholinergic and include vasoactive intestinal polypeptide (VIP), serotonin,

somatostatin, and substance P. Acetylcholine is likely responsible for excitation.

c. **Migrating motor complex (MMC):** The migrating motor complex is a cyclic pattern of spike bursts and muscular contractions present during the fasting state. Four discrete phases are identified that migrate from the duodenum to the terminal ileum:
   Phase I: quiescence, with no spikes or contractions
   Phase II: accelerating irregular spiking activity
   Phase III: activity front, a series of high amplitude, rapid spikes corresponding to strong, rhythmic gut contractions
   Phase IV: subsiding activity

The function of the MMC is unclear. It is thought to propel and remove residual bacteria and cellular debris out of the small intestine to prevent bacterial overgrowth. The cycle lasts approximately 90–120 minutes in humans and is disrupted by feeding. Administration of exogenous motilin, histamine, and metoclopramide can induce the MMC front.

3. **Colon:** Like the stomach and small intestine, the smooth muscle of the colon is arranged in three layers. The inner layer or muscularis mucosa resides beneath the mucosal epithelium. Next is the muscularis propria or middle circular muscle layer. The outer longitudinal muscle layer, however, is grouped into three thick bands, or taenia.

   Similar to the stomach and small intestine, colonic motility is regulated by both myenteric and neurogenic mechanisms. Two groups of plexus exist in the colon. The submucosal (Meissner) plexus lies between the muscularis mucosa and the muscularis propria, and the myenteric (Auerbach) plexus is located between the circular muscle and the outer longitudinal muscle. The Auerbach plexus is intimately involved with colonic motility.

   The primary motor functions of the colon appear to be mixing, slow distal propulsion, and storage. Each segment of the colon appears to have distinct motor activity, independent of each other.

   a. **Myenteric regulation:** Four distinct myoelectric patterns are present that control and regulate the contractile activity of the colon.
      1. **Electrical control activity (ECA):** This is the pacemaker activity of the colon characterized by slow waves. A low-frequency range from 2 to 9 cycles/minute is found in the ascending and sigmoid colon. A higher frequency range, from 9 to 13 cycles/minute, is seen in the transverse and descending colon. ECA alone does not result in a contraction.
      2. **Discrete electrical response activity (DERA)**. Similar to the spike potential in the small bowel, this is a rapid change in the membrane potential. Muscular contraction occurs when a DERA burst is superimposed on ECA. This is thought to be responsible for the mixing action of the colon.
      3. **Continuous electrical response activity (CERA)**. A continuous burst of electrical activity that results in sustained muscular contraction; this also is responsible for mixing.

4. **Contractile electrical complex (CEC)**. Colonic contractions from 25 to 40 cycles/minute; these result in either proximal or distal propagation.

b. **Neural regulation:** Four types of motor nerves have been identified in the colon: cholinergic and noncholinergic *excitatory* nerves and adrenergic and nonadrenergic *inhibitory* nerves. Cholinergic innervation is supplied by the vagus and the sacral nerves. The vagus nerve supplying some of the parasympathetic information is thought to innervate the ascending colon. The main parasympathetic supply arises from nerve roots S2 and S3, innervating the distal colon and rectum. Sympathetic innervation is provided by cell bodies in the dorsal horn of the lumbar spinal cord.

B. Ileus

Ileus is a transient alteration of motility of the gastrointestinal tract following surgery. Clinically this can be defined as the period during which the patient does not pass flatus or stool, characterized by abdominal distension and absence of bowel sounds. After major abdominal surgery the average paralytic state lasts between 0 and 24 hours in the small intestine, from 24 to 48 hours in the stomach, and from 48 to 72 hours in the colon.

1. **Pathogenesis:** Ileus may be caused by peritonitis, spinal cord lesions, electrolyte imbalance, anesthetics, analgesics, surgery, and neural reflexes. Three inhibitory reflexes have been proposed to mediate postoperative ileus. One of these, the long reflex that involves the spinal cord, has been shown to prevent or reduce the development of ileus during spinal anesthesia. Various neurotransmitters and peptides also regulate gastrointestinal motility and may be involved in ileus. Nitric oxide, substance P, and vasoactive intestinal peptide (VIP) are inhibitory neurotransmitters that may prolong ileus. These neurotransmitters may be released systemically following noxious stimuli or local inflammation such as laparotomy.

   Opioids are well-established modulators of the gastrointestinal tract. Mediated by mu receptors, opioids inhibit gastric emptying and cause nonpropulsive smooth muscle contraction that increases intraluminal pressure throughout the gastrointestinal (GI) tract.

2. **Clinical implications:**

   a. **Nasogastric tubes** have been the traditional supportive treatment of postoperative ileus. However, they do not shorten the time to first bowel movement or time to oral diet. It may make those patients with abdominal distension more comfortable. It has demonstrated that the tube is unnecessary in about 85% of patients.

   b. **Ambulation** does not shorten the time of postoperative ileus. Following major abdominal surgery, recovery of intestinal myoelectric activity is similar in patients who began mobilization on postoperative day 1 compared with day 4.

C. Perioperative Management

1. **Analgesia:** As mentioned, **opioid analgesics** have an inhibitory effect on gastrointestinal motility and should be avoided to minimize ileus. Nonsteroidal anti-inflammatory drugs (**NSAIDs**) do not impair overall gastrointestinal motility and are also associated with less nausea and emesis. **Epidural analgesia** has been associated with improved postoperative gastrointestinal function, especially if the epidural catheter is placed above T12; this may be due to blockade of afferent and efferent inhibitory reflexes. In studies where epidural anesthetic administration was compared to systemic opioids, patients who underwent the former had significantly decreased ileus. It also appears that epidural anesthetics plus low-dose opioids offer an advantage over systemic opioids alone.
2. **Early postoperative feeding:** Traditionally, patients were not fed orally until there was evidence, usually in the form of flatus, that the ileus had resolved clinically. There is now evidence that early feeding may, in fact, be beneficial. The presence of food in the intestine leads to the secretion of various intestinal hormones, some of which have a stimulating effect on gut motility. Early feeding may also elicit a reflex response that is propulsive in action. In a select group of colorectal surgery patients, those patients who received early feeding tolerated a regular diet faster and left the hospital 2 days earlier than the patients who were fed late.
3. **Laparoscopy:** Most studies note a shortened postoperative ileus and earlier return to regular diet with laparoscopic procedures when compared to open results. Some have postulated that the reasons for the shortened ileus after minimally invasive surgery are decreased local inflammation and reduced activation of inhibitory reflexes. Wexner has published two randomized prospective studies with conflicting conclusions. The larger study documented an earlier return to normal bowel function after laparoscopic surgery. As a result of the laparoscopic results, to date, most surgeons are feeding their open surgery patients earlier. Fleshman et al. compared the return of bowel function after laparoscopic-assisted and open colon resection done via a small incision (minilaparotomy) and found similar results. The length of the incision may be an important variable in regard to the length of postoperative ileus.
4. **Prokinetic agents: Cisapride** enhances acetylcholine release from the intrinsic neural plexus and acts as a serotonin receptor agonist. Various studies suggest that it significantly reduces ileus when administered intravenously. Adverse cardiac events may occur with cisapride, and it is only available via study protocols presently. **Erythromycin** is a motilin receptor agonist and may induce MMCs. Although erythromycin has been shown to significantly enhance gastric emptying, no clinical advantage related to postoperative ileus has yet been demonstrated. **Metoclopramide** primarily acts as a dopamine antagonist and may alter GI motility; however, it has not been demonstrated to have a significant impact on the length of postoperative ileus.

D. Selected References

Baker R, Senagore AJ, Luchtefeld MA. Laparoscopic-assisted vs. open resection. Dis Colon Rectum 1995;38(2):199–201.

Basse L, Jakobsen DH, Billesbolle P, Werner M, Kehlet H. A clinical pathway to accelerate recovery after colonic resection. Ann Surg 2000;232;51–57.

Bergamaschi RM. Laparoscopic surgery for uncomplicated diverticulitis: advantages? Scand J Gastroenterol 2000;35(5):449–451.

Berthou JC. Elective laparoscopic management of sigmoid diverticulitis: results in a series of 110 patients. Surg Endosc 1999;13:457–460.

Binderow SR, Cohen SM, Wexner SD, Nogueras JJ. Must early postoperative oral intake be limited to laparoscopy. Dis Colon Rectum 1994;37:584–589.

Bohm B, Milsom JW, Fazio VW. Postoperative intestinal motility following conventional and laparoscopic intestinal surgery. Arch Surg 1995;130:415–419.

Brewer DA. Laparoscopic colorectal surgery. Dis Colon Rectum 1995;38:1119.

Bruch HP, Schiedeck THK, Schwandner O. Laparoscopic colorectal surgery: a five-year experience. Dig Surg 1999;16(1):45–54.

Chen HH, Wexner SD, Iroatulam AJN, et al. Laparoscopic colectomy compares favorably with colectomy by laparotomy for reduction of postoperative ileus. Dis Colon Rectum 2000;43(1):61–65.

Davies W. Laparoscopic colectomy shortens postoperative ileus in a canine model. Surgery 1997;121(5):550–555.

Fazio VW, López-Kostner FS. Role of laparoscopic surgery for treatment of early colorectal carcinoma. World J Surg 2000;24(9):1056–1060.

Fleshman JW, Fry RD, Birnbaum EH, Kodner IJ. Laparoscopic-assisted and minilaparotomy approaches to colorectal diseases are similar in early outcome. Dis Colon Rectum 1996;39:15–22.

French Association for Surgical Research, Rouffet F, Hay J-M, Vacher B, et al. Curative resection for left colonic carcinoma: hemicolectomy vs. segmental colectomy: a prospective, controlled, multicenter trial. Dis Colon Rectum 1994;37:651–659.

Gibson M. Laparoscopic colon resections: a five-year retrospective review. Am Surg 2000; 66(3):245–249.

Greenfield L. Surgery: Scientific Principles and Practice. Philadelphia: Lippincott-Raven, 1997.

Holte K, Kehlet H. Postoperative ileus: a preventable event. Br J Surg 2000;87:1480–1493.

Hotokezaka M, Combs MJ, Schirmer BD. Recovery of gastrointestinal motility following open versus laparoscopic colon resection in dogs. Dig Dis Sci 1996;41(4):705–710.

Kockerling F, Scheidbach H, Schneider C, et al. Laparoscopic CSS. Laparoscopic abdominoperineal resection: early postoperative results of a prospective study involving 116 patients. Dis Colon Rectum 2000;43(11):1503–1511.

Kockerling F. Early results of a prospective multicenter study on 500 consecutive cases of laparoscopic colorectal surgery. Surg Endosc 1998;12:37–41.

Kockerling F. Laparoscopic resection of sigmoid diverticulitis: results of a multicenter study. Surg Endosc 1999;13:567–571.

Lacy AM, Garcia-Valdecasas JC, Pique JM, et al. Short-term outcome analysis of a randomized study comparing laparoscopic vs. open colectomy for colon cancer. Surg Endosc 1995;9:1101–1105.

Leung KL. Systemic cytokine response after laparoscopic-assisted resection of rectosigmoid carcinoma: a prospective randomized trial. Ann Surg 2000;231(4):506–511.

Peters W, Bartels T. Minimally invasive colectomy: are the potential benefits realized? Dis Colon Rectum 1993;36:751–756.

Saba AK, Kerlakian GM, Kasper GC, Hearn AT. Laparoscopic assisted colectomies versus open colectomy. J Laparoendosc Surg 1995;5(1):1–6.

Safran DB, Orlando R III. Physiologic effects of pneumoperitoneum. Am J Surg 1994;167:281–286.

Smith AJ, Nissan A, Lanouette NM, et al. Prokinetic effect of erythromycin after colorectal surgery. Dis Colon Rectum 2000;43;333–337.

Steinbrook R. Epidural anesthesia and gastrointestinal motility. Anesth Analg 1998; 86;837–844.

Wexner SD, Johansen OB. Laparoscopic bowel resection: advantages and limitations. Ann Med 1992;24:105–110.

Wexner SD, Johansen OB, Nogueras JJ, Jagelman DG. Laparoscopic total abdominal colectomy. Dis Colon Rectum 1992;35:651–655.

32. Wound Management and Complications

Stanley C. Hewlett, M.D.
Gary C. Vitale, M.D.

There are many advantages of minimal access surgery (MAS) over traditional surgery. In addition to the physiologic benefits associated with avoidance of lengthy incisions, smaller incisions are cosmetically superior. The decreased traumatic insult to the body wall results in less postoperative pain and discomfort as well as decreased narcotic requirement. This minimized traumatic insult is directly related to the shortest, quickest recovery possible followed by an earlier return to the patient's preoperative lifestyle.

Although the incidence of some wound problems may be diminished by avoiding a lengthy incision, MAS wounds are still at risk for traditional wound complications. The MAS surgeon should strive to recognize and treat these complications as early as possible. Further, it should be the goal of the surgeon to minimize the incidence of these complications via meticulous attention to wound management and closure during the operation.

A. Infectious Wound Complications

It has been suggested that one of the advantages of MAS is a decreased rate of wound infection, although there have been no randomized controlled trials that specifically considered this issue. One mechanism by which MAS methods may be associated with fewer infections is better preserved postoperative cell-mediated immune function. It must be remembered that the choice of surgical access method is only one of a number of variables that influence the development of wound infection. To minimize wound infection rates, the MAS surgeon should be well informed of the various factors that may increase the chances of an infection developing.

1. Risk factors
    a. Patient-related
        i. Age
        ii. Chronic illness
        iii. Diabetes
        iv. Malnutrition
        v. Hypoxemia
        vi. Shock
        vii. Untreated active infections (pulmonary/urosepsis)

Table 32.1. Risk of infection in surgical wounds.

Surgical wound classification	Risk of Infection (%)
Clean	1–2
Clean-contaminated	2–4
Contaminated	7–10
Infected	10–40

viii. Hypochlorhydria
ix. Wound classification (Table 32.1)

b. Iatrogenic
i. Steroids or other immunosuppressive medications
ii. Inadequate sterile technique
iii. Excessive operative times
iv. Surgical technical errors. Less than optimal surgical technique may result in hematomas, seromas, and unnecessary tissue trauma, which decrease the size of the bacterial inoculum required to cause a wound infection. Inappropriate cautery use, excessive force in tissue handling, disregard for hemostasis, and unnecessary residual foreign bodies are to be avoided.

2. Prevention
a. Optimize patient and iatrogenic risk factors, where feasible (see above).
b. Appropriate use of systemic perioperative antibiotics (see Chapter 5). A larger bacterial inoculum is necessary for an infection to develop when perioperative antibiotics are used. Routine antibiotic prophylaxis is advised when performing procedures associated with increased rates of simple wound infections, as well as for operations associated with lower rates of infections where the development of an infection can have devastating results (vascular prosthetics).
i. It is important to achieve therapeutic serum levels before making the incision by administering the intravenous antibiotics well before the start of the operation.
ii. Use an antibiotic that will adequately cover the organisms typically found in wound infections that develop after the procedure in question.
iii. Re-dose as needed during surgery depending on the half-life of the antibiotic.
c. Operative site preparation. Consider a preoperative shower treatment. Decreasing excess organic debris (exfoliated skin cells, oils, dirt, etc.) at the skin surface that falls within the operative field facilitates the antiseptic action of iodophor skin prep. The reduction of skin flora bacterial counts at the planned incision site reduces the extent of bacterial contamination of the wound.

i. Avoid unnecessary trauma from hair removal techniques. If hair removal is necessary, use electrical clippers immediately before entering the operating room (OR). Shaving is associated with a 5- to 10-fold increase in wound infection rates, especially if done before the day of surgery. The minute trauma from a razor leads to microexudative wounds with higher bacterial counts as well as an increase in skin surface organic debris. Wet shaving (with soapy water) decreases the amount of trauma and also controls dispersion of loose hair. Loose hair in the operative field can potentially carry resident skin flora into the depths of surgical incisions.

ii. Avoid abrading or massaging the skin after it has been prepped (i.e., wiping off antiseptic) because this decreases the antiseptic activity and, simultaneously, delivers an increased number of bacteria to the skin surface from deep within skin appendages. However, removal of pooled iodophors is recommended to prevent skin irritation.

iii. Strict adherence to the standard principles of sterility. There is always a chance the patient may require conversion to an open approach. Thus, the patient should be prepped widely; this will greatly decrease the probability that the incision required for conversion will extend beyond the prepped area.

iv. Utilize meticulous surgical technique. Poor surgical technique may result in hematomas, foreign bodies, deadspace, and retained necrotic tissue, which impair host immune responses and increase the chances of infection by decreasing the size of bacterial inoculum required to generate a wound infection.

(a) Preoperative local anesthetics that contain epinephrine can increase the wound infection rate due to impairment of local blood flow. Consider avoiding them in patients with multiple risk factors for wound infection.

(b) Make adequate-sized skin incisions. The integrity of the pneumoperitoneum should not be maintained at the skin level via an overly snug port incision that may result in ischemia and marginal wound necrosis. An overt wound infection is more likely to develop in this setting; alternately, a subclinical infection may arise that is related to the pronounced scar that may develop in these wounds.

(c) Dressings. Occlusive dressings are used to increase or maintain wound humidity in order to encourage reepithelialization. This humid setting is also conducive to bacterial overgrowth. After the first 24–48 hours, the wound, which should be reepithelialized by that point, should be left open to the air.

d. Consider visceral preparation. A bowel preparation may reduce perioperative infectious complications in colon surgery. Bowel preparation components include:

        i. Mechanical bowel preparation
        ii. Antibiotic bowel preparation
3. Early postoperative wound infections. These extremely rare infections are associated with particularly high morbidity and mortality rates due to two factors: first, these infections are often aggressive and potentially lethal, and, second, they often go unrecognized until their later stages.
    a. Presentation.
        i. First 24–48 hours after surgery
        ii. Wound signs (may be subtle or absent)
            (a) Erythema
            (b) Edema
            (c) Tenderness
            (d) Dishwater discharge (*Streptococcus*)
            (e) Crepitance (*Clostridia*)
        iii. General signs (usually subtle, if present)
            (a) Anxiety, feeling of impending doom
            (b) Tachycardia
            (c) Tachypnea
            (d) Fever
        iv. Progression beyond these early stages quickly leads to overwhelming sepsis, shock, and death.
    b. Management
        i. Diagnose early.
            (a) Maintain a high index of suspicion.
            (b) Carefully examine all wounds, especially those of patients who manifest a fever in the early postoperative period.
            (c) Gram stain suspicious discharges.
        ii. Immediate surgical treatment: incision and debridement (I&D) emergently at the bedside or in the OR if necessary.
        iii. Use appropriate intravenous antibiotics.
4. Regular postoperative wound infection/abscess
    a. Presentation
        i. 5–10 days postoperative
        ii. Wound signs
            (a) Erythema
            (b) Tumescence
            (c) Tenderness
            (d) Warmth
            (e) Purulent discharge
        iii. General signs
            (a) Fever
            (b) Fatigue
            (c) Hyperglycemia
        iv. Left untreated, these can be life-threatening, particularly in patients with multiple risk factors and compromised host defenses.
    b. Management

- i. Fully open the wound (at the skin and subcutaneous level).
- ii. Drain abscess adequately (break up loculations and all purulent pockets).
- iii. Assiduous wound care (debridement, where necessary, and frequent dressing changes).
- iv. Antibiotics in patients with the following risk factors:
  - (a) Diabetes
  - (b) Immunosuppression
  - (c) Prosthetic heart valves or murmurs requiring prophylaxis
  - (d) Those with multiple risk factors
- v. Antibiotics in wounds that manifest:
  - (a) Necrotic fascia
  - (b) Necrotic subcutaneous tissue

B. Port Site Bleeding Complications

Bleeding complications of surgical wounds either occur during or after surgery (see Chapter 21).

All patients are at some risk for bleeding complications; however, those with hemostatic disorders are at increased risk. Such conditions may be the result of a disease process (e.g., cirrhosis-induced liver dysfunction), an inherited disorder (hemophilia, factor deficiencies, or von Willebrand's disease) or related to a medication [aspirin, selected nonsteroidal antiinflammatory drugs (NSAIDs), coumadin, or heparin]. The surgeon should strive to limit and, hopefully, prevent perioperative bleeding. Preoperative identification of the high-risk patient population is a critical step in this process.

1. Prevention
   - a. Identification of patients at risk for perioperative bleeding.
     - i. History and physical examination. Pertinent questions in regard to bleeding and coagulation:
       - (a) Easy bruisability
       - (b) Voluminous bleeding with incidental trauma or during menses
       - (c) Bleeding gums on tooth brushing
       - (d) Personal or family history of bleeding disorders
       - (e) History of unusual hemarthroses
       - (f) Jaundice
       - (g) Liver/spleen disorders
       - (h) Medication history: use of anticoagulants, NSAIDs, or other medications that may interfere with hemostasis
     - ii. Patients with a suggestive history or physical examination findings should undergo a laboratory analysis.
       - (a) Standard quantitative evaluation
         - (i) Prothrombin time (PT/INR)
         - (ii) Partial thromboplastin time (APTT)
         - (iii) Platelet count

(b) Specialized evaluations
(i) Bleeding time: assesses platelet function
(ii) Factor assays: quantitative functional assay of the various clotting factors
(iii) Thromboelastography: analyzes the dynamics of functional clotting

b. Optimize patients documented to have abnormal hemostasis.

i. Self-correction of a medication-induced therapeutic coagulopathy.

(a) Coumadin (warfarin): stop warfarin 4–5 days before surgery. Depending on the indication for anticoagulation and the recommendations of the patient's physicians, in-hospital intravenous heparin for 2–3 days immediately before the operation (after the coumadin has been stopped) may be advised (a so-called heparin window). The heparin anticoagulates the patient but is rapidly reversible (within 3–4 hours time) once stopped before the operation. Furthermore, warfarin should be withheld from patients in the early postoperative period, or the dose reduced initially if general anesthetics that affect liver drug metabolism were administered to the patient (e.g., Propofol). An exaggerated warfarin effect due to increased drug half-life secondary to decreased hepatic metabolism can be anticipated in this setting.

(b) Aspirin (ASA): aspirin has an **irreversible** effect on platelets. The induced platelet dysfunction is "corrected" only when new platelets are released. For this reason, ASA-containing medications should be stopped 10 days before surgery.

(c) Ibuprofen: this drug's antiplatelet effect is reversible. Although most authorities advise stopping ibuprofen 5 days before surgery, a 6- to 12-hour period off this medication should be adequate.

ii. Active reversal of a medication-induced therapeutic coagulopathy: in situations where it is not possible to delay surgery while the medication-induced coagulopathy autocorrects, it is usually necessary to give vitamin K or to replace the clotting factors via transfusion of fresh frozen plasma or other blood products. Although minimizing the coagulopathy is almost always appropriate, it should be recognized that there is a risk of possibly overshooting the baseline and rendering a patient hypercoagulable. Thrombotic complications are sometimes a greater concern than the risk of bleeding complications. A recommendation from a hematologist or other specialist managing the patient's antithrombotic treatment in regard to reversing the coagulopathy can be helpful. However, when faced with active or uncontrolled bleeding, reversal is always necessary.

(a) Warfarin
   (i) Parenteral vitamin K.
   Effects are unpredictable, require a functional liver, and need several hours to days for complete correction of coagulopathy.
   (ii) Fresh frozen plasma (FFP) transfusion (factors II, VII, IX, X).
   FFP effects are temporary (due to the 4-hour half-life of factor VII), and therefore repeated administration of FFP or other blood products is required.

iii. Correction of a naturally occurring coagulopathy, possibly of unknown etiology.
   (a) Consult a hematologist if needed.
   (b) Use FFP, vitamin K, and/or other blood products.
   (c) A minimum of 30% clotting factor activity is necessary for adequate perioperative hemostasis.

c. Meticulous operative technique: abdominal wall vascular injuries may occur during port insertion. Most commercially available ports utilize a sharp trocar of some type to penetrate the abdominal wall. Trocar designs vary considerably; the surgeon should be familiar with the mechanics of a given trocar before using it in humans. There are certain basic guidelines that should be followed when inserting a port, regardless of the specific type of port/trocar system that is being used.
   i. Abdominal wall penetration should never be tangential. The trocar and port should enter the abdomen at a 90° degree angle to the skin surface. Angled or tangential insertion toward the intended operative field has been erroneously recommended to facilitate the insertion of instruments into the proper quadrant. However, angled insertion increases the volume of tissue that the trocar must traverse and thereby increases the chances of vascular injury. Further, when an injury does occur, the bleeding is more difficult to control when the path of the port is angled.
   ii. Complete the dermal incision before utilizing the trocar to penetrate the fascia. Although using the trocar to divide the dermis does not increase the chances of a major abdominal wall vascular injury, it does increase the chances of incurring a visceral injury because of the increased force required to traverse the dermis. Trocar penetration of the dermis may also result in subcutaneous bleeding from a dermal or subdermal vessel (usually a vein).
   iii. The used of preincisional local anesthetics with epinephrine may delay the onset of bleeding. The port, when in place, may also prevent bleeding via direct pressure against the wound's circumference. At the end of the case, the ports should be removed under videoscopic guidance. After removal, the port wound should be briefly observed from the inside and outside for bleeding.

d. Avoid injury to named vessels of the body wall.
   i. Epigastric artery
      (a) Any trocar placed within the rectus sheath in the paramedian anterior abdominal wall risks injury to this vessel. Ports should be placed either in the midline or lateral to the edge of the rectus sheath to eliminate the possibility of epigastric injury. When it is necessary to insert a port through the rectus muscle, an open cut-down technique is best employed.
      (b) Caution should be used in cases where a patient may have had an interruption in collateral epigastric flow [previous Kocher incision, or coronary artery bypass graft (CABG) with internal mammory artery (IMA) graft]. In these cases, an injury to an uncollateralized epigastric can result in abdominal wall ischemia with poor wound healing and even complete necrosis of the affected portions of the abdominal wall between the injury and the site of disruption of the collateral epigastric artery.
   ii. Intercostal arteries
      (a) Thoracic ports should be placed over ribs to avoid injury to these vessels, which run below each rib.
      (b) Blunt-tipped ports should be used instead of sharp cutting ports.

2. Management of bleeding
   a. Intraoperative abdominal wall bleeding. Significant bleeding that occurs as a result of trocar insertion can be controlled via definitive or temporizing measures when recognized. If the latter course is chosen, it must be remembered that definitive control must be obtained at the end of the case.
      i. Immediate external direct approach
         Remove port, enlarge port incision, and identify and ligate the injured vessels.
      ii. Temporary MAS techniques
         (a) Port manipulation
            (i) Torquing of port so as to tamponade the bleeding vessel (most often not successful for transected epigastric vessels)
            (ii) Use of conically shaped port anchoring device to tamponade the bleeding
               1. Similar to Hasson trocar shape
               2. Often threaded
         (b) Foley occlusion (via inflated balloon) of wound
         (c) Transabdominal wall horizontal mattress sutures (port left in place)
            (i) Two sutures placed: one cephalad and the other caudad to the port site so as to encircle the epigastric vessels in two places (thus blocking inflow and outflow to the injured vessels).

(ii) Number 2 nylon or similar heavy monofilament suture with largest curved needle (2.5–3 inches long, usually used for placement of retention sutures).
(iii) Needle straightened.
(iv) Needle passed from outside to inside via laparoscopic visualization just lateral to the vessel location.
(v) Needle grasped via laparoscopic instrument, pulled into the abdomen, carefully turned around, and then passed back outside at a more medial point to encircle the vessel.
(vi) Two external ends are tied snugly over a gauze buttress to occlude the injured vessel.

(d) Endo-Kitner pressure (intercostal vessels)

iii. Definitive MAS techniques (employed at the time injury is recognized)
(a) Endoclose (USSC) hemostatic stitch
(b) Bipolar cauterization of smaller vessels
(c) Endoclip

iv. Delayed definitive control at the end of the case (via external means, 2.a.i. above)

b. Postoperative bleeding and hematoma

i. Hemodynamically significant postoperative bleeding requires rapid and definitive surgical control no matter the source (intraabdominal or abdominal wall). Such control should be obtained in the OR setting.
(a) Substantial abdominal wall bleeding may dissect in the abdominal wall to the flank, back, or groin if the peritoneal and skin incisions have been well closed. In this case, large ecchymoses and purple-colored discoloration of the abdominal wall, flank, or back may be noted.
(b) Abdominal wall bleeding may also collect in the abdomen. In this case, physical examination may reveal mild to moderate distension and, at worst, minimal tenderness because blood is often not irritating and is relatively innocuous to the peritoneum.
(c) At the time of reoperation, clotted and extravascular blood should be evacuated from the patient (consider using a cell-saver device where reasonable).
(d) Postthoracoscopy port site bleeding usually presents as a hemothorax.

ii. Significant abdominal wall bleeding should be controlled via ligation, cauterization, or other direct means through the open wound (often enlarged). Temporarily, external direct pressure can be used to control the bleeding. Bleeding from the abdominal wall may track between the fascial sutures to the subcutaneous planes and then to the outside via the skin incision, in which case the dressing will be stained or saturated.

iii. Oozing from multiple surgical sites (and possibly I.V. sites) should raise the suspicion of an undiagnosed bleeding disorder.
   (a) Apply pressure in 5-minute intervals.
   (b) Warm the patient.
   (c) Initiate a laboratory evaluation and correct the coagulopathy once it has been documented.

C. Port Site Seroma

This unusual complication of port wounds can be difficult to distinguish from a wound infection, hematoma, or even an early postoperative hernia. The typical presentation is a painless ballotable swelling at a healing port site (usually 1–5 days postoperatively). If a hernia is suspected, transcutaneous ultrasonography via an appropriate transducer (8–10 MHz) should reveal if the fascial closure is intact. Signs of inflammation should be absent in an uncomplicated seroma; if present, a wound infection should be ruled out with aspiration and gram stain, or even an I&D of the wound. Obviously, this should be done only if a hernia is not present. Seromas usually resolve spontaneously within days unless complicated by a superinfection. On occasion, however, they may persist for weeks or longer. Repeated aspiration of simple seromas followed by pressure dressings may enhance resolution but introduces the possibility of bacterial seeding. Close observation, provided the patient has been well educated as to what are the worrisome signs and symptoms, seems to be just as effective.

A feared complication related to the presence of ascites has been uncontrolled leakage of ascitic fluid from the wound. This rare complication can be avoided by closing all fascial port sites, combined with aggressive medical management of ascites perioperatively. However, infectious and bleeding complications occur more frequently in patients with ascites.

D. Poor Cosmesis

Some patients clearly are interested in the cosmetic benefits that MAS approaches offer in regard to avoiding a lengthy incision. However, the cosmetic results can be further improved if the location and orientation of the port incisions are carefully considered and care is taken when closing the wounds.

1. Incision placement
   a. Orientation of the axis of incision should be in the direction of Langer's lines of tension. This will minimize the intrinsic potential of the wound to gape. This also facilitates adequate skin edge apposition during wound closure and decreases the tension needed to close the wound, no matter which method is used (Steri-strip, adhesives, staples, or suture).

   b. Placement of the incisions in prominent skin creases makes them less apparent. Using the recessed superior aspect of the umbilicus, or even the base, rather than the inferior skin trough will obscure this incision from normal view. This is a bikini-friendly umbilical incision.
2. Incision size. In regard to port wound size, smaller is not necessarily better. The incision should be large enough to accept the selected trocar size (3, 5, 10, or 15 mm, etc.) easily, without any marginal incisional pressure. There should not be a pneumoperitoneal seal at the level of the skin. Excessive pressure of the trocar against the skin will result in compromised wound circulation and possible marginal necrosis of the skin wound. This is manifested as a postoperative incision that appears excessively reddened and hypertrophic.
3. Incision closure.
   a. Closure of a well-developed or pronounced Scarpa's fascia will reduce the incidence of a divit scar. The sutures used for closing these deeper layers should not entangle the subcutaneous tissue.
   b. Several options are available for skin closure. Simple tape, wound adhesives, staples, and sutures each have unique advantages. Familiarity with more than one technique is recommended. Of course, the use of meticulous surgical technique when closing the wound yields the best results. The care of the abdominal wound should not be left to chance. The surgeon's recommendation for the wound dressings should be clearly communicated to the ancillary staff as well as the patient.

E. Neuralgia

This disappointing complication can be very difficult to manage for the surgeon. Before referral to a pain center, the surgeon should evaluate the patient to ensure that there is no other local wound process to account for the patient's symptoms such as infection, hernia, or tumor recurrence. Initial treatment includes reassurance and oral nonnarcotic analgesics. Trigger point injections can help define the potential benefit of neuroma excision or permanent neurolysis injections. In regard to thoracoscopy, neuromas can be prevented by avoidance of the subcostal neurovascular bundle during trocar insertion.

F. Selected References

Balli JE, Franklin ME, Almeida JA, Glass JL, Diaz JA, Reymond M. How to prevent port-site metastases in laparoscopic colorectal surgery. Surg Endosc 2000;14(11): 1034–1036.

Fry DE. Surgical Infections. Philadelphia: Lippincott-Raven, 1995.

33. Postoperative Restrictions After Laparoscopic Operations

Robert N. Cacchione, M.D.
Gerald M. Larson, M.D.

The postoperative restrictions and limitations for seven frequently performed laparoscopic procedures are described in this chapter. For each operation, we give guidelines for six activities of daily living usually covered in the doctor's discharge instructions. Although there are increasing amounts of data to guide the surgeon in managing patients before and during operative procedures, there are few published data to assist in managing patients postoperatively. The information we present here represents what we believe to be reasonable discharge guidelines based on our experience and judgment. We note instances where published data exist.

A. Laparoscopic Cholecystectomy

1. Diet: After leaving the recovery room, the patient can start on liquids and be advanced to a regular diet as tolerated. Most patients tend to stay on liquids or a light diet the first day. An occasional patient experiences nausea related to either anesthesia or the procedure and needs intravenous fluids and an antiemetic for a variable period of time. There is also a 3%–10% incidence of a postoperative ileus, which will postpone the onset of appetite and eating.

2. Bath/shower: Wait 24 hours for skin incisions to seal and then bathe as patient's activity level allows.

3. Activity: There is no restriction to walking and stair climbing. The patient should use incisional pain as an endpoint to exertion. We instruct our patients that if a particular activity hurts, do not do it. Moderate lifting is not harmful and should be governed by incisional discomfort. Most patients can easily lift 25 pounds by the first week and resume preoperative activity by 2 weeks.

4. Exercise/sport: Walking is preferred to running for the first 10–14 days, but running would not interfere with patient healing if this activity is not painful. We usually advise patients against weight lifting and contact sports for 4 weeks in most instances; after 4 weeks, normal activity and exercise are encouraged.

5. Driving: Resumption of driving depends on mobility, reaction time, and the patient's ability to respond to any road hazard. Before driving, the patient should sit in the car, behind the steering wheel, and go through the motions of

stepping on the gas and brake pedals and should also use the shift. Similarly, the patient should turn to the right and look out the rear window of the car. Driving can be resumed provided that these activities are not painful. For most patients who were driving before the operation, their reflexes and faculties will be back to baseline in 1–2 weeks.

6. Return to work: The decision to return to work is multifactorial and based on the physical demands of the job, the patient's motivation, and the duration of sick time allowed by the employer or the insurer. If the patient follows an uncomplicated course and has a sedentary or nonlifting job, there is no physiologic basis for not working during the first week postoperatively. Frequently fatigue is a factor and patients often choose to resume work on a half-time basis or on light duty. In a comparative study of American and French patterns of postoperative care regarding this question, we found that after laparoscopic cholecystectomy 63% of the Americans and 25% of the French returned to work within 14 days of the operation.

B. Inguinal Hernia Repair

1. Diet: Laparoscopic inguinal hernia repair is performed on an outpatient basis at our institution, and as such, most patients are discharged within several hours following their procedure. These patients may begin a liquid diet immediately upon discharge from the recovery room. Their diet is advanced to regular food as tolerated. Nevertheless, most patients tend to have some degree of nausea related to the anesthesia, and for the first postoperative day tend to stay on a liquid or light diet after which they return to a regular diet. Unless pain/medication-related, it is unusual for hernia patients to develop an ileus or dietary issues.

2. Bath/shower: Nearly all patients are closed with subcuticular stitches. They are instructed to wait 24 hours before removal of bandages and then are allowed to bathe or shower.

3. Activity: This is certainly the most controversial area following laparoscopic inguinal hernia repair. Our practice is to not restrict walking or stair climbing. We instruct patients to use their incisional pain as an endpoint to exertion. Patients are instructed to slowly introduce physical activity into their daily routine over the first week. They are instructed not to engage in physical activity that causes an increase in incisional pain. Most patients are able to lift moderate amounts (i.e., 5–10 pounds) by the end of the first week. By the end of the second week, patients should have resumed nearly the full range of their daily activities.

A recent study compared laparoscopic to open repair of inguinal hernias in which patients completed a 6-minute treadmill test. The results suggest that it is reasonable to expect patients to return to usual daily activity in 1 week. This level of activity is separate from maximally strenuous physical activity.

4. Exercise/sport: For the first 2 weeks following laparoscopic inguinal hernia repair, we encourage the patients to engage in walking and stair climbing. Lifting during this period should be limited to 5–10 pounds. Patients may resume graded increases in activity as the incisional discomfort permits. After 2 weeks of a limited exercise regimen, patients may resume running, likewise

on a graded schedule of introduction. After 1 month, a gradual schedule of weight lifting and contact sports may be resumed. There are only occasional patients who, because of continued discomfort, are unable to resume full activity at the end of 1 month following laparoscopic inguinal hernia repair.

5. Driving: Resumption of driving depends on mobility, reaction time, and the patient's ability to respond to any road hazard. For most patients who were driving before the operation, their reflexes and faculties will be back to baseline by 1–2 weeks. As a general rule, patients who require narcotic analgesia should not be operating motor vehicles while under the influence of these prescription medications. As mentioned in the previous section, the patient should not begin driving if the physical activities required (movements of feet, arms, and upper torso) are painful.

6. Return to work: As with laparoscopic cholecystectomy, the decision to return to work is multifactorial and based on not only the operation performed but also the patient's desire to return to work as well as the nature of the patient's job. Those patients who work at sedentary or nonlifting jobs are often able to return to work during the first week postoperatively. Those patients who have occupations that require more vigorous activities, such as restaurant waiters/waitresses or store clerks, may be comfortable enough to return to work at the end of 2 weeks. For those patients who have highly physically demanding jobs, such as construction workers, police officers, and fire-fighters in whom good physical conditioning is necessary for the safe execution of their job, we sometimes recommend longer periods of abstinence from work, ranging up to 4 weeks.

As a general rule, however, most patients are able to return to work when they are largely painfree. Frequently this occurs at approximately 2 weeks postoperatively. This notion is supported by many of the studies comparing laparoscopic and open inguinal hernia repairs in which return to work is studied as a parameter.

C. Ventral Hernia Repair

1. Diet: At what point the patient is ready for liquids and solid food after ventral hernia repair depends on the function of the gastrointestinal tract and whether an ileus is present. In our experience, this time interval is quite variable because it is related to the size of the hernia(s), the difficulty of the dissection, the extent of adhesions, and the duration of the operation. Most of these patients will be admitted to the hospital for 1 day or more, except those with small (3–5 cm) hernias that are readily repaired on an outpatient basis. If ileus and nausea are not present, these patients can be started on liquids the night of surgery and rapidly advanced to a regular diet.

2. Bath/shower: Size of the hernia and the extent of the repair usually correlate with incisional pain and patient discomfort postoperatively; therefore, although in theory a patient can bathe and shower at 24 hours, he or she may not actually be interested in doing so. If a patient has an abdominal drain in place, bathing such that the drain site is submerged should be avoided until the drain is removed.

3. Activity: For the patient who has an outpatient ventral hernia repair, walking, climbing stairs, and lifting up to 10 pounds are allowed for the first 2 weeks. We repair these defects with a mesh placed in the peritoneal cavity and anchored at the periphery with interrupted suture and spiral tacks. For the first 2 weeks, the strength of the repair depends on the sutures and for that reason lifting is restricted. From 2 to 4 weeks, increased activity and lifting are permitted as described with inguinal hernia repair. At 4 weeks the patient can often resume normal activity and lifting. The level of incisional pain and abdominal wall discomfort should be the gauge to temper the patient's activity. For patients with ventral hernias larger than 5 cm or multiple hernias who spend 1 or 2 days in the hospital, the return to normal activity is likely to take longer. We encourage walking the evening of surgery and recommend progressive walking from the first day on. Lifting is limited to 10 pounds, and at 4 weeks we allow the patients to lift as they did preoperatively.

4. Exercise/sport: For the first month exercise is limited to walking and stair climbing. After 4 weeks, those patients who had small hernias and an uncomplicated course may gradually increase their activity to include running and weight lifting. Patients who have had difficult repairs, or multiple, large, or recurrent hernias, probably should avoid contact sports altogether.

5. Driving: Resumption of driving depends on mobility, reaction time, and the patient's ability to respond to any road hazard. For most patients who were driving before the operation, their reflexes and faculties will be back to baseline by 1–2 weeks. As mentioned above, the patient should not begin driving if the physical activities required (movements of feet, arms, and upper torso) are painful.

6. Return to work: From a wound healing and surgical point of view, patients with smaller ventral hernias could return to work as early as 7–10 days postoperatively. Whether they do return to work early is a multifactorial decision modified in large part by the patient's motivation and energy level in the postoperative period. Patients with office jobs and limited physical activity certainly could return to work at 2 weeks, at least on a part-time basis.

Patients with large or multiple hernia repairs who spend several days in the hospital sometimes need a longer recovery period and may require 3–4 weeks before returning to work.

The laparoscopic approach decreases the incidence of wound complications after hernia repair. This may shorten the hospital stay and recovery time for these patients and may also allow them to return to work sooner than with the traditional open approach.

D. Laparoscopic Antireflux Procedures: Fundoplications

1. Diet: These patients are frequently kept in the hospital at least 1 night after surgery. There are two popular philosophies to which surgeons ascribe with regard to feeding. One practice is to obtain a barium or gastrograffin swallowing study to rule out an esophageal injury before feeding the patient. This study

is usually performed on the first postoperative day, and if the study is normal, the patient is started on a liquid diet. The other school of thought determines suitability for feeding on a clinical basis, and patients may be started on liquids the night of surgery.

Often the combination of fundoplication and postoperative swelling may make certain solid foods difficult to swallow. We warn our patients to expect a small degree of postsurgical dysphagia. We instruct them to be certain to eat small bites of food and to chew well. We also caution them against eating breads and dry meats such as turkey or roast beef during the first postoperative week.

2. Bath/shower: Wait 24 hours for the incisions to seal and then the patient may shower or bathe as desired.

3. Activity: As with laparoscopic cholecystectomy, abdominal wall pain and incision discomfort determine the level of each patient's activity. Walking and stair climbing are encouraged, and lifting 5–10 pounds is allowed as tolerated. Usually abdominal discomfort is the limiting factor, but by 4 weeks the patient should be back to normal preoperative capabilities.

4. Exercise/sport: There is no reason not to participate in noncontact sports such as running or swimming after 1–2 weeks. Again, incision discomfort should be the guide by which activities are reintroduced. It seems prudent to avoid weight lifting and contact sports for the first 4 weeks to allow the cannulation sites to fully heal.

If the patient had a particularly large hiatus hernia, we typically ask them to refrain from any lifting whatsoever during the first month following surgery. We worry that strenuous activity that would result in Valsalva maneuvers might cause the hernia to recur in the early postoperative period.

5. Driving: Resumption of driving depends on mobility, reaction time, and the patient's ability to respond to any road hazard. For most patients who were driving before the operation, their reflexes and faculties will be back to baseline by 1–2 weeks. As mentioned above, the patient should not begin driving if the physical activities required (movements of feet, arms, and upper torso) are painful.

6. Return to work: The decision to determine when to return to work depends on the type of work and how physically demanding it is, patient motivation, energy level, and length of sick time allowed by the employer and/or the insurance company. From a physiologic and anatomic point of view, it is possible and safe for a person with a nonlifting job to return to work after 1 week. As with many other major surgical procedures, fatigue is not unusual and therefore resumption of work on a part-time or light duty basis is appropriate. We commonly recommend longer periods off work (up to 4 weeks) for those patients who have more strenuous jobs, such as construction workers or truck drivers.

E. Gastric Bypass/Bariatric Procedures

1. Diet: The schedule for feeding a patient varies from surgeon to surgeon. Patients with a gastrojejunostomy frequently have a barium or gastrograffin swallowing study before starting a diet. Patients are then advanced from clear

liquids to full liquids over the next 3–5 days and then switched to regular diet eaten in small amounts several times a day. This schedule is also often followed for patients who have had a vertical banded gastroplasty or a laparoscopic gastric band placed. In each case the pouch is quite restrictive, and therefore in the first weeks eating small amounts several times a day is recommended. Because of the limited size of the gastric outlet in these patients following surgery, we caution them against eating breads and dry meats such as turkey or roast beef during the first 4 postoperative weeks. Food must be cut into small pieces (about the size of a pencil eraser) and chewed well.

2. Shower/bathing: Wait 24 hours for the incisions to heal and then the patient may shower or bathe. If an abdominal wall drain is in place, wait until the drain is removed before bathing.

3. Activity/lifting: Pain and incisional discomfort are the usual limitations to postoperative activity. Walking and stair climbing are encouraged. Many of these patients have significant comorbidities such as degenerative joint disease, dyspnea on exertion, and hypoventilation syndrome. Consequently, their postoperative activity will be less than that of patients after cholecystectomy or inguinal hernia repair. Nonetheless, the risk of incisional hernia is small, and walking and stair climbing are encouraged.

4. Exercise/sport: These patients have not engaged in running, contact sports, or active exercises because of their obesity preoperatively, and participation in sports thus will not be an immediate goal or question in the postoperative period. Walking, stair climbing, and swimming are the preferred forms of exercise for these patients, and competitive sports will be an option down the road as their weight gets closer to the ideal.

5. Driving: Resumption of driving for these patients will depend on their driving skills before the operation, their mobility and response time, and their overall energy level. General guidelines here are a bit difficult, and we would recommend that the doctor and the patient decide this on a case-by-case basis.

6. Return to work: The decision to return to work will largely be determined by the patient's energy level, the activity and mobility of the individual, disabilities caused by comorbid conditions, and the type of work the patient performs. White-collar workers often are able to return to work within 2–3 weeks if their disabilities are limited to hypertension and diabetes. If patients were significantly disabled before their operation, their fitness for the workplace in many cases will improve as they lose weight and the comorbid problems become less of a burden. These patients experience more fatigue in the first month postoperatively, and it may be necessary for them to start work on a part-time basis.

F. Splenectomy

1. Diet: After laparoscopic splenectomy, most patients resume a liquid and then a solid diet within a day or two. The limiting factors will be nausea or postoperative ileus, which occurs in 5%–10% of patients. Because there is no intestinal anastomosis, there is no concern about intestinal leak and, therefore, patients

can more rapidly resume their normal eating habits. In addition, patients can take their preoperative medicines right away. We generally hold anticoagulation for 24 hours.

2. Bath/shower: Wait 24 hours for the incisions to seal and then the patient may shower or bathe as desired.

3. Activity: We encourage walking and allow stair climbing. The amount of activity is generally determined by any incisional pain or abdominal discomfort that the patient may experience. Moderate lifting of 5–10 pounds is not harmful, and most patients can easily resume preoperative activity by 2 weeks.

4. Exercise/sport: Walking is preferred to running for the first 10–14 days, but running would not interfere with healing if this activity is not painful. Some patients require a longer incision for extraction of the specimen in certain disease states. In these patients we restrict weight lifting and contact sports for 4 weeks; after 4 weeks, full activities can be resumed as tolerated.

5. Driving: This decision should be individualized for each patient. There are many factors to consider, including the patient's age, mobility, reaction time, and ability to respond to any road hazard or emergency. For most patients who were driving before the operation, their reflexes and motor skills will be back to baseline by 1–2 weeks. As for the other operations discussed above, the patient should not begin driving until the physical activities required (movements of feet, arms, and upper torso) are not painful.

6. Return to work: After splenectomy, the patient's general medical condition and indications for the operation are the most important determinants of when the patient returns to work. These patients often suffer from chronic illness and have serious medical conditions that preclude work before and after surgery. However, if the patient is interested in working, and feels well, then return to nonstrenuous work can be expected 2 weeks after splenectomy.

G. Laparoscopic Colectomy

1. Diet: In most cases after colectomy, the patient will have either an anastomosis or a colostomy. As with open surgery, there is a postoperative ileus that must resolve before we feed these patients. The ileus usually resolves within 1 to 4 days. The usual guidelines for diet and feeding after open colectomy apply here as well.

2. Bath/shower: From the wound healing perspective, patients can shower 24 hours after surgery.

3. Activity: Walking the evening of surgery is allowed and certainly encouraged. Incisional pain and abdominal discomfort will largely determine how much a patient walks. Many of these procedures require incisions of varying length to facilitate specimen removal. Moderate lifting of 5–10 pounds is not harmful, and in an uncomplicated case the patient can usually resume normal daily activity within 1–2 weeks.

4. Exercise/sport: Walking is preferred to running for the first 10–14 days, but running would not interfere with healing if this activity is not painful. We

tend to restrict weight lifting and contact sports for 4 weeks in most patients; after 4 weeks, normal activity and exercise are encouraged on a gradual schedule.

5. Driving: Resumption of driving depends on the patient's energy level, mobility, reaction time, and ability to respond to any road hazard as well as their general condition. For most patients who were driving before colectomy, driving should be possible in 3–4 weeks. The patient should not begin driving until the physical activities required (movements of feet, arms, and upper torso) are not painful.

6. Return to work: After colectomy, the patient's general medical condition is the most important determinants of when the patient returns to work. These patients often suffer from chronic illness and have serious medical conditions that preclude work before surgery. If the patient is interested in working, feels well, and has a good energy level, resumption of a nonlifting job or light duty work within 2 weeks after colectomy is reasonable.

H. Selected References

Gibson M, Byrd C, Pierce C, et al. Laparoscopic colon resections: a five-year retrospective review. Am Surg 2000;66(3):245–248.

Hotokezaka M, Dix J, Mentis EP, Minasi JS, Schirmer BD. Gastrointestinal recovery following laparoscopic vs open colon surgery. Surg Endosc 1996;10(5):485–489.

Johansson B, Hallerback B, Glise H, et al. Laparoscopic mesh versus open properitoneal mesh versus conventional technique for inguinal hernia repair: a randomized multicenter trial (SCUR Hernia Repair Study). Ann Surg 1999;230(2):225–231.

Liem MS, van der Graaf Y, van Steensel CJ, et al. Comparison of conventional anterior surgery and laparoscopic surgery for inguinal-hernia repair. N Engl J Med 1997; 336(22):1541–1547.

Matthews BD, Sing RF, DeLegge MH, Ponsky JL, Heniford BT. Initial results with a stapled gastrojejunostomy for the laparoscopic isolated Roux-en-Y gastric bypass. Am J Surg 2000;179:476–481.

Nguyen NT, Ho HS, Palmer LS, Wolfe BM. A comparison study of laparoscopic versus open gastric bypass for morbid obesity. J Am Coll Surg 2000;191(2):149–157.

Ramshaw B, Shuler FW, Jones HB, Duncan TD, et al. Laparoscopic inguinal hernia repair. Surg Endosc 2001;15:50–54.

Rosen M, Garcia-Ruiz A, Malm J, et al. Laparoscopic hernia repair enhances early return of physical work capacity. Surg Laparosc Endosc Percutan Tech 2001;11(1): 28–33.

Schauer PR, Ikramuddin S, Gourash W, Ramanathan R, Luketich J. Outcomes after laparoscopic Roux-en-Y gastric bypass for morbid obesity. Ann of Surg 2000;232(4): 515–529.

Schlachta CM, Mamazza J, Poulin EC. Laparoscopic sigmoid rcscction for acute and chronic diverticulitis. An outcomes comparison with laparoscopic resection for non-diverticular disease. Surg Endosc 1999;13(7):649–653.

Tobin G. Personal clinical experience and concepts of wound healing.

Vitale GC, Collet D, Larson GM, et al. Interruption of professional and home activity after laparoscopic cholecystectomy among French and American patients. Am J Surg 1991; 161:396–398.

Part IV
Physiologic Implications of CO_2 Pneumoperitoneum and Minimally Invasive Methods

34. Cardiovascular Effects of CO_2 Pneumoperitoneum

Lee L. Swanström, M.D., F.A.C.S.

Any surgical procedure elicits a physiologic response from the patient. This response is both acute, occurring during the procedure, and of intermediate duration, during the healing/recovery phase. The causes of the host response are multifactorial and include the psychological stress induced by the need for surgery, the effects of medication and anesthetic agents, the hormonally mediated stress response to the surgical insult, and mechanical effects peculiar to the procedure. These mechanical effects include, but are not limited to, volume shifts from positioning, compression from retraction and exposure, induced transient organ ischemia, hypovolemia from blood and fluid loss, hypothermia, and a myriad of other factors. Perioperative surgical stress can affect any of the major organ systems. Of primary concern is its impact on the cardiovascular system, as this can be difficult to control and may be potentially dangerous for the patient.

Minimally invasive surgical techniques, as defined by access via small incisions, operative imagery by videoscopy, and exposure by instillation of insufflated gas, offer some physiologic advantage to patients (e.g., a lessened surgical stress response) at the cost of introducing other unique cardiovascular variables.

Cardiovascular changes in minimally invasive surgery can be categorized as those resulting from patient positioning, neurologically mediated responses, hypothermia, and absorption of insufflated gas as well as the pressure effects of insufflating a body compartment.

A. Effects of Positioning

In minimally invasive surgery, organ retraction and manipulation are compromised by the small size of laparoscopic instruments. This drawback is, to a large extent, overcome by creative and sometimes radical positioning of the patient during surgery. In effect, the laparoscopic surgeon uses gravity to retract solid organs, viscera, or lungs away from the operative field. Various positions are described for different procedures and include Trendelenburg, reverse Trendelenburg, lateral decubitus, and even prone. Some procedures such as colon resections may even require several changes of position during a single case. These unusual position changes result in significant fluid shifts that are frequently amplified by positive-pressure insufflation. These position-related alterations should be foreseen and compensated for by the anesthetist.

For the most part, patients in exaggerated reverse Trendelenburg position have a decreased cardiac preload and subsequent decreased cardiac output (CO). This should primarily be treated with volume replacement, although simple compression stockings or sequential pneumatic compression devices have been postulated to help as well. Patients in steep Trendelenburg position have the opposite problem, with dramatically increased right heart pressures secondary to increased central venous pressure. This can lead to right heart failure in susceptible patients and should be treated with fluid restriction and even afterload reduction (nitrates, nitroprusside) in severe cases. Acute intraoperative changes are best handled initially by simply decreasing the acute angle of the positioning, even if additional access ports need to be inserted to maintain exposure.

B. Neurologically Mediated Cardiac Effects

Although rare, cardiac output can be affected indirectly by pneumoperitoneum via central nerve stimulation. The most common cause is a vasovagal reaction to peritoneal stretch. Although this is usually benign and self-limited, on occasion it can lead to profound bradycardia and even asystole and cardiovascular collapse. Treatment consists of immediate desufflation of the abdomen, atropine administration, and CPR if necessary. A rarer cause of bradycardia is the increased intracranial pressure associated with pneumoperitoneum. In head-injured patients, this effect can result in a Cushing's response in which the heart rate decreases but blood pressure increases. This can be further compounded by the acidosis associated with CO_2 insufflation, which indirectly contributes to brain swelling and can even lead to cerebral herniation. For these reasons, a CO_2 pneumoperitoneum should probably be avoided in patients with increased intracranial pressure.

C. Hypothermia

Unless insufflated gas is heated and humidified, it invariably induces hypothermia. Total body cooling can be surprisingly rapid because of the large area of exposed serosa and peritoneum as well as the vasodilation that occurs from the increased PCO_2. If the core temperature drops below 34°, marked cardiac alterations such as bradycardia and decreased cardiac output may develop. These cardiac responses are attributed to direct myocardial depression as well as to the contradictory effects of peripheral vasoconstriction (the body's compensatory response to hypothermia) and venous dilation (related to the systemic acidosis caused by the CO_2 pneumoperitoneum). These cardiovascular alterations can be corrected by restoring the normal body temperature. It is best to avoid hypothermia by using warm blankets, "bear huggers," and by warming and humidifying the CO_2 gas used to create the pneumoperitoneum.

D. Biologic Effect of Insufflated Gas

Although some have advocated the use of abdominal wall lifting devices (isobaric exposure techniques), positive-pressure pneumoperitoneum has long been recognized as the most effective and widely applicable method of abdominal exposure. Thoracoscopy, on the other hand, because of the bony chest, can be carried out without positive-pressure insufflation although some surgeons prefer low-pressure pneumothorax. The most commonly used insufflation gas is CO_2. CO_2 is inexpensive, inhibits combustion, is readily available, and is rapidly absorbed and metabolized by the patient. It is this rapid absorption and metabolism that gives CO_2 its safety profile. It takes large amounts of intravascular CO_2 gas to cause an embolic event because the body has a large buffering capability and is able to excrete excess absorbed CO_2. These same biologic factors can also impact the cardiovascular system, however, and can lead to anesthesia management problems. CO_2 is rapidly absorbed into the intravascular space because of its high solubility quotient.

Hypercarbia is associated with multiple cardiovascular alterations (Table 34.1). In general, CO_2 excess is well managed by humans because of the inherent buffering system of the intravascular and extravascular spaces. In addition, the pulmonary exchange mechanism whereby CO_2 is exchanged for oxygen via transalveolar diffusion is incredibly efficient. This ability to compensate, however, can be compromised in several instances.

CO_2 pneumoperitoneum has direct and indirect cardiovascular effects. These effects and alterations are amplified in patients whose homeostatic protective mechanisms are compromised (Table 34.2).

Once absorbed, CO_2 combines with H_2O to form carbonic acid, which dissociates into bicarbonate (HCO_3^-) and hydrogen ions (H^+). The body's impressive buffering capability helps limit the acidosis that ensues. CO_2 is also efficiently eliminated from the body by the lungs; however, the pneumoperitoneum impairs ventilation to a varying extent. Furthermore, the acidosis results in profound vasodilation, which lowers the systemic vascular resistance and elevates the pulmonary vascular resistance. These alterations typically result in a lower blood pressure and an increased cardiac output. These effects are balanced by the sympathomimetic response that occurs as a result of peritoneal stretch and irritation and other alterations associated with pneumoperitoneum.

Table 34.1. The cardiovascular effects of absorbed CO_2 from abdominal or thoracic insufflation.

Parameter	Metabolic acidosis
Cardiac output	Increased from lowered systemic vascular resistance Decreased from myocardial depression and elevated pulmonary vascular resistance Net effect = slight decrease
Blood pressure	Slight decrease from diminished cardiac output and vasodilation
Stroke volume	Decreased due to myocardial depression
Pulmonary vascular resistance	Increased

Table 34.2. Patients who are at increased risk of cardiovascular complications with standard CO_2 pneumoperitoneum.

- Pulmonary hypertension
- Congestive heart failure or gross fluid overload
- Sepsis
- Hypovolemia/anemia (chronic or acute)
- Myocardiopathy
- Pulmonary dysfunction (chronic or acute)

E. Cardiovascular Effects of Positive-Pressure Pneumoperitoneum

Positive-pressure insufflation provides the best exposure for intraabdominal and thoracic procedures as well as for operations where CO_2 is intentionally insufflated into subcutaneous tissue planes (e.g., for inguinal hernia repair). The size or, more correctly stated, the volume of the intracorporeal operative field to a large extent varies directly with the insufflation pressure (the higher the pressure, the better the exposure). Unfortunately, the untoward physiologic manifestations of CO_2 pneumoperitoneum (both gas- and pressure related) also directly correlate with the insufflation pressure. In general, pneumoperitoneum in excess of 15 mmHg has deleterious effects on the cardiovascular system. The pneumoperitoneum compresses the vena cava and thus decreases venous return to the heart; this results in blood pooling in the lower half of the body and a decrease in cardiac output. Higher insufflation pressures also further impair ventilation by pushing up on the diaphragms. Last, the higher insufflation pressures also increase the systemic absorption of CO_2. Under these circumstances the systemic acidosis worsens and, ultimately, the cardiac output decreases. This can, in extreme cases (in compromised patients or with very high insufflation pressures), lead to cardiovascular collapse or death.

Saffran et al. documented a 15% decrease in cardiac output and a 30% increase in mean arterial pressure in patients undergoing CO_2 pneumoperitoneum at 15 mmHg pressure. Clinically, this studied patient population showed no adverse outcomes from pneumoperitoneum.

In normal patients, the effect of positive-pressure pneumoperitoneum or pneumothorax relates directly to decreased pulmonary efficiency and gas exchange. This, in turn, leads to an increase in acidosis with its well-known cardiac effects. Higher insufflation pressures can also compress the vena cava, which decreases venous return to the right heart and leads to a decreased cardiac output. The pressures generated by insufflation can therefore amplify the biologic activity of the absorbed CO_2.

F. Conclusion

In general, CO_2 pneumoperitoneum and pneumothorax are well tolerated. The cardiac depressive effects of acidosis, decreased preload, and decreased systemic vascular resistance are usually mitigated by the sympathomimetic effects of surgical intervention and by anesthesia management (primarily hyperventilation and intravascular volume replacement). The net effect in a normal patient is therefore negligible. This homeostatic balance can be easily upset, however, by underlying patient disease: acidosis from other causes, respiratory failure, hypovolemia, or hypothermia. In such cases insufflation with CO_2 can lead to marked hypotension, decreased cardiac output, and even death. Awareness of the physiologic effects of CO_2 pneumoperitoneum and pneumothorax on cardiovascular function is critical for the surgeon. Such awareness allows for the safe application of this important surgical tool in appropriate patients.

G. Selected References

Andrus CH, Wittgen CM, Naunheim KS. Anesthetic and physiological changes during laparoscopy and thoracoscopy: the surgeon's view. Semin Laparosc Surg 1994;1: 228–240.

Cuschieri A. Adverse cardiovascular changes induced by positive pressure pneumoperitoneum. Surg Endosc 1998;12:93–94.

Gray RI, Ott DE, Henderson AC, Cochran SA. Severe local hypothermia from laparoscopic gas evaporative jet cooling: a mechanism to explain clinical observations. J Soc Laparosc Surg 1999;3:171–177.

Greene FL. Pneumoperitoneum in the cancer patient: advantages and pitfalls. Semin Surg Oncol 1998;15:151–154.

Halverson A, Buchanan R, Jacobs L, et al. Evaluation of mechanism of increased intracranial pressure with insufflation. Surg Endosc 1998;12:266–269.

Hardacre JM, Talamini MA. Pulmonary and hemodynamic changes during laparoscopy: are they important? Surgery 2000;127:241–244.

Peden CJ, Prys-Roberts C. Capnothorax: implications for the anaesthetist. Anesthesia 1993; 48:664–666.

Reed DN, Duff JL. Persistent occurrence of bradycardia during laparoscopic cholecystectomy in low-risk patients. Dig Surg 2000;17:513–517.

Safran D, Orlando R. Physiologic effects of pneumoperitoneum. Am J Surg 1994;167: 281–286.

35. Pulmonary Implications of CO_2 Pneumoperitoneum in Minimally Invasive Surgery

Karen E. Deveney, M.D.

Laparoscopic methods are associated with intraoperative pulmonary alterations in all patients, even those who are young and healthy. Factors that affect pulmonary function during laparoscopic procedures include the pneumoperitoneum-related (secondary to increased pressure) elevation of the diaphragms, carbon dioxide-related physiologic changes, and the radical body positions that are usually required to facilitate performance of the procedures (Table 35.1). Obesity and certain other patient comorbidities may further affect pulmonary function. Finally, intraoperative complications of the procedures can produce abrupt, life-threatening changes in pulmonary function.

A. Effects of the Pneumoperitoneum

Creating a pneumoperitoneum increases the abdominal pressure that pushes the diaphragm cephalad and decreases the volume of the chest cavity. The functional residual volume is thereby diminished and the work of breathing is increased. Lung compliance is decreased. If the patient is under a general anesthetic with a fixed tidal volume, the peak inspiratory pressure will be increased. If the patient is ventilating spontaneously without neuromuscular blockade, the tidal volume will be decreased and atelectasis will generally occur. Pulmonary shunting then occurs and contributes to a decrease in arterial oxygenation.

The use of abdominal wall lifting devices to provide laparoscopic exposure avoids the pneumoperitoneum and CO_2-related deleterious pulmonary effects. The cardiopulmonary alterations are, therefore, minimal when the position is neutrally positioned. However, when the patient is placed in the Trendelenburg position, deleterious pulmonary function abnormalities are noted that are similar to those observed in similarly positioned CO_2 pneumoperitoneum patients. Largely because abdominal wall lifting methods provide inferior exposure, they have not gained widespread acceptance.

The anesthesiologist who is taking care of laparoscopic patients, especially those undergoing a CO_2 pneumoperitoneum, must be ready to increase the respiratory rate, which will increase the minute ventilation and, if need be, increase the oxygen concentration during the procedure. Appropriate intraoperative monitoring techniques are discussed in a later section.

Table 35.1. Effects of laparoscopy on pulmonary function.

Factor	Immediate result	Effect on pulmonary function
Pneumoperitoneum	↑ Abdominal volume ↑ Abdominal pressure (resulting in elevation of diaphragms)	↓ Lung volumes • Decreases the functional residual capacity • Decreases the tidal volume • Decreases the vital capacity ↓ Lung compliance ↑ Peak inspiratory pressure • Atelectasis → alveolar-arteriolar • O_2 mismatch → resulting in ↓PaO_2
CO_2 insufflation	Hypercarbia	Hyperventilation (in spontaneously breathing patient)
	Acidosis	Increased minute ventilation (in spontaneously breathing patient)

B. Physiologic Effects of CO2 Insufflation

Carbon dioxide is almost universally employed to create and maintain pneumoperitoneum during laparoscopic procedures. Although air, helium, nitrogen, oxygen, nitrous oxide and argon have been considered as gases for insufflation, CO_2, in the final analysis, has been found to be superior because it is extremely soluble, nonflammable, inert, and nonirritating. CO_2 is rapidly absorbed across the peritoneal membrane into the bloodstream and equilibrates quickly, with a diffusion coefficient 20 times that of oxygen or helium and 40 times that of nitrogen. Thus, the risk of gas embolism is far less with CO_2 than with the other gases mentioned. Most of the absorbed carbon dioxide is eventually eliminated by the lungs. The high solubility of CO_2 has several important negative ramifications.

The rapid equilibration of carbon dioxide results in significant hypercarbia and acidosis, which, in turn, may influence cardiac and pulmonary function. Aortic and carotid body chemoreceptors normally respond to hypercarbia by relaying afferent impulses to respiratory centers that result in hyperventilation and the increased elimination of CO_2 through the lungs. Because most laparoscopic procedures are performed with controlled ventilation under general anesthesia, the normal compensatory hyperventilation does not occur and hypercarbia persists unless the respiratory rate or tidal volume is increased by the anesthesiologist.

C. Effects of Patient Position

Patient positioning during surgery can also significantly affect pulmonary function. Due to a cephalad shift in the abdominal viscera and upward pressure on the diaphragm, the Trendelenburg position causes further decreases in lung volume, functional residual capacity, and pulmonary compliance beyond that seen with pneumoperitoneum alone. Overall, the Trendelenburg position further increases the work of breathing. The trachea also shifts in the cephalad direction with the patient in the head-down position so that the tip of an endotracheal tube that is secured at the mouth may advance into the right main-stem bronchus. The simultaneous increased intraabdominal pressure further exacerbates this shift in position of the tracheal bronchial tree. The reverse Trendelenburg position improves pulmonary mechanics by increasing lung volumes and lessening the work of breathing.

D. The Impact of Comorbid Conditions

In general, the mechanical work of breathing is increased and pulmonary compliance is decreased in obese patients. This is partly because obese patients at baseline have increased intraabdominal pressures. In this population, laparoscopic procedures done under a CO_2 pneumoperitoneum not surprisingly result in more dramatic pulmonary function alterations than are noted in the general population. Similarly, body position changes during surgery in this population are associated with more striking pulmonary function alterations. The Trendelenburg and even the supine position further impair pulmonary function whereas the reverse Trendelenburg position, which is commonly employed during upper abdominal procedures, lessens the deleterious pulmonary effects of both obesity and pneumoperitoneum.

Individuals with severe preexisting lung or heart disease are at the greatest risk for serious CO_2 pneumoperitoneum-related pulmonary function alterations. The pulmonary effects of pneumoperitoneum are often noted earlier and are more dramatic in this patient population. In this population, especially those with restrictive lung disease, it is also harder to correct these changes by increasing the minute ventilation or inspiratory pressures; therefore, conversion to open surgical methods is necessary more often than in the general population. As is the case for obese patients, the Trendelenburg position impact on pulmonary function is accentuated in patients with severe cardiopulmonary disease.

The principal effects of preexisting lung disease are to exacerbate the hypercarbia and acidosis associated with the CO_2 pneumoperitoneum. Although the increased intraabdominal pressure contributes to these alterations, it is probably the CO_2 gas itself that is the main cause of the dramatic hypercarbia and acidosis often noted in these patients. Chronic obstructive pulmonary disease (COPD) patients with chronic carbon dioxide retention, at baseline, have nearly or fully saturated their body's CO_2 storage sites, such as the bone and skeletal muscle, and have a limited ability to accommodate additional CO_2 during a laparoscopic procedure. These individuals often manifest an exaggerated hypercarbia when compared to patients with normal lung function and require more time to eliminate the CO_2 through their lungs after desufflation. As mentioned above, increasing the minute ventilation in patients with chronic pulmonary disease may not adequately compensate for the hypercarbia and acidosis; in these cases conversion to traditional open methods may be necessary (see Section F).

E. Effects of Anesthetic Method on Pulmonary Function

The anesthetic technique chosen for a given laparoscopic procedure has important ramifications in regard to intraoperative pulmonary function. Local anesthetics with sedation are satisfactory only for brief lower abdominal procedures in motivated healthy patients because insufflation of the abdominal cavity irritates the diaphragm and restricts the patient's voluntary inspiratory efforts. Similarly, the high level of spinal or epidural anesthetic required to achieve adequate abdominal wall muscle relaxation and eliminate diaphragmatic irritation prevents the patient from increasing spontaneous ventilation to the extent that CO_2 levels are maintained within normal limits. Therefore, a general anesthetic with endotracheal intubation and positive-pressure mechanical ventilation is necessary for most laparoscopic procedures. Endotracheal intubation decreases the risk of aspiration of gastric acid when regurgitation occurs as a result of insufflation-related elevated intraabdominal pressure. Controlled ventilation allows the respiratory rate and tidal volume to be adjusted in response to hypercarbia and changes in patient position. Peak inspiratory pressures can be increased as necessary to counteract the effects of pneumoperitoneum on lung volumes. Muscle paralysis minimizes the volume of insufflated gas and the peak insufflation pressure needed to provide adequate abdominal exposure. The lower the peak insufflation pressure, the smaller the lung volume alterations and the less extreme the hypercarbia.

Careful monitoring of the patient during CO_2 pneumoperitoneum provides the anesthesiologist with the information needed to make respiratory rate, volume, or pressure changes to adequately ventilate and oxygenate the patient. All patients undergoing general anesthesia routinely have the following functions monitored: arterial blood pressure, heart rate, body temperature, ECG, O_2 saturation, and end-tidal CO_2 levels. The latter measurement is critical for laparoscopic procedures because it gives the anesthesiologist moment-to-moment indirect data regarding the Pa CO_2. Arterial blood gases (ABGs) are the "gold standard" in regard to determining arterial oxygen and CO_2 levels as well as the blood pH during an operation; however, these tests are done sporadically during a case. End-tidal CO_2 monitors reveal the CO_2 concentration of the expired gas in a continuous fashion. It is important to note that there is always a gradient between the Pa CO_2 and the end-tidal CO_2; the latter is always lower than the former. The size of this gradient varies from patient to patient (as little as 5 mmHg to 20 mmHg or higher). Those with significant pulmonary disease manifest a larger gradient than patients with normal lungs. For the anesthesiologist to correctly extrapolate the $PaCO_2$ from the end-tidal CO_2, the size of the gradient needs to be determined at the start of the procedure via correlation of the end-tidal value and a blood gas-derived Pa CO_2. The arterial–end-tidal CO_2 gradient may be altered when lung perfusion suddenly changes and alters the volume of alveolar deadspace. Decreased lung perfusion will increase the alveolar deadspace, which, in turn, dilutes the CO_2 in the expired gas and hence results in a lower end-tidal CO_2 level. These changes may occur when the cardiac output suddenly decreases as a result of high inflation pressures, reverse Trendelenburg position, or gas embolism. Therefore, it is recommended that reassessment of the CO_2 gradient, via repeat ABGs, be carried out periodically during a long laparoscopic case, especially for patients with significant pulmonary disease.

In patients with pulmonary impairment, preoperative ABGs should be obtained as a baseline for comparison with intraoperative values. Formal pulmonary function tests are also useful preoperatively in this population. Evidence of decreased flow rates, limited vital capacity and inspiratory capacity, and decreased diffusion capacity correlate with intraoperative acidosis. If the forced expiratory volume (FEV) is significantly compromised (less than 70%) and diffusion capacity is less than 88% of predicted values, the patient is at increased risk of developing hypercarbia and acidosis. Patients with significantly compromised pulmonary function should have an arterial line placed before the start of the surgical procedure and, as mentioned above, have frequent blood gas analysis. The anesthesiologist needs to closely monitor these patients intraoperatively and to frequently update the surgeon as to the patient's end-tidal CO_2, the tidal volume, and minute ventilation, as well as the size of the CO_2 gradient.

F. Minimizing Insufflation Pressures and Pneumoperitoneum "Holiday"

The surgeon must strive to use as low an insufflation pressure as possible during all laparoscopic cases. Reducing the pressure limit from 15 to 12 or to 10 mmHg will decrease the mechanical pulmonary function and blood gas alterations. A sizable percentage of cases can be successfully completed using a reduced peak insufflation pressure. Another useful tool or strategy when attempting to complete a laparoscopic case in a patient who is retaining CO_2 despite all the usual maneuvers is to simply stop the dissection, fully desufflate the abdomen, and place the patient in reverse Trendelenburg for 5–10 minutes. This pneumoperitoneum "holiday" removes the iatrogenic source of the problem and permits the patient to lower their $PaCO_2$. Once the end-tidal CO_2 has fallen sufficiently, the pneumoperitoneum can be reestablished and the procedure recommenced.

G. Selected References

Brampton WJ, Watson RJ. Arterial to end-tidal carbon dioxide tension difference during laparoscopy. Anaesthesia 1990;45:210–214.

Chough EK, Andrus CH. Physiology of pneumoperitoneum. In: Andrus CH, Cosgrove JM, Longo WE (eds) Minimally Invasive Surgery: Principles and Outcomes. Amsterdam: Harwood, 1998:13–18.

Fitzgerald SD, Andrus CH, Baudendistel LJ, et al. Hypercarbia during carbon dioxide pneumoperitoneum. Am J Surg 1992;163:186–190.

Joris JL. Anesthetic management of laparoscopy. In: Cucchiara RF, Miller ED Jr, Reves JG, et al. (eds) Anesthesia, 4th edition. New York: Churchill Livingstone, 1994:2011–2029.

McMahon AJ, Baxter JN, Murray W, et al. Helium pneumoperitoneum for laparoscopic cholecystectomy: ventilatory and blood gas changes. Br J Surg 1994;81:1033–1036.

Neuberger TJ, Andrus CH, Wittgen CM, et al. Prospective comparison of helium versus carbon dioxide pneumoperitoneum. Gastrointest Endosc 1996;43:38–41.

Ortega AE, Peters JH. Physiologic alterations of endosurgery. In: Peters JH, Demeester TR (eds) Minimally Invasive Surgery of the Foregut. St Louis: Quality Medical, 1994: 23–37.

Schauer PR, Luna J, Ghiatas AA, et al. Pulmonary function after laparoscopic cholecystectomy. Surgery 1993;114:389–399.

Wittgen CM, Andrus CH, Fitzgerald SD, et al. Analysis of the hemodynamic and ventilatory effects of laparoscopic cholecystectomy. Arch Surg 1991;126:997–1001.

Wittgen CM, Naunheim KS, Andrus CH, et al. Preoperative pulmonary function evaluation for laparoscopic cholecystectomy. Arch Surg 1993;128:880–886.

36. Renal Ramifications of CO_2 Pneumoperitoneum

Ayal M. Kaynan, M.D.
Sherry M. Wren, M.D.

The changes in renal physiology that occur during carbon dioxide insufflation of the abdomen are complex and most likely include both mechanical and neurohumoral mechanisms. At times, these factors may together result in profound oliguria (urine output <0.5 mL/kg/hr), which may develop soon after insufflation and persist for several hours following surgery. Thus, it is incumbent upon the surgeon and anesthesiologist to recognize this fact so that an appropriate intraoperative fluid management plan can be devised and implemented. This chapter focuses on the direct and indirect renal effects of carbon dioxide pneumoperitoneum, the mechanisms by which oliguria occurs, and a logical approach to fluid management in laparoscopic patients.

A. Direct Renal Effects of CO2 Pneumoperitoneum

Multiple animal and clinical studies have documented 20%–40% decreases in glomerular filtration rate (GFR) and a 60%–80% decrease in urine output during laparoscopic procedures carried out via CO_2 pneumoperitoneum [1–3]. These effects are most often noted when the intraabdominal pressure is above 10 mmHg [4] and are exacerbated by the reverse Trendelenburg position [5]. Diminished renal function is usually noted soon after insufflation and may persist for several hours following desufflation [3]. Ultimately, in otherwise healthy individuals, there is full recovery of renal function to preinsufflation levels [2, 6, 7] (Table 36.1).

Renal blood flow is also significantly affected by pneumoperitoneum. Measurements of renal blood flow during pneumoperitoneum in dogs have shown decreases of the order of 26% [2]. Elevation in the intraabdominal or renal venous pressure causes blood to shift from the outer cortex to the juxtamedullary zone [8]. The drop in renal cortical perfusion increases with increasing intraabdominal pressures, such that at an insufflation pressure of 20 mmHg renal flow is decreased by as much as 60%. Filtration is thereby compromised because the majority of glomeruli reside in the cortex. To the extent that intraabdominal pressure is uniform in the abdomen, it is intuitive that intravascular pressure gradients would favor centralization of blood flow to the larger vessels within the

Table 36.1. Summary of renal effects of CO_2 pneumoperitoneum.

Increased	Decreased
Antidiuretic hormone	Renal blood flow
Renin	Glomerular filtration rate (GFR)
Aldosterone	Urine output
FE_K	FE_{Na}
Epinephrine	Cardiac index
Endothelin	
Systemic vascular resistance (SVR)	
Mean arterial pressure (MAP)	

FE, Fractional Excretion.

juxtamedullary zone. The result of these alterations in renal perfusion are diminished overall renal blood flow, glomerular filtration rate, and urine output.

Creatinine clearance is known to be decreased during CO_2 insufflation and for several hours afterward. Despite this, plasma creatinine levels usually normalize soon after desufflation [6]. Fortunately, histologic sections of kidneys taken both immediately following and long after CO_2 pneumoperitoneum demonstrate no identifiable anatomic defects. This is true despite the fact that it has been demonstrated that pneumoperitoneum may result in elevations in the enzyme *N*-methyl-beta-D-glucosaminidase (NAG), a marker of proximal renal tubular cell damage. Thus, whatever toxic effect CO_2 pneumoperitoneum has upon normal renal parenchyma, the physiologic changes are transient and the long-term effects appear to be insignificant. In fact, there are no reports, to date, of pneumoperitoneum-induced renal failure in the setting of normal preoperative renal function.

What impact does the type of gas used for insufflation have on renal function? There is evidence that oliguria develops regardless of the gas used to establish pneumoperitoneum. CO_2, however, has been associated with increased mean arterial pressure when compared to blood pressures observed with other gases such as N_2O [9]. CO_2 pneumoperitoneum has also been associated with elevated systemic vascular resistance whereas the effect of N_2O has been unclear. At very high blood concentrations, CO_2 can result in cardiac toxicity. Thus, in addition to the direct effects of CO_2 pneumoperitoneum on renal blood flow [decreased renal blood flow (RBF) and glomerular filtration rate (GFR)], CO_2-related cardiovascular effects, via alterations in systemic blood pressure, vascular resistance, or cardiac output, may, indirectly, have an impact on renal function. The cardiovascular impact on renal function is discussed in greater detail below.

B. Purported Mechanisms for Oliguria

There are three putative explanations for pneumoperitoneum-induced oliguria: (1) renal parenchymal compression and associated renal blood flow alterations, (2) cardiac output and arterial blood pressure alterations, and (3) central venous congestion. To test whether direct renal compression had any effect on renal function, canine renal parenchyma was compressed using a pressure cuff inflated to 15 mmHg in vivo, sparing involvement of the hilar vasculature, ureter, and contralateral kidney. For the treated kidney, glomerular filtration rate decreased 21%, estimated renal blood flow decreased 26%, and urine output decreased 63% [2]. In a similar study, rat kidneys were studied ex vivo in CO_2 chambers pressurized to 15 mmHg. The renal hilar vasculature and ureters were catheterized and excluded from the pressurized chambers, thereby avoiding the potentially confounding direct effects of the CO_2 pneumoperitoneum on these structures. When the kidneys were perfused with blood/Ringer's solution at 37°C in the CO_2 environment, significant oliguria was noted. Therefore, pneumoperitoneum-related direct renal compression most likely contributes to the oliguria observed during laparoscopic cases. Further, when the blood pressure and inflow perfusion rate of the system were controlled, it was found that reduced intraparenchymal cortical blood flow accounted for much of the reduction in urine output. Thus, ***increased*** pre- and postglomerular resistance were thought to be significant secondary factors [10].

The extent to which pneumoperitoneum-related cardiovascular alterations contribute to the development of oliguria is less certain and more controversial. In the setting of CO_2 pneumoperitoneum, the main systemic hemodynamic systemic effects, as mentioned above, are increased systemic vascular resistance, increased mean arterial pressure, and decreased cardiac index [11]. Cardiac output may decrease by more than 10% as a result of increases in intraabdominal pressure [12]. Hypercarbia, if it should ensue, may further impair cardiac function. A decrease in cardiac output in and of itself is a well-established physiologic cause for oliguria. Prolonged cardiac dysfunction and hypoperfusion can, of course, result in acute tubular necrosis and renal failure. In a canine study that assessed the effects of intraabdominal pressure at 0, 20, and 40 mmHg on cardiac output and renal function, it was found that renal blood flow and GRF were decreased. When compared to the measurements at 0 mmHg, an increase to 20 mmHg decreased both variables to less than 25% of control values. Increasing to a level of 40 mmHg decreased renal blood flow and GFR to 0 in some animals and 7% in the others. This was accompanied by a drop in cardiac output of 37% compared to dogs with 0 mmHg intraabdominal pressures. Expansion of volume via administration of the plasma expander dextran-40 corrected the drop in cardiac output but only restored the renal blood flow and GFR to 25% of the normal level. The measured renal vascular resistance increased 555% when the pressure was elevated from 0 to 20 mmHg in test subjects, suggesting the changes in renal blood flow and GFR are a local renal phenomenon, probably from renal compression, and are not as influenced by changes in cardiac output [4]. Thus, these results suggested that relatively small impairment in cardiac output is not a significant factor in the development of renal dysfunction seen with increased intraabdominal pressure in a euvolemic animal. Nevertheless, cardiac output is reduced with pneumoperitoneum, and it is difficult to ignore the associated deleterious renal effects.

Increasing the intraabdominal pressure via pneumoperitoneum increases the renal vein pressures via compression [13]. This increased pressure, in turn, results in a significant reduction in blood flow through this vessel [6]. Several investigators have examined the effects of pneumoperitoneum-induced renal vein compression in greater detail. It has been demonstrated that unilateral renal vein compression decreases the glomerular filtration rate and urine output of both kidneys; of note, the effects are much more pronounced on the compressed side [1]. These results suggest that neurohumoral factors are also at play in addition to the more obvious compression-related decreased renal blood flow. Therefore, venous compression may impair renal function via several different mechanisms.

Ureteral compression may also contribute to pneumoperitoneum-related oliguria; however, the available evidence does not support this position. Intravenous pyelograms [6] and ultrasound examinations (personal experience) performed during laparoscopic procedures have not revealed hydronephrosis. It is conceivable that increased intraabdominal pressure may limit distension of the renal pelvis or that a longer period of ureteral compression is required before hydronephrosis becomes evident. However, ureteral catheterization, which should ensure that the ureter remains patent, has failed to mitigate oliguria during pneumoperitoneum [4]. To better define the effects of increased intraabdominal pressure on the ureter and renal function, selective ureteral compression studies need to be performed. At worst, ureteral compression is a minor contributor to pneumoperitoneum-related oliguria.

C. Neurohumoral Components

The very fact that oliguria persists after desufflation suggests that direct pressure-related renal effects do not fully account for the functional impairment that has been observed. Although direct compression could, in theory, result in transient occult renal parenchymal injury that might account for early postoperative oliguria, it is likely that neurohumoral factors also play a role. Indeed, it has been shown that antidiuretic hormone (ADH) levels rise early during laparoscopic surgery and remain significantly elevated for at least 30 minutes to an hour afterward [14, 15]. This finding is surprising if one considers that mean arterial pressure is elevated and sodium and water are retained during pneumoperitoneum. However, the following pneumoperitoneum-related alterations might account for increased ADH release in this setting: decreased cardiac output, increased release of catecholamines, or increased renin production. Regardless of the cause, persistent ADH elevation immediately after release of the pneumoperitoneum may explain, at least in part, the oliguria observed early after laparoscopic surgery.

Other pneumoperitoneum-related humoral factors may also have profound effects on renal blood flow. The release of epinephrine, which causes vasoconstriction and reduces renal blood flow, has been shown to be increased during laparoscopic surgery [14, 16]. Endothelin, one of the most potent vasoconstrictors known, is also released during pneumoperitoneum [1]. The use of nonselective endothelin antagonists has been shown to attenuate the surgery-related reduction in GFR by 35%; however, interestingly, oliguria persisted despite the better preserved GFR.

The documented activation of the renin-angiotensin-aldosterone system (RAAS) during laparoscopic procedures is another curious phenomenon. Renin levels have been shown to increase up to 400% during CO_2 pneumoperitoneum [3, 17–19] and to return to baseline on desufflation [13]. Renin elevation in this setting may be the result of changes in intrarenal blood flow [20]. The typical electrolyte alterations associated with increased aldosterone levels have been noted during laparoscopic procedures carried out under CO_2 pneumoperitoneum: hypernatremia, decreased fractional excretion of sodium, and increased fractional excretion of potassium [1]. The use of angiotensin-converting enzyme inhibitors, however, does not reverse pneumoperitoneum-related oliguria [13]. Activation of the RAAS, although not the primary cause of oliguria during laparoscopy, in all likelihood contributes to the decreased urine output observed during these procedures.

D. Exacerbating Risk Factors for Renal Dysfunction

Preexisting renal insufficiency must be considered when assessing the potential impact of pneumoperitoneum on renal function. As mentioned previously, pneumoperitoneum is associated with elevation of the enzyme NAG (*N*-methyl-beta-D-glucosaminidase), which is a marker of proximal renal tubular damage. Although histologic sections following pneumoperitoneum show no signs of necrosis, there is evidence to suggest that the kidneys undergo strain during laparoscopy [21]. In the living-related kidney donor literature, creatinine nadirs in recipients of laparoscopically harvested kidneys have been noted to be slightly higher than those observed in patients who received kidneys obtained via open methods. Despite this, graft survival and long-term creatinine levels are equivalent between the two groups [22]. In an animal study carried out to assess the fate of subjects with abnormal renal function, renal insufficiency was surgically induced, after which the animals were subjected to CO_2 pneumoperitoneum. Transient florid renal failure resulted; however, with time, the renal function of the animals returned to baseline levels [23]. Thus, abdominal insufflation does cause more marked, albeit transient, renal dysfunction in those with preexisting renal disease.

Hemodynamic instability, a well-established cause of renal dysfunction and morbidity during and after open surgery, would be expected to exacerbate the renal effects of CO_2 pneumoperitoneum. Cardiac dysfunction from any cause (e.g., decreased venous return, CO_2 toxicity, pneumothorax, pneumomediastinum) may result in reduced cardiac output and decreased renal blood flow. In this setting, reductions in glomerular filtration rate and urine production may be predicted; in extreme cases, renal failure may ensue.

It has been suggested by some that aminoglycosides be avoided in patients undergoing laparoscopic surgery. It has been shown, however, that there is no synergistic toxicity associated with their administration in the setting of CO_2 pneumoperitoneum [24].

E. Intraoperative Fluid Management

As for open surgery patients, the preoperative volume status of the patient must be taken into consideration when formulating a fluid management plan for a given patient who is to undergo a laparoscopic procedure. Most patients go into surgery a bit hypovolemic because they have taken nothing by mouth (NPO) for at least 8 hours. Patients who have completed a full mechanical bowel preparation in anticipation of a large bowel resection, however, are usually much more dehydrated. It is important that the anesthetist adequately hydrate the patient before surgery such that the patient is euvolemic. The cardiovascular effects of pneumoperitoneum and anesthetic induction will be more dramatic in a hypovolemic patient. Although 1–2 L isotonic fluid is all that is necessary to compensate for preoperative NPO status in most patients, patients who have undergone a mechanical bowel preparation usually require additional fluid.

In one study, moderate hydration with 500 mL fluid has been shown to improve cardiac index and reduce systemic vascular resistance when compared to the results of "nonhydrated" controls [13]. In experimental models of pneumoperitoneum-related renal dysfunction, hypervolemia attained via the administration of hypertonic fluids has been shown to reverse changes in renal blood flow and urine output. Interestingly, despite these improvements, impairment in creatinine clearance persists [25].

Having noted the importance of adequate hydration, it is a common mistake to overhydrate patients during laparoscopic surgery. Anesthesiologists often treat low intraoperative urine output with aggressive hydration because they wrongly attribute oliguria to hypovolemia. Likewise, anesthetists and surgeons often set the baseline I.V. rates based on the typical insensible losses incurred during an open procedure. In most instances, the insensible loss from abdominal insufflation and mechanical ventilation during a laparoscopic case is less than the losses observed during a comparable open case. In one study, water vapor content following dry gas insufflation was assessed; insignificant insensible water loss was demonstrated [26]. Although patients with normal cardiopulmonary function tolerate the additional fluid without difficulty, overhydration in patients with impaired or marginally adequate cardiopulmonary reserve may lead to significant problems. Therefore, accounting for maintenance plus insensible losses, intraoperative fluids generally should be approximately 125 mL/hr for a 70-kg male.

F. Conclusions

Carbon dioxide pneumoperitoneum directly and indirectly reduces renal function during surgery and for several hours after the procedure. The main effects are decreased renal blood flow, glomerular filtration rate, and urine output. The most important causes of these effects are renal parenchymal compression, decreased cardiac output, and central venous compression. Elevated blood levels of antidiuretic hormone, epinephrine, endothelin, and renin contribute to these transient dysfunctions. In patients with normal renal function before surgery, full recovery of renal function to baseline levels after surgery is almost always the rule. Those with significant preexisting renal dysfunction are the subgroup most likely to develop more serious renal problems during and after laparoscopic surgery. To minimize the negative impact of CO_2 pneumoperitoneum, it is important that preoperative fluid deficits be corrected. During the operation, however, for most patients conservative intraoperative fluid administration is advised because insensible losses are usually minimal. As always, each patient must be individually assessed and scrutinized to formulate a plan that takes into account their particular situation (preoperative renal function, fluid status, and anticipated operative insensible and blood losses).

G. References

1. Hamilton BD, Chow GK, Inman SR, Stowe NT, Winfield HN. Increased intra-abdominal pressure during pneumoperitoneum stimulates endothelin release in a canine model. J Endourol 1998;12:193–197.
2. Razvi HA, Fields D, Vargas JC, Vaughan ED Jr, Vukasin A, Sosa RE. Oliguria during laparoscopic surgery: evidence for direct renal parenchymal compression as an etiologic factor. J Endourol 1996;10:1–4.
3. Koivusalo A, Kellokumpu I, Ristkari S, Lindgren L. Splanchnic and renal deterioration during and after laparoscopic cholecystectomy: a comparison of the carbon dioxide pneumoperitoneum and the abdominal wall lift method. Anesth Analg 1997;85:886–891.
4. Harman RK, Kron IL, McLachlan HD, Freedlender AE, Nolan SP. Elevated intra-abdominal pressure and renal function. Ann Surg 1982;196:594–597.
5. Junghans T, Bohm B, Grundel K, Schwenk W, Muller JM. Does pneumoperitoneum with different gases, body positions, and intraperitoneal pressures influence renal and hepatic blood flow? Surgery 1997;121:206–211.
6. Kirsch AJ, Hensle TW, Chang DT, Kayton ML, Olsson CA, Sawczuk IS. Renal effects of CO_2 insufflation: oliguria and acute renal dysfunction in a rat pneumoperitoneum model. Urology 1994;43:453–459.
7. Hunter JG. Laparoscopic pneumoperitoneum: the abdominal compartment syndrome revisited [editorial]. J Am Coll Surg 1995;181:469–470.
8. Chiu AW, Azadzoi KM, Hatzichristou DG, Siroky MB, Krane RJ, Babayan RK. Effects of intra-abdominal pressure on renal tissue perfusion during laparoscopy. J Endourol 1994;8:99–103.
9. Rademaker BM, Odoom JA, de Wit LT, Kalkman CJ, ten Brink SA, Ringers J. Haemodynamic effects of pneumoperitoneum for laparoscopic surgery: a comparison of CO_2 with N_2O insufflation. Eur J Anaesthesiol 1994;11:301–306.
10. Stowe NT, Sung GT, Soble JJ, Hamilton BD, Winfield HN, Gill IS. Effect of constant renal perfusion pressure versus blood flow on urine output during simulated pneumoperitoneum in an isolated rat kidney model. J Endourol 1998;12:s97.
11. Joris JL. Anesthesia for laparoscopic surgery. In: Miller R, Miller E, Reves J, eds. Anesthesia, Vol. 2. San Francisco: Churchill Livingstone, 2000:2003–2023.

12. Cisek LJ, Peters CA. Pneumoperitoneum is associated with acute but not chronic alteration of renal function. J Endourol 1997;11:s54.
13. Vukasin A, Lopez M, Shichman S, Horn D, Vaughan ED Jr. Oliguria in laparoscopic surgery. J Urol 1994;151:343A.
14. Ortega AE, Peters JH, Incarbone R, et al. A prospective randomized comparison of the metabolic and stress hormonal responses of laparoscopic and open cholecystectomy. J Am Coll Surg 1996;183:249–256.
15. LeRoith DL, Bark H, Nyska M, et al. The effect of abdominal pressure on plasma antidiuretic hormone levels in the dog. J Surg Res 1982;32:65–69.
16. Massry S, Glassock R. Renal physiology. In: Massry S, Glassock R, eds. Massry & Glassock's Textbook of Nephrology. Philadelphia: Lippincott Williams & Wilkins, 2001:43.
17. O'Leary E, Hubbard K, Tormey W, Cunningham AJ. Laparoscopic cholecystectomy: haemodynamic and neuroendocrine responses after pneumoperitoneum and changes in position. Br J Anaesth 1996;76:640–644.
18. Bloomfield GI, Blocher CR, Fakhry IF, Sica DA, Sugerman HJ. Elevated intra-abdominal pressure increases plasma renin activity and aldosterone levels. J Trauma 1997;42:997–1004; discussion 1004–1005.
19. Diebel LN, Wilson RF, Dulchavsky SA, Saxe J. Effect of increased intra-abdominal pressure on hepatic arterial, portal venous, and hepatic microcirculatory blood flow. J Trauma 1992;33:279–282; discussion 282–283.
20. Kishimoto T, Maekawa M, Abe Y, Yamamoto K. Intrarenal distribution of blood flow and renin release during venous pressure elevation. Kid Int 1973;4:259–266.
21. Lee BR, Cadeddu JA, Molnar-Nadasdy G, et al. Chronic effect of pneumoperitoneum on renal histology. J Endourol 1999;13:279–282.
22. Jacobs SC, Cho E, Dunkin BJ, et al. Laparoscopic live donor nephrectomy: the University of Maryland 3-year experience. Urology 2000;164:1494–1499.
23. Cisek LJ, Gobet RM, Peters CA. Pneumoperitoneum produces reversible renal dysfunction in animals with normal and chronically reduced renal function. J Endourol 1998;12:95–100.
24. Beduschi R, Bedusci MC, Williams AL, Wolf JS Jr. Pneumoperitoneum does not potentiate the nephrotoxicity of aminoglycosides in rats. J Endourol 1998;12:s94.
25. London ET, Ho HS, Neuhaus AM, Wolfe BM, Rudich SM, Perez RV. Effect of intravascular volume expansion on renal function during prolonged CO_2 pneumoperitoneum. Ann Surg 2000;23:195–201.
26. Biegner A, Anderson D, Olson R, Vacchiano C. Quantification of insensible water loss associated with insufflation of non-humidified CO_2 in patients undergoing laparoscopic surgery. J Laparoendosc Adv Surg Tech A 1999;9:325–329.

37. The Systemic Oncologic Implications of Surgery

Sang W. Lee, M.D.

The use of minimally invasive methods for the curative resection of malignancies has been and remains a highly controversial indication. Legitimate concerns regarding the extent and adequacy of resection, port wound tumor recurrences, and the lack of long-term outcome data were raised by many surgeons early after the introduction of advanced laparoscopic methods. However, a decade after the introduction of laparoscopic-assisted colectomy, the first two of these issues, for the most part, have been addressed, at least in regard to colon cancer. It has been demonstrated through both prospective and retrospective studies that an equivalent oncologic colorectal resection can be performed laparoscopically [1, 2]. Reasonably sized prospective series have demonstrated that, in experienced hands, the incidence of port wound tumors is comparable to the rate of incisional recurrences after open tumor resection [3, 4]. Most importantly and to the surprise of most surgeons, the interim results of a single center randomized trial of colorectal cancer patients, summarized at the end of this chapter, suggest that there might be a long-term oncologic benefit associated with the use of minimally invasive methods. Despite these encouraging clinical findings, some critics still believe that there may be something inherently dangerous about minimal access surgery in the setting of malignancy, especially when carried out under a CO_2 pneumoperitoneum.

It is interesting to note that at the same time reports regarding port site tumors were raising fears regarding the safety of laparoscopic cancer operations, the results of a number of animal studies suggested that minimally invasive surgery may be associated with distinct systemic oncologic benefits when compared to open methods. This chapter briefly reviews the existing data regarding the systemic oncologic impact of both open and closed surgical approaches.

A. Animal Data

It had been well established in small animal models, before the introduction of advanced minimally invasive methods, that laparotomy was associated with accelerated tumor growth and an increased rate of metastatic tumor formation in the early postoperative period when compared to anesthesia control animals [5, 6]. In an effort to determine the impact of laparoscopic methods on tumor behavior, a number of investigators carried out a series of experiments in mice and rats.

Allendorf et al. demonstrated, in a murine study, that preexisting subcutaneous adenocarcinomas, distant from the abdominal incision, grew significantly larger following laparotomy than after peritoneal insufflation with carbon dioxide gas [7]. In the same study it was shown that, when intradermal tumor cell inoculation was carried on the day of surgery, tumors were more easily established and grew larger after laparotomy than after CO_2 insufflation. Subsequent investigations by the same group demonstrated similar results for two additional tumor cell lines [8]. DaCosta et al., in a similar experiment comparing sham procedures, noted that the open group tumors were significantly larger than the tumors of the CO_2 insufflation or the anesthesia control groups [9]. Of note, although smaller than the open group tumors, the insufflation group tumors were found to be significantly larger than those of the control group. Allendorf et al., in a later study, demonstrated that the differences in tumor establishment and growth between the open and laparoscopic groups persisted in the setting of a bowel resection [10]. Similar to the DaCosta et al. study, there was a stepwise increase in the mass of the tumors from the control group to the CO_2 insufflation and, finally, the laparotomy group.

Lee et al. determined the proliferation and apoptotic rates of murine dorsal tumors, established on the day of surgery, via high-dose subcutaneous injection of tumor cells, 14 days after sham laparotomy or CO_2 insufflation [11]. Tumors from the laparotomy group mice had significantly greater proliferation rates than those of the insufflation group, which in turn were significantly greater than the results of the control groups tumors. Conversely, the laparotomy group tumors demonstrated significantly lower rates of apoptosis than the tumors from the CO_2 group, which in turn were significantly lower than the control group tumor apoptotic rates.

A murine study that compared tumor growth after laparotomy, CO_2 insufflation, and anesthesia alone in nude (athymic) and immunocompetent mice sought to determine the impact of cell-mediated immune function on postoperative tumor growth. It had been shown previously that full sham laparotomy is associated with a period of cell-mediated immunosuppression. In the immunocompetent mice, after laparotomy, subcutaneous tumors were shown to grow significantly larger than in mice that underwent CO_2 insufflation, similar to the results mentioned previously. In the athymic mice, however, following surgery there was no significant difference in tumor size between the laparotomy and the CO_2 insufflation groups. This result suggested that the differences in tumor growth that were noted between open and laparoscopic groups in the immunocompetent mice were due, at least in part, to differences in postoperative immune function. Although there was no difference in tumor size between the open and the laparoscopic athymic mice groups, tumors of both groups were significantly larger than those of the anesthesia control group. This finding suggested that after surgery, in addition to immune function considerations, other tumor growth-altering factors are at work [12].

Lee et al. examined the possibility that a surgery-related plasma factor may exist that influences tumor growth [13]. It was determined that cancer cells incubated in vitro with plasma from mice that had undergone sham laparotomy proliferated significantly faster than cells incubated with plasma from the insufflation group. In the same study, Lee et al. determined that the factor responsible for this increase in tumor growth was heat labile and nondialyzable. These results suggested that a plasma-soluble factor was responsible, in part, for the increase in tumor growth after laparotomy. In a subsequent study, the same group of investigators attempted to isolate and characterize the factor(s) responsible for increased systemic tumor growth following laparotomy [14]. The results suggested that the plasma level of a heparin-binding growth factor consistent with platelet-derived growth factor (PDGF) is significantly higher after laparotomy and that this increase in PDGF may account for the noted increase in in vitro tumor growth. A human study was next carried out to determine if major abdominal surgery was associated with oncologically relevant plasma compositional changes.

B. Human Studies

Kirman et al. assessed in vitro tumor growth in cultures to which either preoperative or postoperative plasma samples had been added. Plasma samples were obtained from a total of 84 patients undergoing either colorectal resection or gastric bypass. Comparable numbers of open and laparoscopic patients for each type of operation were evaluated. Postoperative day 1 plasma from open surgery patients was associated with significantly greater in vitro tumor growth when compared to results obtained with their preoperative plasma. The rate of tumor cell proliferation correlated with the length of incision. No in vitro tumor growth differences were noted when the laparoscopic group preoperative and postoperative plasma were likewise assessed. The investigators next sought to determine the mechanism of the observed effect. Despite the murine study results, no differences in PDGF levels were noted. However, the plasma levels of a tumor inhibitory protein, insulin-like growth factor-binding protein 3 (IGF-BP3), were noted to be appreciably diminished 1 day following surgery in the great majority of open surgical patients. (The laparoscopic group's IGF-BP-3 levels were similar before and after surgery.) The addition of IGF-BP3 to the postoperative plasma samples prevented the increase in tumor growth observed with "raw" postoperative plasma; further, the supplementation of preoperative plasma with antibodies to IGF-BP3 increased in vitro tumor proliferation rates [15]. To summarize, major open surgery is associated with a decrease in a protein normally found in the blood that inhibits tumor growth. It is not clear whether this difference will have any clinical relevance in regard to long-term outcome.

Both open and laparoscopic abdominal surgical methods influence tumor growth and behavior in the postoperative period. Tumors are more readily established, grow more rapidly, and demonstrate lower rates of apoptosis after surgery than after anesthesia alone. Full laparotomy is associated with the greatest changes. Laparoscopy is associated with similar, but significantly less marked, effects on tumor behavior. Surgery-related immunosuppression and one or more alterations in the makeup of the plasma may be responsible for these postsurgical tumor growth alterations. The possibility exists that minimally invasive approaches may be associated with improved survival and recurrence rates. The intermediate oncologic results of the Lacy et al. single center randomized trial of colon cancer patients, published in Lancet in June 2002, support this conclusion.

This study involved 208 patients; the demographics, extent of resection, and stage distribution were similar between the open and laparoscopic-assisted groups. When all the patients in each group were considered, with a mean follow-up of 43 months, the laparoscopic group had a significantly higher disease free survival rate than the open group. Furthermore, a significantly lower rate of tumor recurrence was noted for the minimally invasive group. When each stage of disease was independently assessed, it was noted that the stage 3 open and laparoscopic subgroups manifested the greatest differences in recurrence and survival [16]. Obviously, it is not possible to make definitive conclusions on the basis of a single study. Nonetheless, the results of Lacy et al. have far-reaching implications. The multicenter randomized trials that are underway worldwide will, hopefully, settle this question.

C. Summary

Most published animal studies that have assessed postoperative tumor growth have noted that laparotomy is associated with a period of accelerated tumor growth. Of note, CO_2 pneumoperitoneum and laparoscopic procedures have been found to be associated with significantly smaller increases in tumor growth in animal studies when compared to open procedures. Although unproven, the greater immunosuppression that is attendant to open procedures may be the cause, at least in part, of the accelerated tumor growth noted after laparotomy. Similarly, both animal studies and one human study suggest that surgery-related changes in the plasma protein composition are likely to account for part of the tumor growth alterations. From a basic science point of view, the avoidance of a large incision and the use of minimally invasive methods, in theory, may be associated with oncologic benefits. The results of a single center randomized human trial of colon cancer patients support these conclusions. The long-term results of the ongoing randomized and prospective colectomy trials will, it is hoped, shed further light on this matter.

D. References

1. Lacy AM, Delgado S, Garcia-Valdecasas JC, et al. Port site metastases and recurrence after laparoscopic colectomy: a randomized trial. Surg Endsoc 1998;12:1039–1042.
2. Milsom JW, Bartholomaus B, Hammerhofer KA, et al. A prospective randomized trial comparing laparoscopic versus conventional techniques in colorectal cancer surgery: a preliminary report. J Am Coll Surg 1998;187:46–57.
3. Fielding GA, Lumley J, Nathanson L, et al. Laparoscopic colectomy. Surg Endosc 1997;11:745–749.
4. Franklin ME, Rosenthal D, Abrego-Medina D, et al. Prospective comparison of open vs. laparoscopic colon surgery for carcinoma: five year results. Dis Col Rectum 1996;39:s35–s46.
5. Ergomont AM, Steller EP, Marquet RL, et al. Local regional promotion of tumor growth after abdominal surgery is dominant over immuno therapy with interleukin-2 and lymphokine activated killer cells. Cancer Detect Prevent 1988;12:421–429.

6. Goshima H, Saji S, Furata T, et al. Experimental study on preventive effects of lung metastases using LAK cells induced from various lymphocytes: special references to enhancement of lung metastasis after laparotomy stress. J Jpn Surg Soc 1989;90: 1245–1250.
7. Allendorf JDF, Bessler M, Kayton ML, et al. Increased tumor establishment and growth after laparotomy vs. laparoscopy in a murine model. Arch Surg 1995;130: 649–653.
8. Southall JC, Lee SW, Allendorf JD, et al. Colon adenocarcinoma and B-16 melanoma grow larger following laparotomy vs. pneumoperitoneum in a murine model. Dis Colon Rectum 1998;41(5):564–569.
9. DaCosta ML, Redmond P, Finnegan N, et al. Laparotomy and laparoscopy differentially accelerate experimental flank tumor growth. Br J Surg 1998;85:1439–1442.
10. Allendorf JD, Bessler M, Horvath KD, et al. Increased tumor establishment and growth after open versus laparoscopic bowel resection in mice. Surg Endosc 1998;12: 1035–1038.
11. Lee SW, Gleason NR, Blanco I, et al. Higher colon cancer tumor proliferative index and tumor cell death rate in mice undergoing laparotomy versus insufflation. Surg Endosc 2002;16(1):36–39.
12. Allendorf JD, Bessler M, Horvath KD, et al. Increased tumor establishment and growth after open versus laparoscopic surgery in mice may be related to differences in post operative T-cell function. Surg Endosc 1999;13:233–235.
13. Lee SW, Gleason NR, Southall JC, et al. A serum soluble factor(s) stimulates tumor growth following laparotomy in a murine model. Surg Endosc 2000;14(5):490–494.
14. Lee SW, Gleason NR, Stapleton GS, et al. Increased platelet-derived growth factor (PDGF) release after laparotomy stimulates systemic tumor growth in mice. Surg Endosc 2001;15(9):981–985.
15. Kirman I, Cekic V, Poltaratskaia N, et al. Plasma from patients undergoing major open surgery stimulates in vitro tumor growth; lower IGF-BP3 levels may, in part, account for this change. Surgery 2002;132:186–192.
16. Lacy AM, Garcia-Valdecasas JC, Delgado S, et al. Laparoscopically-assisted colectomy versus open colectomy for treatment of non-metastatic colon cancer: a randomized trial. Lancet 2002;359:2224–2229.

38. Liver Function and Portal Blood Flow

Michael W. Potter, M.D.
Shimul A. Shah, M.D.
Mark P. Callery, M.D., F.A.C.S.

The effect of CO_2 pneumoperitoneum on hepatic function is clinically insignificant in most patients. Given the number of laparoscopic procedures performed each day, this is fortunate. Theoretically, some patients, such as those with diminished hepatic reserve, may require an alternative to pneumoperitoneum to recover most effectively from surgery.

A. Liver Physiology

The liver is the largest organ in the peritoneal cavity, weighing between 1200 and 1600 g in the average adult. Blood supply to the liver is from both the portal vein (70%) and hepatic artery (30%). The portal vein is a low-pressure, thin-walled vessel, receiving almost all the venous drainage from the digestive tract between proximal stomach and upper rectum, as well as the spleen and pancreas. Drainage of blood from the liver occurs through the hepatic veins, which drain directly into the inferior vena cava.

The liver has a broad range of functions, which reflect its key location interposed between the abdominal viscera and the systemic circulation. It is essential for maintenance of energy homeostasis in the body. It is the first organ to be exposed to pancreatic endocrine secretions, and its sensitivity to these polypeptides can determine the overall catabolic or anabolic balance in the body. A large number of proteins including plasma proteins, acute-phase proteins, and coagulation factors are synthesized by the liver. The liver is also responsible for the detoxification and secretion of various substances, including exogenous substances such as drugs and endogenous substances such as heme. Finally, the liver's reticuloendothelial cell system provides surveillance of the bloodstream and produces cytokines important to the systemic immune response [1]. Therefore, any insult to such a complex organ could affect the overall well-being of the patient and induce morbidity.

B. Pneumoperitoneum

Carbon dioxide pneumoperitoneum is the usual method for achieving laparoscopic access. It is achieved by insufflation of the abdominal cavity to a pressure in the range of 10–15 mmHg. CO_2 is preferred because it is abundant, inexpensive, rapidly absorbed, and does not support combustion. This latter quality is also a drawback because it becomes biologically active when dissolved in the blood and can affect acid-base status and other physiologic functions. Other gases have been investigated as alternatives to CO_2 including room air, oxygen, nitrous oxide, nitrogen, helium, and argon, which prevent the hemodynamic changes associated with CO_2 absorption but still result in elevated intraabdominal pressure. Abdominal wall lifting devices may enable the surgeon to minimize hemodynamic changes altogether, although at this point the visualization provided by these lift devices is substandard.

C. The Effect of Pneumoperitoneum on Hepatic Function

Insufflation of the abdomen applies a direct pressure to the liver parenchyma because it is a solid organ and is not easily compressed. The actual total pressure exerted on the liver may be higher than the insufflation pressure because its location just beneath the right hemidiaphragm subjects the liver to pressures from above during positive-pressure ventilation. This mechanical pressure alone may be enough to produce some damage to the liver. The serum markers commonly known as "liver function tests" are good indicators of damage to hepatocytes. Routine laparoscopic cholecystectomy (LC), in patients who had neither preoperative hepatic dysfunction nor intraoperative bile duct injury, causes significant increases in aspartate aminotransferase (AST) and alanine aminotransferase (ALT). In one study, AST was increased in 79% of patients and ALT in 82%. Levels were as high as 1.8 and 2.2 times the mean preoperative levels, respectively, returning to normal within 72 hours. Alkaline phosphatase (ALP) and total bilirubin were elevated in 53% and 12% of patients, respectively, although the differences when compared to preoperative levels were not statistically significant [2]. Elevation of these liver enzymes is not specific for damage caused by pneumoperitoneum alone, because use of the electrocautery, tension on the liver due to gallbladder retraction, transient elevation of biliary pressures as a result of kinking of the extrahepatic biliary tree, and other sorts of minor liver trauma that occur during surgery may contribute.

Some evidence implicating pneumoperitoneum-related increased intraabdominal pressure as a cause of liver enzyme elevation was provided by Morino et al., who examined 32 patients randomly assigned to undergo LC under insufflation pressures of 10 or 14 mmHg. All patients developed an increase in AST, ALT, bilirubin, and prothrombin time postoperatively, although only the levels of AST and ALT attained statistical significance. There were differences between the two intraabdominal pressure groups; the higher enzyme levels were noted in the 14 mmHg group. Additionally, the liver function of a group of 20 laparoscopic cases insufflated to 14 mmHg that did not involve the liver was compared to the results of the cholecystectomy patients. In this group, AST and ALT were found to be elevated to levels higher than in the 10 mmHg LC group but not as high as the 14 mmHg LC group [3]. In a different study that compared patients receiving LC to those undergoing open cholecystectomy (OC), a significant increase in AST and ALT was found only in the laparoscopic group [4]. These data suggest that the hepatic damage is related to the CO_2 pneumoperitoneum, perhaps due to compression of the relatively low pressure portal venous system. This damage does not manifest itself as clinically notable liver dysfunction, as there was no morbidity attributable to the liver reported in these studies. The markers more specific for true liver function (total bilirubin, prothrombin time) rather than liver damage were also not significantly increased in these studies.

D. The Effect of Pneumoperitoneum on Hepatic Blood Flow

The effects of increased intraabdominal pressure on blood flow in general have been well characterized and include increases in mean arterial blood pressure and systemic vascular resistance. Splanchnic blood flow is affected by pneumoperitoneum as well. In dogs subjected to an elevated intraperitoneal pressure, blood flow to the liver, spleen, and intestines decreases, likely due to compression of the portal vein [5, 6]. In pigs, portal venous flow is decreased by two-thirds with higher levels of intraabdominal pressure [7]. In humans undergoing LC, portal blood flow, as measured by duplex doppler ultrasound, decreased by 53% during insufflation of the abdomen to 14 mmHg [8]. Whether pneumoperitoneum causes compression of the hepatic artery and decrease in arterial blood flow is controversial. Most studies have found that there is little change with increased intraabdominal pressure (IAP); however, Klopfenstein et al. found a 49% increase in hepatic arterial flow using transit-time ultrasound [9].

This overall decreased blood flow correlates with liver dysfunction. Hepatic clearance of indocyanine green (ICG) is impaired in pigs undergoing laparoscopic surgery or simple CO_2 pneumoperitoneum as compared to animals undergoing open surgery [10]. This diminished blood flow could conceivably contribute to alterations in the ability of the liver to process various anesthetic agents, as it does ICG. Additionally, CO_2 insufflation of the rat abdomen leads to decreased particle elimination by the liver mononuclear phagocyte system as compared to open surgery or endoscopic surgery without pneumoperitoneum [11].

E. The Effect of CO_2 on the Liver

Changes in hepatic blood flow may not be caused entirely by the effects of the pressure of the pneumoperitoneum on the portal vein and inferior vena cava (IVC). Local microcirculatory changes may occur as a result of increased PCO_2

caused by CO_2 pneumoperitoneum, and this could be a mechanism for hepatic dysfunction; however, this does not seem to be a predominant factor. In a study of dogs insufflated to 14 mmHg with CO_2 or helium (He), all hemodynamic measurements that were made were equivalent between the two groups, except that the PCO_2 measured at the IVC was higher in the CO_2 group [5]. On the other hand, a similar study showed that helium was associated with a greater decrease in hepatic blood flow than CO_2 pneumoperitoneum [12].

There is some concern regarding the use of CO_2 in laparoscopic liver resection. Because of pressure differences between the hepatic venous system, which normally has a pressure of 5–10 mmHg, and the elevated intraabdominal pressure due to the pneumoperitoneum (10–14 mmHg), there is the potential for gas embolism when the hepatic venous system is injured and thus directly exposed to the pneumoperitoneum. During laparoscopic liver resection, CO_2 microbubbles seem to form in the hepatic circulation [13]; these microbubbles could conceivably travel to the vena cava and right atrium, creating a gas lock. The benefit of using a physiologic gas such as CO_2 rather than an inert gas like helium might come in to play in this situation because CO_2 can be rapidly dissolved and absorbed in the blood, producing only transient and minor symptoms [14]. Abdominal wall lift devices have been employed due to concern for CO_2 embolism [15, 16], but laparoscopic hepatic resection under pneumoperitoneum has been well described without significant changes [14, 17].

F. Special Considerations

As is clear from the preceding studies, the liver is affected by pneumoperitoneum, but not usually to a clinically evident level. Are there cases in which this liver dysfunction can become clinically important? The most obvious situation in which this might occur is in patients who have preexisting limitations of hepatic reserve. Cirrhotic livers or those with chronic hepatitis may not have the functional capacity to recover from the insult that pneumoperitoneum incurs. One study addresses this question by evaluating the liver's ability to convert amino nitrogen in the blood to urea nitrogen in patients with cirrhosis as a measure of the metabolic stress response. There was no significant difference, in this value, between the metabolic stress response of those patients who underwent OC and those who had a laparoscopic procedure [18]. In these patients with limited reserve, it may be that any impairment of hepatic function that may be induced by CO_2 pneumoperitoneum is well compensated for by the decreased need for a metabolic stress response afforded by minimally invasive surgery.

Another area in which pneumoperitoneum might affect the liver is laparoscopic cancer surgery. Decreasing morbidity, patient comfort, and hospital stay would be a boon to patients requiring cancer resection. There is some concern, however, that the presence of pneumoperitoneum may increase the chances for tumor dissemination and metastases. Tumor cells that are shed hematogeneously during resection are likely to find their way into the portal vein. In a study of tumor cells injected directly into the portal veins of rabbits, Ishida et al. found a significant increase in the subsequent amount of tumor found in the livers of those animals that were exposed to pneumoperitoneum when compared to the results in animals that underwent laparotomy [19]. In a similar model, although in mice, Chen et al. found that the number of tumor cells initially localized to the liver was higher in the pneumoperitoneum group, although this increase lessened over time [20]. These authors propose that impaired hepatic blood flow may create an environment more conducive to tumor cell implantation, that oxygen-derived free radicals created following restoration of blood flow might induce endothelial cell damage and thus allow better tumor cell localization, or that hypercapnia might induce the growth of tumor cells directly. Impaired reticuloendothelial cell function may also play a role during or following pneumoperitoneum. These hypotheses have not been adequately investigated in human subjects.

G. Conclusion

Clearly, pneumoperitoneum, whether with CO_2 or other gases, causes some hepatic damage although effects on hepatic function are limited. Blood flow to the liver is altered, and this affects hepatic clearance of some drugs. These changes are small and clinically insignificant in most situations. As our repertoire of laparoscopic procedures increases, it will be necessary to consider in what ways pneumoperitoneum can have an effect on the liver and whether alternatives to insufflation would be appropriate. New technologies such as abdominal lift devices with minimal insufflation could minimize any hepatic damage and help to placate worries about impaired hepatic reserve or metastases to the liver.

H. References

1. Vittemberga FJ, Foley DP, Meyers WC, et al. Laparoscopic surgery and the systemic immune response. Ann Surg 1998;227:326–334.
2. Halevy A, Gold-Deutch R, Negri M, et al. Are elevated liver enzymes and bilirubin levels significant after laparoscopic cholecystectomy in the absence of bile duct injury? Ann Surg 1994;219:362–364.
3. Morino M, Giraudo G, Festa V. Alterations in hepatic function during laparoscopic surgery. Surg Endosc 1998;12:968–972.
4. Saber AA, Laraja RD, Nalbandian HI, et al. Changes in liver function tests after laparoscopic cholecystectomy: not so rare, not always ominous. Am Surg 2000;66:699–702.
5. Kotzampassi K, Kapanidis N, Kazamias P, et al. Hemodynamic events in the peritoneal environment during pneumoperitoneum in dogs. Surg Endosc 1993;7:494–499.
6. Caldwell CB, Ricotta JJ. Changes in visceral blood flow with elevated intraabdominal pressure. J Surg Res 1987;43:14–20.
7. Rasmussen I, Berggren, Arvidsson D, et al. Effects of pneumoperitoneum on splanchnic hemodynamics: an experimental study in pigs. Eur J Surg 1995;161:819–826.

8. Jakimowicz J, Stultiëns G, Smulders F. Laparoscopic insufflation of the abdomen reduces portal venous flow. Surg Endosc 1998;12:129–132.
9. Klopfenstein CE, Morel DR, Clergue F, et al. Effects of abdominal CO_2 insufflation and changes of position on hepatic blood flow in anesthetized pigs. Am J Physiol 1998;275:H900–H905.
10. Tunon MJ, Gonsalez P, Jorquera F, et al. Liver blood flow changes during laparoscopic surgery in pigs. Surg Endosc 1999;13:668–672.
11. Gutt CN, Heinz P, Kaps W, et al. The phagocytosis activity during conventional and laparoscopic operations in the rat: a preliminary study. Surg Endosc 1997;11:899–901.
12. Sala-Blanch X, Fontanals J, Martinez-Palli G, et al. Effects of carbon dioxide vs. helium pneumoperitoneum on hepatic blood flow. Surg Endosc 1998;12:1121–1125.
13. Takagi S. Hepatic and portal vein blood flow during carbon dioxide pneumoperitoneum for laparoscopic hepatectomy. Surg Endosc 1998;12:427–431.
14. Hashizume M, Takenaka K, Yanaga K, et al. Laparoscopic hepatic resection for hepatocellular carcinoma. Surg Endosc 1995;9:1289–1291.
15. Watanabe Y, Sato M, Ueda S, et al. Laparoscopic hepatic resection: a new and safe procedure by abdominal wall lifting method. Hepatogastroenterology 1997;44:143–147.
16. Huscher CGS, Lirici MM, Chiodini S. Laparoscopic liver resections. Semin Laparosc Surg 1998;5:204–210.
17. Kaneko H, Takagi S, Shiba T. Laparoscopic partial hepatectomy and left lateral segmentectomy: technique and results of a clinical series. Surgery 1996;120:468–475.
18. Lausten SB, El-Sefi T, Marwan I, et al. Postoperative hepatic catabolic stress response in patients with cirrhosis and chronic hepatitis. World J Surg 2000;24:365–371.
19. Ishida H, Murata N, Yamada H, et al. Pneumoperitoneum with carbon dioxide enhances liver metastases of cancer cells implanted into the portal vein in rabbits. Surg Endosc 2000;14:239–242.
20. Chen WS, Lin W, Kou YR, et al. Possible effect of pneumoperitoneum on the spreading of colon cancer tumor cells. Dis Colon Rectum 1997;40:791–797.

39. Port Site Tumors: Local Oncologic Effect

James W. Fleshman Jr., M.D.

A. Problem

Laparoscopic procedures for malignancy may be associated with an unexpected and untoward late development referred to as "port site tumor recurrences." These are metastatic tumors of the abdominal wall that can develop at the extraction wound (for specimen removal) or at one of the port wounds remote from the specimen extraction site. These tumors have been noted to develop after a variety of intraabdominal malignancies including colon and gallbladder adenocarcinoma as well as gynecologic tumors. The latter are associated with the highest reported rates of port site recurrences; this is most likely due to the diffuse nature of ovarian cancer. The true incidence is unknown but has been reported to be as high as 16% in one report regarding patients undergoing laparoscopic exploration for metastatic gynecologic malignancy [1]. In regard to the gynecologic population, this serious complication has been noted most often in the setting of ovarian cancer and to a lesser extent in patients with endometrial cancer; these recurrences are rare in cervical cancer patients. Advanced stages of disease clearly predispose to port site recurrences regardless of tumor type.

The first report regarding a port site recurrence in the setting of colorectal cancer was published in 1993. In the years to follow reports concerning at least an additional 50 of these abdominal wall tumors were added to the literature. In large part, it was fear of port wound tumors that led to the development and organization of the numerous randomized and prospective trials of colon cancer patients that are presently underway worldwide. It is important to note that wound tumors can also develop after open cancer operations. Two large retrospective reviews of colon cancer patients undergoing open colectomy noted incisional wound recurrences in between 0.6% and 0.69% of patients [2, 3]. The incidence of port site recurrences after colectomy in reported series containing more than 50 patients is 0%–2.5%. The majority of these series have reported incidences less than 1%. The three randomized controlled trials on colorectal cancer and laparoscopy that have published interim papers reported no port site recurrences [4–6].

Gallbladder cancer is a rare (less than 1%) finding after laparoscopic cholecystectomy and is usually unsuspected. However, port site recurrence occurs in 10%–14% of patients with gallbladder cancer who undergo laparoscopic surgery, probably due to inadvertent perforation and spillage of cells during manipulation or extraction. Gallbladder ultrasonography (either transabdominal or laparoscopic) would be expected to alert the surgeon as to the possibility of gallbladder cancer (finding of a mass in the gallbladder wall). In those circumstances, open cholecystectomy should be performed.

Laparoscopic nephrectomy and lymphadenectomy for renal cell cancer and prostate cancer, respectively, have not been associated with a high incidence of port site recurrences despite morselization of specimens after nephrectomy and piecemeal extraction of retroperitoneal lymph nodes. Direct laparoscopic biopsy of bladder cancer has resulted in a port site recurrence.

Diagnostic laparoscopy for the staging of upper gastrointestinal malignancies (pancreas, duodenal, gastric, liver, bile duct, and esophageal) has resulted in a remarkably low rate of port site recurrences. The majority of the recurrences that have been noted after such procedures were found in patients with disseminated or locally advanced disease. Muensterer et al. [7] recommended midline placement of trocars to facilitate excision of the port sites during subsequent cytoreductive surgery.

B. Etiology

For a port tumor recurrence to develop, viable tumor cells must somehow separate from the primary lesion after which the cells must be transported to one of the incisions. Provided the conditions for tumor establishment and growth are met in the wound, a metastasis develops. Most laparoscopic surgeons agree that traumatic handling of a tumor during mobilization, resection, and extraction may liberate tumor cells from the primary. The stage of the lesion is also an important variable. Tumor shedding into the peritoneal cavity is far less likely to occur with a small T1 lesion (invasion limited to submucosa) than with a large T3 lesion (invasion through the entire bowel wall). Thus, poor technique, especially in the setting of a more advanced tumor, is likely to increase the chances of wound tumor formation whereas meticulous oncologic technique should decrease the chances of port wound tumor formation.

It is important to realize that in certain, thankfully rare, situations (in regard to colorectal cancer), tumor cells spontaneously separate from the primary tumor and are able to successfully implant in a wound or on an uninjured peritoneal surface. This highlights the fact that the "biology" of a tumor, which may vary tremendously from lesion to lesion, is also an important variable. Although the surgeon can have an impact on the chances of tumor cell shedding related to resection by using sound technique, he cannot alter the genetic makeup of the tumor or its tendency to spontaneously spread. Tumor cells from aggressive tumors are more likely to survive and implant once separated from the primary.

It is likely that, at the start of a case, there are often cancer cells free-floating in the abdominal cavity in patients with tumors invading through the serosal or visceral peritoneal covering. Surgery, as already mentioned, also may result in the liberation of tumor cells. Cytologic and immunohistologic analyses of cells recovered from the abdominal cavity of cancer patients undergoing surgery and blood from tumor specimens have documented that tumor cells are shed in this manner. The precise incidence of such shedding, the number of cells shed, and the viability of these cells, which is likely to vary widely from tumor to tumor and from case to case, is not known. Obviously, it must be very difficult for these cells to survive and implant and form metastases because the incidence of intraabdominal and wound recurrences, after both open and closed resection, is low.

The surgeon must focus on the variables in the equation on which they can have an impact. As mentioned, traumatic handling of the tumor will greatly increase the chances of shedding cells. A skilled surgeon is much less likely to disrupt the tumor than an inexperienced one. Therefore, the laparoscopic skill level of the surgeon is a critical factor when dealing with intraabdominal cancer. Proper cancer technique, that is, minimal handling of the tumor, containment, complete mesenteric removal, proximal vascular ligation, and adequate proximal and distal bowel margins, should guarantee a low rate of tumor spillage and thus a low rate of port site recurrence. Many of the reports of port site recurrence in patients with colorectal cancer were published within the first 2 years after the first laparoscopic colectomies for cancer were attempted in 1991. Thus, the majority of these tumor recurrences were noted in the period when general and colorectal surgeons were performing their initial cases and were gaining laparoscopic experience. As surgeons have become more familiar and adept with minimally invasive approaches, fewer such reports have been published. Port site tumor recurrences have not been a major concern, thus far, in the randomized trials that are ongoing. Furthermore, published reports concerning large prospective or retrospective series of patients from experienced surgeons have, with few exceptions, reported wound tumor recurrence rates of less than 1%.

The presence of a 10 to 15 mmHg pneumoperitoneum may facilitate the dispersion of liberated tumor cells throughout the abdomen and to the port sites via desufflation events or, in theory, because of the CO_2 gas. However, port site recurrences can develop after gasless laparoscopy as well; therefore, it is not clear how large a role the CO_2 pneumoperitoneum plays in the development of port site tumors. The current opinion of most laparoscopic experts is that surgical technique and the spontaneous shedding of tumor cells by some tumors are much more important variables than the CO_2 pneumoperitoneum.

C. Research Results

Numerous mouse, rat, and human tumor cell lines have been used in a variety of tumor models to investigate incisional tumor recurrences and the effect of laparoscopy on cancer development. These areas of investigation are categorized below. Then, a brief review of some of these studies is provided.

1. Studies that assessed the rate of wound tumor formation after laparoscopy. The majority of investigations in this category have simultaneously studied incisional recurrence rates after laparotomy and anesthesia alone.
2. Investigation of the mechanism(s) of tumor cell transport to the wounds and the establishment of tumor at port sites.
3. Determination of the impact of laparoscopic conditions (for example, elevated intraabdominal pressure and the specific type of gas used) on wound tumor formation.

4. Identification of preventative maneuvers or strategies to reduce port wound tumors.
5. Studies that have assessed the systemic oncologic and immunologic impact of open and closed surgical techniques are reviewed separately, in another chapter in this manual. (See Chapters 37 and 41.)

Wound Tumors After Laparoscopic and Open Procedures: Rodent Studies

The initial report documenting a role for pneumoperitoneum in the development of port site recurrence came from Jones et al. [8] in a hamster study that utilized a human colon cancer cell suspension model. This model assessed the rate of port wound tumor formation after injecting a solution containing a large number of viable tumor cells (in this case, 1.6×10^6 GW39 tumor cells) into the abdominal cavity and then subjecting half the animals to a 10 mmHg pneumoperitoneum. A threefold increase in port site recurrence was found in the pneumoperitoneum group compared to laparotomy controls. Subsequent studies with the same model confirmed the role of pneumoperitoneum but also found that reduced tumor inoculums resulted in much lower rates of wound tumor formation than noted with the high-dose inoculums [9, 10]. At an inoculum half that used in the original study, no significant difference was found in the number of animals with at least one port tumor recurrence. This latter study highlighted the fact that, in tumor cell suspension studies, the size of the inoculum was critical. One of the drawbacks to the tumor cell suspension model is that it did not permit assessment of how tumor cells become separated from the primary lesion or how good and bad surgical technique influenced wound tumor formation.

Lee et al. [11] developed a solid tumor model that allowed surgical technique to be studied. Splenic tumors were established by carefully injecting tumor cells into the spleen 10 days before an operation at which time a splenectomy was carried out. In the first study done with this model, it was demonstrated that intentional crushing of the tumor capsule during the removal of the spleen, as compared to splenectomy done with minimal touching of the tumor, resulted in a significantly higher port wound tumor formation rate. The presence or absence of a CO_2 pneumoperitoneum did not significantly alter the results. A later study, using the same model, assessed the ability of one surgeon to perform a meticulous laparoscopic-assisted splenectomy. The study was made up of five different groups of both open and laparoscopic mice that underwent surgery on different days. Regarding the first group to be operated on, significantly more port wound tumors were noted in the laparoscopic group than in the open group. However, in the subsequent surgical groups the rate of port wound tumors decreased in the closed groups such that there was no significant difference between the open and closed groups when the entire cohort of animals was considered. Of note, the time it took to complete the laparoscopic splenectomy and the number of times the surgeon grasped the tumor during mobilization of the spleen decreased from group to group. The results suggest that as the surgeon gained experience the incidence of port tumors fell until it was similar to the rate of wound tumors after open splenectomy. The results of these studies support the concept that traumatization of the tumor and surgical technique are critical risk factors in regard to the development of wound tumors.

Different Gases and Pneumoperitoneum Conditions and Lifting Devices

Numerous authors have studied the impact of different insufflation gases and of abdominal wall lifting methods on the rate of port wound tumor formation. Jacobi et al. [12] performed a cell suspension study in a rat model that examined abdominal wound tumor growth after CO_2 or helium pneumoperitoneum. Significantly more animals in the CO_2 pneumoperitoneum group developed tumors at the abdominal wounds than in either the helium or anesthesia control groups. Bouvy et al. [13], in a cell suspension study, showed that gasless laparoscopy was associated with fewer port site recurrences and less tumor spread than laparotomy or CO_2 pneumoperitoneum. Watson et al. [14], utilizing a retroperitoneal solid tumor model, compared CO_2 pneumoperitoneum and lifting methods and found fewer tumors with the latter. The same investigators also compared different gases with the same model and found the lowest rate of tumor formation after helium was used [15]. It should be noted that the conditions chosen for these studies were not realistic in that there was a very high volume CO_2 leak maintained during the pneumoperitoneum; the equivalent in a human would be at least 5–10 L/min. This rapid leakage of CO_2 may have influenced the results.

Some small animal studies have found that laparoscopy is associated with smaller or fewer wound recurrences when compared to laparotomy. Bouvy et al. [16], utilizing a rat tumor cell suspension model, compared CO_2 pneumoperitoneum, gasless laparoscopy (abdominal wall lifting), and sham laparotomy. After 4 weeks, a significantly greater volume of abdominal wall tumor was noted in the laparotomy group than in the other groups. Paik et al. [17] actually demonstrated a protective effect of laparoscopy on wound implantation in a rat colon cancer model.

Transport of Tumor Cells to the Wounds

Do aerosols of free tumor cells form during pneumoperitoneum? Matthew et al. [18] found that rat to rat transfer of tumor cells through a connecting tube was related more to large tumor cell inoculums and high CO_2 flow rates between the animals (due to an intentional leak) than to aerosolization. Sellers et al. [19], utilizing an in vitro model, were unable to demonstrate that aerosols formed in high-pressure CO_2 environments. The latter investigators did demonstrate that rapid desufflation could propel droplets of fluid containing tumor cells to the mouth of the in vitro apparatus that they utilized.

Hewett et al. [20] were the first to suggest that the removal of tumor cell-contaminated laparoscopic instruments was an important potential means of seeding port wounds. Using video scintigraphy they have also demonstrated that injected tumor cells are more rapidly distributed throughout the abdominal cavity during pneumoperitoneum than during laparotomy. Allardyce et al. [21], using a porcine model, suggested that the "chimney effect" of gas leaking around trocar sites during instrument passage, torquing of the port, and port removal may transport tumor cells to the wounds.

Prevention of Port Wound Tumors

The employment of sound oncologic surgical technique is probably the best way to avoid port tumors. The use of wound protectors or specimen bags is also recommended. Local treatment to prevent or destroy implanted cells and intraperitoneal chemotherapy are potential means of limiting port site recurrence. A variety of tumoricidal solutions have been tested as abdominal and wound irrigants; several have been found to lower the rate of wound tumor formation in animal studies. None of these agents has yet been tested in a randomized, controlled trial in humans. The reader is referred to Chapter 40 of this manual for an in-depth discussion on this topic.

D. Summary

Port wound tumor recurrences after laparoscopy in the setting of malignancy are a potential problem, as are incisional tumors after open surgery. In regard to colorectal cancer, the feared high incidence of port wound tumors that laparoscopic critics anticipated and predicted has not materialized. The most recent human data suggest that there is no difference in the rate of wound tumor formation after open and closed colectomy for colon cancer.

In regard to the animal literature on this subject, the results are conflicting and difficult to interpret. The models used for these studies are imperfect and, in some cases, have little relevance to the human setting. The conditions of pneumoperitoneum tested as well as the size of the tumor cell inoculums, in some studies, were unrealistic. Aerosols of tumor cells do not commonly form. However, the CO_2 environment, under rare conditions (very high rate of tumor spillage), may have some influence on port wound tumor development. Further, the CO_2 pneumoperitoneum, via desufflation events, may transport viable free tumor cells to the abdominal wounds. Contaminated instruments may also carry tumor cells to the wounds. Finally, the inherent ability of the tumor cells in question to survive once separated and to implant in a wound and form a tumor is also a critical variable, one over which the surgeon has little control.

In the final analysis, tumor cell liberation, either spontaneous or via traumatization of the tumor at surgery, is probably a far more important factor in the human setting than the CO_2 pneumoperitoneum. The human results to date support this hypothesis. In many cases, wound tumors may be preventable provided that sound oncologic surgical technique is employed. The surgeon may be able to further lower the rate of wound tumor formation by irrigating with tumoricidal solutions or using other perioperative measures. The author advises that surgeons performing laparoscopic procedures in patients with intraabdominal malignancies should do so in the setting of protocols that monitor cancer outcome.

E. References

1. Kadar N. Port-site recurrences following laparoscopic operations for gynecological malignancies. Br J Obstet Gynecol 1997;104:1308–1313.
2. Hughes ESR, McDermott FT, Polglase AL, et al. Tumor recurrence in the abdominal wall scar after large-bowel cancer surgery. Dis Colon Rectum 1983;26(9):571–572.
3. Reilly WT, Nelson H, Schroeder G, Wieand HS, Bolton J, O'Connell MJ. Wound recurrence following conventional treatment of colorectal cancer. Dis Colon Rectum 1996;39:200–207.
4. Lacy AM, Garcia-Valdecasas JC, Pique JM, et al. Short-term outcome analysis of a randomized study comparing laparoscopic vs. open colectomy for colon cancer. Surg Endosc 1995;9:1101–1105.
5. Milsom JW, Bohm B, Hammerhofer KA, Fazio V, Steiger E, Elson P. A prospective, randomized trial comparing laparoscopic versus conventional techniques in colorectal cancer surgery: a preliminary report. J Am Coll Surg 1998;187:46–57.
6. Stage JG, Schulze S, Moller P, et al. Prospective randomized study of laparoscopic versus open colonic resection for adenocarcinoma. Br J Surg 1997;84:391–396.
7. Muensterer OJ, Averbach AM, Jacquet P, Otero SE, Sugarbaker PH. Malignant peritoneal mesothelioma. Case-report demonstrating pitfalls of diagnostic laparoscopy. Int Surg 1997;82:240–243.
8. Jones DB, Guo LW, Reinhard MK, et al. Impact of pneumoperitoneum on trocar site implantation of colon cancer in hamster model. Dis Colon Rectum 1995;38:1182–1188.
9. Wu JS, Brasfield EB, Guo LW, et al. Implantation of colon cancer at trocar sites is increased by low pressure pneumoperitoneum. Surgery 1997;122:1–7.
10. Wu JS, Jones DB, Fuo LW, et al. Effects of pneumoperitoneum on tumor implantation with decreasing tumor inoculum. Dis Colon Rectum 1998;41:141–146.
11. Lee SW, Southall J, Allendorf J, Bessler M, Whelan RL. Traumatic handling of the tumor independent of pneumoperitoneum increases port-site implantation rate of colon cancer in a murine model. Surg Endosc 1998;12:828–834.
12. Jacobi CA, Sabat R, Bohm B, Zieren HU, Volk HD, Muller JM. Pneumoperitoneum with carbon dioxide stimulates growth of malignant colonic cells. Surgery 1997;121:72–78.
13. Bouvy ND, Giuffrida MC, Tseng LNL, et al. Effects of carbon dioxide pneumoperitoneum, air pneumoperitoneum, and gasless laparoscopy on body weight and tumor growth. Arch Surg 1998;133:652–656.

14. Watson DI, Mathew G, Ellis T, Baigrie CF, Rofe AM, Jamieson GG. Gasless laparoscopy may reduce the risk of port-site recurrences following laparoscopic tumor surgery. Arch Surg 1997;132:166–169.
15. Neuhaus SJ, Watson DI, Ellis T, et al. Wound metastasis after laparoscopy with different insufflation gases. Surgery 1998;123:579–583.
16. Bouvy ND, Marquet RL, Jeekel H, Bonjer HJ. Impact of gas(less) laparoscopy and laparotomy on peritoneal tumor growth and abdominal wall metastases. Ann Surg 1996; 224:694–701.
17. Paik PS, Misawa T, Chiang M, et al. Abdominal incision tumor implantation following pneumoperitoneum laparoscopic procedure vs. standard open incision in a syngeneic rat model. Dis Colon Rectum 1998;41:419–422.
18. Mathew G, Watson DI, Ellis T, DeYoung N, Rofe AM, Jamieson GG. The effect of laparoscopy on the movement of tumor cells and metastasis to surgical wounds. Surg Endosc 1997;11:1163–1166.
19. Sellers GJ, Whelan RL, Allendorf JD, et al. An in vitro model fails to demonstrate aerosolization of tumor cells. Surg Endosc 1998;12:436–439.
20. Hewett PJ, Thomas WM, King G, Eaton M. Intraperitoneal cell movement during abdominal carbon dioxide insufflation and laparoscopy: an in vivo model. Dis Colon Rectum 1996;39:62–66.
21. Allardyce RA, Morreau P, Bagshaw PF. Operative factors affecting tumor cell distribution following laparoscopic colectomy in a porcine model. Dis Colon Rectum 1997;40:939–945.

40. Port Site Tumors: Means of Prevention

Marc A. Reymond, M.D.
Hans Lippert, M.D.
Morris E. Franklin, M.D.

> *"Tumor grafts in wounds are of particular interest for the surgeon. After laparotomy for malignant ascites, it is not rare to find small cancer nodules within drainage sites, on the contrary such findings are exceptional—if ever present—in laparotomy wounds."*
>
> —Peterson, 1904

Possible means of prevention of port site recurrences have been identified on the basis of the contamination pathways and the local conditions identified in clinical observations and animal experiments. After reading this chapter, the reader should be able to understand the potential for the implantation of tumor cells into port site and other wounds during laparoscopic procedures. The reader should also gain knowledge of the prophylactic countermeasures that are available to surgeons performing laparoscopic procedures.

The suggested means of prevention include preoperative measures, as well as technical tips to be applied before, during, and after tumor resection has been completed (Table 40.1). Collectively, these measures, when applied alone or in combination, should result in a lower incidence of port wound recurrences.

A. Preoperative Measures

Preoperative measures include proper patient selection, adequate training of the surgeon and of the operating team, and adequate surgical technique as well as complete and adequate equipment for advanced laparoscopic surgery.

Tumor infiltration into adjacent structures is present in about 10% of all colorectal cancers. There is an increased risk of iatrogenic traumatization of such tumors, in part because these tumors are usually bulky and difficult to manipulate laparoscopically. In locally advanced tumors, to adhere to accepted oncologic principles, en bloc multivisceral resection with tumor-free resection margins is recommended. This type of resection for a locally advanced lesion is best performed via an open approach.

Traumatic manipulation of a tumor is one mechanism whereby viable tumor cells may be shed during a cancer resection; however, in some patients, usually

Table 40.1. Suggested techniques for the prevention of port wound tumor recurrences.

Before resection:
Proper patient selection (exclude patients with very large lesions or lesions invading adjacent organs)
Adequate training and experience of surgeon and assistants
Careful tumor localization (tattoo, barium enema, etc.)
Proper port placement (position, angle, incision size, etc.)
Anchor all ports (grips, threaded ports, or skin sutures)
During resection:
Avoid gas leaks
Identify tumor-bearing segment (intraoperative colonoscopy if needed)
Avoidance of direct tumor handling or manipulation
Sound surgical techniques
Respect of oncologic principles (closed resection, en bloc resection with lymphatic drainage, proximal vessel control, clearance of resection margin)
Thorough irrigation and suctioning of abdomen
After resection:
Adequate-sized incision for removal of specimen
Wound protector or specimen bag
Macroscopic and, if need be, microscopic analysis of resected specimen
Thorough irrigation of ports and abdomen before closure (cytotoxic solution or saline)
Fascial and peritoneal wound closure (for ports 10 mm or larger)

those with advanced lesions, tumor cells may be spontaneously shed into the peritoneal cavity [3]. Regardless of how the tumor cells are liberated, once free-floating in the peritoneal cavity, they may give rise to a port wound recurrence or a local recurrence elsewhere in the abdomen [7]. In animal models that utilized tumor cell suspension models, the development of port wound recurrences appeared to be dose dependent [7]. In a review of all port site recurrences published after the introduction of laparoscopic colectomy, three-fourths occurred in patients with advanced tumor stages (TNM/Jass stages III and IV) [19]. Thus, in the opinion of the authors, large tumors that invade through the serosa or into adjacent organs are best not operated on using the laparoscope. This implies that all patients scheduled for curative oncologic laparoscopic surgery should be staged preoperatively with computerized tomography and, when indicated, endoultrasonography.

It is a known fact in surgery that the experience of the surgeon correlates directly with their results. Thus, a laparoscopic oncologic resection, in particular when performed with a curative intent, should not be carried out by a surgeon with little minimally invasive experience; the same is true for an open cancer resection [8, 10]. In laparoscopic surgery, it is widely accepted that surgeons wishing to perform curative operations must first demonstrate minimally invasive proficiency by performing colorectal resections for benign indications [12].

The location of the tumor must be precisely identified or the lesion containing the tumor clearly marked before the start of the operation. It is not reasonable to rely solely on the gastroenterologist's impression of the location of the lesions with the exception of tumors at or within site of the ileocecal valve. A variety of endoscopic and radiologic techniques have been described that serve to identify the tumor-bearing segment. Tattooing is the most reliable endoscopic method; India ink, the most widely used agent, results in a long-lasting and probably permanent tattoo. Endoscopic clips are less reliable and remain cumbersome to use [6]. If these methods fail to definitively identify the tumor location, then intraoperative endoscopy must be performed. Colonoscopy can also be used if there is any question as to what constitutes an adequate margin of resection.

Tissue trauma has been shown to enhance tumor growth in experimental studies [1, 17], and clinical observations confirm the paramount significance of raw surfaces in the development of intraperitoneal and intrapleural recurrences. Thus, parietal trauma should be minimized by proper placement of trocars; ideally, ports should be placed so as to provide adequate access to the segment in question without requiring heavy torquing or levering of the port. Moreover, trocars should be placed perpendicularly to the abdominal wall to avoid tearing the peritoneum [2].

CO_2 leakage around trocars should be prevented. There is experimental evidence that tumor growth at trocar sites is enhanced in the presence of massive gas leaks [17]. Although a "chimney effect" has been postulated, the effect of gas leaks on port site recurrences is probably indirect, because it has been fairly well demonstrated that aerosolization of tumor cells (stable suspension of tumor cells in the CO_2 pneumoperitoneum) only occurs during grossly contaminated and prolonged surgery, and does not commonly lead to the seeding of port wounds [9, 13, 15]. Massive gas leaks, however, may transport tumor cells by propelling fluid microdroplets that contain tumor cells out of the abdomen and into the wound. Ports may also become contaminated during desufflation events; these ports may seed the wound when they are removed at the end of the case. Regardless of the precise mechanism by which CO_2 leaks facilitate port tumors in experimental models, such leaks can be prevented or minimized via a variety of measures. The incisions for ports should be carefully made so as to avoid an overly large skin opening that would encourage gas leakage. The use of some type of port-anchoring method will also prevent accidental port dislodgement and sudden desufflation (Figure 40.1A).

B. During Resection

We have shown that during oncologic surgery in animal models the instruments often become highly contaminated with tumor cells [13]. Rinsing of the tip of the instrument before its withdrawal is recommended (Figure 40.1B) and, conversely, the extracorporeal cleansing or decontamination of an instrument before its reinsertion is advised. The latter can be done by dipping the instrument into a plastic bag partially filled with a cytotoxic solution off the surgical field [11]. For example, the surgeon can use an iodine povidone (Betadine) solution, which has been shown to be tumoricidal in vitro, as well as in vivo, in most studies [5, 14, 21]. Alternately, a solution of taurolidine can also be used. Mechanical cleansing of the instruments by thoroughly wiping them should also reduce the chances of seeding port wounds by this mechanism.

During surgical manipulation, ports are progressively loaded with tumor cells, as shown not only in the pig model with radioactivity studies [16], but also

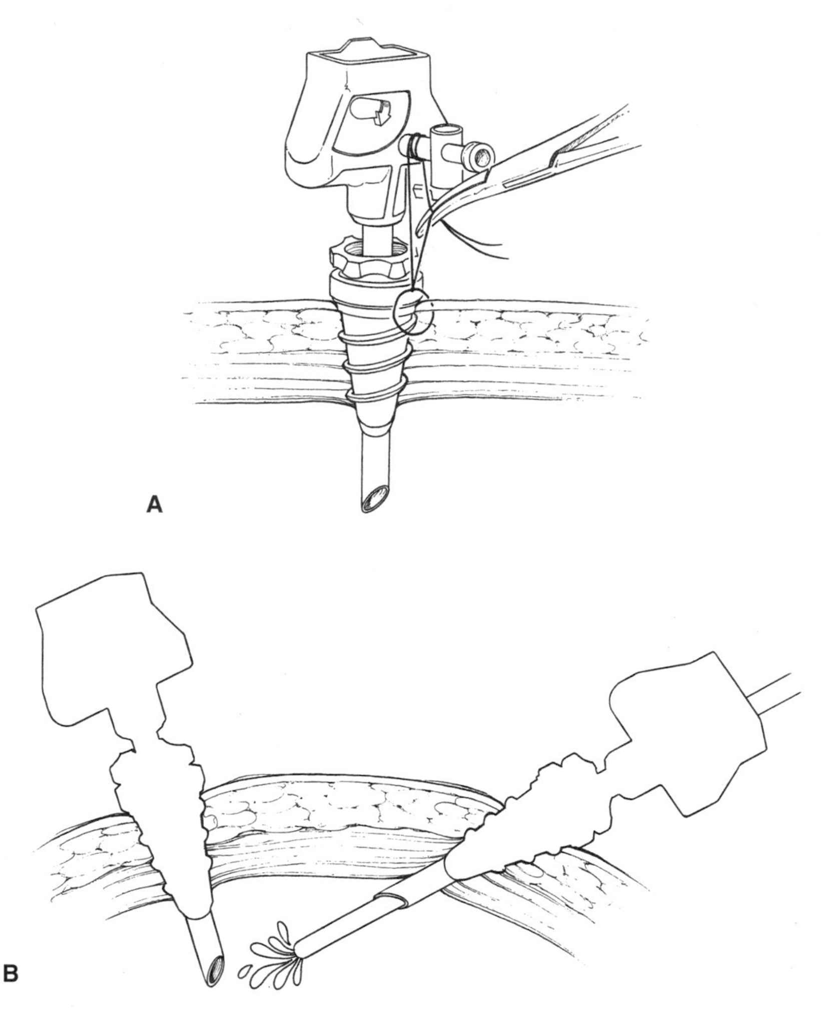

Figure 40.1. (A) Laparoscopic port "anchored" to the abdominal wall with a conically shaped "port grip." (B) Irrigation of laparoscopic port intracorporeally. Irrigation should be followed by thorough suctioning of intraperitoneal fluid. (C) Removal of resected cancer via specimen bag. (D) Fascial and peritoneal closure of all ports 10 mm in size or bigger via a suture passer with port still in place.

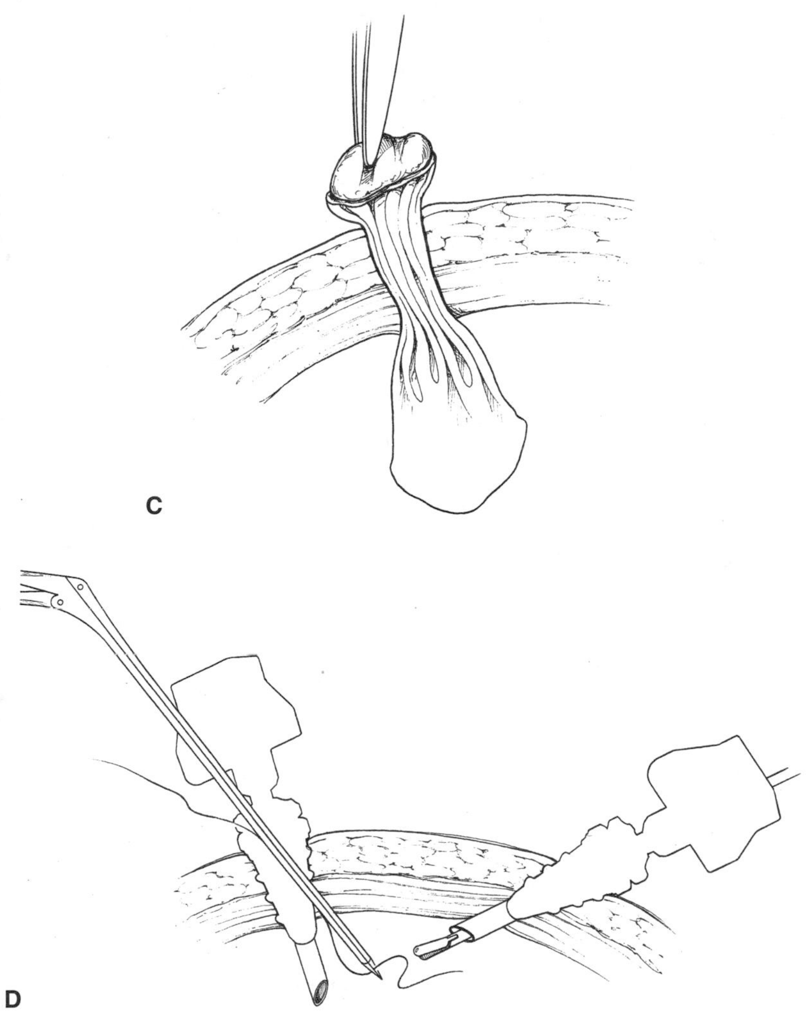

Figure 40.1. *Continued*

in the human setting [13]. Thus, trocar exchange, such as the introduction of a larger-diameter trocar via a smaller port wound, is prohibited in cancer surgery. As mentioned above, port dislodgement should be prevented by making an adequate incision, by selecting well-designed ports, and by securely fixing the ports to the abdominal wall [14].

In addition to careful handling of the colon, resection must follow the same oncologic principles observed in open surgery, namely, en bloc resection with removal of the corresponding lymphatics, use of "no-touch" technique, proximal transsection of blood vessels, adequate bowel and mesenteric margins, and avoidance of intraoperative tearing or perforation of the tumor [12].

Spillage of colonic contents into the abdominal cavity should be prevented. It is important to achieve proximal control of the colon with intracorporeal intestinal clamps (bulldog clamps or other noncrushing clamps) and to ligate the open end of the resected colon immediately after the colon is divided (if a totally intracorporeal technique is being used) or to divide the colon intracorporeally with a G.I.A.-type (Gastro Intestinal Anastomotic) linear stapler [2].

Tumor cells are carried across and through the peritoneal cavity by peritoneal fluid currents. These peritoneal fluids, including ascites and blood, are influenced by physical factors, such as the position of the patient, the laparoscopic instruments, and also by gas flow [16]. Ports, at the end of a cancer resection, have been shown to be highly contaminated with tumor cells, as already mentioned [13]. Circumstances in which the port site is brought into contact with peritoneal fluid (such as desufflation for smoke removal or during port removal) facilitate wound contamination with tumor cells. Ports should be thoroughly irrigated prior to being removed at the end of the case.

Sodium hyaluronate carboxymethylcellulose-based bioresorbable membrane (Seprafilm), used to prevent adhesion formation, has not been shown to affect the rate of tumor implantation at abdominal wound sites [18].

C. After Resection

After resection is an important time in a laparoscopic oncologic resection because most mistakes appear to occur at this point [2]. Most surgeons remove the specimen through a small abdominal wound. The wound used to extract the tumor should be protected in some manner. If the segment being resected has been fully detached, then the specimen is best placed in a plastic specimen bag, which is then tightly closed and then pulled out through the wound (Figure 40.1C). If the bowel segment remains attached at one end, usually the proximal end in the case of left or sigmoid colectomy, then it is not possible to put the entire specimen in a bag. In this case, a wound protector should be employed that will prevent contamination of the wound during removal of the tumor. Some advocate the use of both a bag and a wound protector. The incision should be large enough to allow a smooth extraction of the specimen. Another option, which avoids the "assisted" incision altogether, is to remove the specimen transanally [2]. In this case, the specimen must be fully detached and placed into a bag that is then pulled out via the anus.

Immediately after extraction, macroscopic assessment of the specimen should be performed by the surgeon himself, and frozen section analysis of the resection margins by a pathologist is strongly advised if there is any question as to the completeness of resection.

There is some evidence that closure of the port site's peritoneal wound might be of importance in preventing local recurrence (Figure 40.1D). In an experimental model, repair of injured peritoneum at port sites reduced the frequency of wound metastases in laparoscopic surgery for gallbladder carcinoma [1].

In an experimental model, excision of the laparoscopic abdominal port wound sites significantly, but not completely, reduced the wound tumor implantation rate compared with simple wound closure [20], suggesting that port site contamination occurs after completion of the surgical procedure, perhaps by tumor cell-containing peritoneal fluids. This rather drastic measure has not been utilized in humans thus far; however, these data do behoove the surgeon to make an effort to reduce the chances of port wound contamination. Thus, before extraction, the trocars inside the abdominal cavity should be thoroughly irrigated with a cytotoxic solution to kill any viable tumor cells that may be present [2, 14]. In the case of dilute poviodine irrigation, it is important to thoroughly irrigate the abdomen with saline after the poviodine has been allowed to dwell for several minutes. The abdomen should be desufflated with the ports in place to avoid creating a chimney effect through a port site. The previously placed fascial sutures are immediately tied to avoid spillage of abdominal liquid through the port wounds. Irrigation of the subcutaneous tissues of the port and extraction wound with a dilute Betadine solution or other tumoricidal solution before skin closure is also advised [2].

If the surgeon decides to drain the abdomen when performing laparoscopic cancer surgery, a closed suction device is highly recommended. Capillarity-based drains will lead to a contamination of the wound.

D. Conclusions

Port site tumor recurrences are a potential complication of laparoscopic colorectal cancer surgery. In the final analysis, they have to be considered local recurrences. As is the case with other intraabdominal "local" tumor recurrences, the surgical technique utilized and the surgeons themselves are important variables. Wound tumor recurrences, in many instances, are probably the aftermath of poor surgical technique. However, the biology of the tumor likely also plays an important role [4]. It is hoped that after studying this chapter the reader understands the potential for the implantation of tumor cells into port-wounds associated with the various steps of a laparoscopic cancer resection. It is further hoped that the reader will adjust their technique so as to make use of the prophylactic measures that are believed to reduce the chances of port wound tumor formation.

E. References

1. Aoki Y, Shimura H, Li H, Mizumoto K, Date K, Tanaka M. A model of port-site metastases of gallbladder cancer: the influence of peritoneal injury and its repair on abdominal wall metastases. Surgery 1999;125:553–559.
2. Balli JE, Franklin ME, Almeida JA, Glass JL, Diaz JA, Reymond MA. How to prevent port-site metastases in laparoscopic colorectal surgery. Surg Endosc 2000;14:1034–1036.

3. Buchmann P, Christen D, Moll C, Flury R. Intraperitoneal tumor cell spread during colorectal cancer surgery: a comparison of laparoscopic versus open surgery. Langenbeck Arch Chir 1996;381(SII):573–576.
4. Cuschieri A. Foreword. In: Reymond MA, Bonjer HJ, Koeckerling F, eds. Port-Site and Wound Recurrences in Cancer Surgery. New York: Springer-Verlag, 2000:v–vi.
5. Docherty JG, McGregor JR, Purdie CA, Galloway DJ, O'Dwyer PJ. Efficacy of tumoricidal agents in vitro and in vivo. Br J Surg 1995;82:1050–1052.
6. Ellis KK, Fennerty MB. Marking and identifying colon lesions. Tattoos, clips, and radiology in imaging the colon. Gastrointest Endosc Clin N Am 1996;7:401–411.
7. Fleshman JW. Pathogenesis: tumor cell lines and application in experimental animal studies. In: Reymond MA, Bonjer HJ, Koeckerling F, eds. Port-Site and Wound Recurrences in Cancer Surgery. New York: Springer-Verlag, 2000:29–43.
8. Hermanek P, Wiebelt H, Staimmer D, Riedel ST. The German Study Group Colo-rectal Carcinoma (SGCRC). Prognostic factors of rectum carcinoma. Experience of the German Multicenter Study SGCRC. Tumori 1995;81(SI):60–64.
9. Ikramuddin S, Lucus J, Ellison EC, Schirmer WJ, Melvin WS. Detection of aerosolized cells during carbon dioxide laparoscopy. J Gastrointest Surg 1998;2:580–583.
10. Johnstone PAS, Rohde DC, Swartz SE, Fetter JE, Wexner SD. Port site recurrences after laparoscopic and thoracoscopic procedures in malignancy. J Clin Oncol 1996; 14:1950–1956.
11. Koeckerling F, Reymond MA, Schneider C, Hohenberger W. Mistakes and hazards in oncological laparoscopic surgery. Chirurg 1997;68:215–224.
12. Koeckerling F, Reymond MA, Schneider C, et al. Prospective multicenter study of the quality of oncologic resections in patients undergoing laparoscopic colorectal surgery for cancer. The Laparoscopic Colorectal Surgery Study Group. Dis Colon Rectum 1998; 41:963–970.
13. Reymond MA, Wittekind C, Jung A, Hohenberger W, Kirchner TH, Koeckerling F. The incidence of port-site metastases might be reduced. Surg Endosc 1997;11:902–906.
14. Schneider C, Jung A, Reymond MA, et al. Efficacy of surgical measures in the prevention of port-site recurrences in a porcine model. Surg Endosc 2001;15(2):121–125.
15. Texler ML, Hewett PJ. Pathogenesis: transportation of tumor cells in animal studies. In: Reymond MA, Bonjer HJ, Koeckerling F, eds. Port-Site and Wound Recurrences in Cancer Surgery. New York: Springer-Verlag, 2000:44–51.
16. Texler ML, Luck A, Hewett PJ, King G, Anderson D, Chatterton B. A real time in vivo model of intraperitoneal movement of tumor cells during laparoscopy. Surg Endosc 1998;12:518 [abstract].
17. Tseng LNL, Berends FJ, Wittich P, et al. Port-site metastases. Impact of local tissue trauma and gas leakage. Surg Endosc 1998;12:1377–1380.
18. Underwood RA, Wu JS, Wright MP, et al. Sodium hyaluronate carboxymethylcellulose-based resorbable membrane (Seprafilm)—does it affect tumor implantation at abdominal wound sites? Dis Colon Rectum 1999;42:614–618.

19. Wittich P, Bonjer HJ. Port-site recurrences in laparoscopic surgery. In: Reymond MA, Bonjer HJ, Koeckerling F (eds) Port-site and wound recurrences in cancer surgery. New York: Springer-Verlag, 2000:12–20.
20. Wu JS, Guo LW, Ruiz MD, Pfister SM, Connett JM, Fleshman JW. Excision of trocar sites reduces wound implantation in an animal model. Dis Colon Rectum 1998;41: 1107–1111.
21. Wu JS, Pfister SM, Ruiz MD, Connett JM, Fleshman JW. Local treatment of abdominal wound reduces tumor implantation. J Surg Oncol 1998;69:9–13.

41. Immunologic Consequences and Considerations of the Laparoscopic Approach

Daniel L. Feingold
Joseph Carter
Richard L. Whelan

The introduction of advanced laparoscopic operations in the early 1990s led to a close examination of the immunologic consequences of both open and closed surgical methods. This scrutiny has significantly increased our understanding of the impact of surgery on the body and will, it is hoped, lead to new perioperative pharmacologic therapies that will lessen the deleterious immunologic effects of all types of surgery. Before the laparoscopic era, it had been well established that major open surgery is associated with the temporary suppression of a variety of cells that are involved with both innate and specific immunity, including lymphocytes, neutrophils, monocytes, and macrophages. Interactions between cells, chemotaxis, expression of surface antigens, the ability to produce cytokines, and other functions of these immune system cells are negatively influenced by open surgical trauma. Further, the ability to mount a positive response to a delayed-type hypersensitivity (DTH) recall antigen challenge is suppressed after surgery [1–5].

The relative contribution of each part of an abdominal procedure (abdominal wall access incision versus intraabdominal dissection and resection) to postsurgical immunosuppression had not been assessed before the advent of advanced laparoscopic methods. The results of recent studies suggest that the method of entry into the abdomen is the most important determinant of postoperative immune function. Minimally invasive methods, for a variety of immune parameters, have been shown to be associated with significantly better preserved function when compared to the equivalent open procedure. Of note, in many cases the differences are small and short lived, on the order of a day, and sometimes less for several variables. For a number of parameters no differences have been noted.

It should be realized that the clinical significance, if any exists, of the immune function differences that have been found has not been determined. Better preserved postoperative cell-mediated immune function, in theory, may have an impact on the rate of infections and, possibly, tumor recurrence rates and survival.

This chapter reviews the available literature in this area and also speculates on how our improved understanding of surgery's impact on the immune system may lead to novel perioperative treatments in the future.

A. Delayed-Type Hypersensitivity

One of the simplest methods of evaluating immune function is via delayed-type hypersensitivity (DTH) testing. The ability to mount a DTH response to an intradermally injected antigen to which the subject has been previously exposed verifies that several important elements of the immune system are functioning. A positive response, as indicated by the development of an indurated area at the site of injection, requires (1) that the antigen be processed and presented to a specific CD4+ T lymphocyte by an antigen-presenting cell (APC), (2) activation and replication of the CD4+ T lymphocyte and cytokine elaboration, and (3) accumulation of "effector" cells as well as deposition of fibrin at the challenge site. In the perioperative setting, serial DTH challenges, done both before and after surgery, provide the observer with some idea of the functional status of the immune system at different time points and permit comparison of postoperative responses to the patient's baseline preoperative response. Although a diminished DTH reaction is believed to correlate with a decrease in the functional status of the cell-mediated immune system, thus far it has not been demonstrated that patients with significantly decreased postoperative DTH responses have an increased rate of complications.

In mice, it has been shown that both sham laparotomy and open bowel resection via a full laparotomy are associated with a significant decrease in the size of the DTH responses for at least 5 days after surgery. The equivalent laparoscopic procedures, in contrast, were associated with significantly better preserved DTH responses [7, 8]. Two human DTH studies have been done, a cholecystectomy and a colectomy study; both were fairly small and nonrandomized. Both studies demonstrated that the open procedure was associated with a significant drop in the size of the response whereas the minimally invasive groups had smaller nonsignificant decreases [9, 10]. These studies, and others, suggest that early after surgery cell-mediated immune function is better preserved after laparoscopic procedures.

B. Lymphocyte Proliferation

Inherent to cellular immunity is lymphocyte function, which can be assessed in a number of ways. One method is to perform lymphocyte proliferation assays (LPA). In an LPA, lymphocytes from peripheral blood samples are exposed, in vitro, to a mitogen such as lipopolysaccharide, and their degree of proliferation measured. A decreased proliferation rate suggests that cellular immune function is suppressed. In a pig model, Nguyen et al. demonstrated decreased lymphocyte proliferation after both open and laparoscopic cholecystectomy; however, the open group was significantly more suppressed than the minimally invasive group [11]. Horgan et al. carried out an LPA study on mice undergoing sham full laparotomy, CO_2 pneumoperitoneum, or anesthesia alone [12]. Proliferation was significantly depressed postoperatively in the open group mice only. Lee et al., also in mice, confirmed the Horgan et al. results but also determined the time course of the depressed lymphocyte proliferation following laparotomy [13].

Significantly decreased proliferation rates were noted on postoperative days 2, 3, and 4 whereas the results had normalized by day 8 (the next sampling point). Griffith et al., in a nonrandomized human study, showed that there was significant reduction in lymphocyte proliferation the day after open cholecystectomy when compared to the results after laparoscopic removal of the gallbladder [14]. To summarize, the small number of animal and human LPA studies that have been done demonstrate short-lived, relatively small, yet statistically significant differences in proliferation rates between open and closed surgery groups. These results suggest that the lymphocytes from laparoscopic patients may be more easily activated early after surgery than those from open patients.

C. Lymphocyte Subpopulation Studies

Studies assessing the number of circulating lymphocytes of different subtypes have, with rare exception, found no significant differences between open and closed groups [9, 15, 16]. A randomized cholecystectomy study that indirectly assessed the ratio of Th-1/Th-2 lymphocytes by measuring levels of interferon-γ (Th-1) and interleukin-4 (IL-4) (Th-2) that were elaborated by peripheral blood monocytes in vitro, after stimulation, found a significant difference between the laparoscopic and open groups only 2 hours after the operation; all other sampling points yielded similar result between groups [16]. They suggested that this shift in cytokine release was a manifestation of downregulated cell-mediated immunity and upregulated humoral immunity. A recent colectomy study analyzed CD31 expression on circulating T lymphocytes before and after surgery. Efficient killing of tumor cells or other pathogens depends on, among other things, T-cell migration from the circulation to peripheral tissues. T cells migrating from the circulation to the peripheral tissues express the CD31 antigen. CD31 expression was found to be significantly decreased from preoperative baseline levels in the open group but not in the laparoscopic group. Furthermore, there was a significant correlation between the decrease in CD31 expression and the incision length in the open group [17]. These results suggest that there are more circulating T cells able to migrate to the periphery after laparoscopy than following open surgery.

D. Monocytes and Neutrophils

Monocytes, which play a central role in cell-mediated immune function, have also been studied perioperatively. Monocytes present antigens to lymphocytes in the context of major histocompatibility (MHC) restriction via class II human leukocyte antigen (HLA) molecules such as HLA-DR. Decreases in the percentage of circulating monocytes that express HLA-DR are associated with a worse short-term outcome after major elective surgery and trauma [18–20]. Kloosterman et al. reported a significant decline in the expression of HLA-DR 1 day after open cholecystectomy whereas laparoscopic removal was not associated with a change from baseline [9]. Ordemann and colleagues reported the results of a prospective, randomized clinical trial of patients with colorectal cancer [21]. Their group found that both procedures resulted in significant reductions in postoperative HLA-DR expression compared with preoperative levels. When the two groups' results were compared, a significantly lower level of HLA-DR expressions was noted in the open group only on the fourth postoperative day.

Studies involving in vitro stimulation of peripheral blood mononuclear cells (PBMCs) followed by measurement of cytokine elaboration have also been carried out. Open cholecystectomy has been shown to be associated with significantly higher tumor necrosis factor (TNF)-alpha and superoxide anion elaboration from PBMCs following stimulation. Therefore, PBMCs are more readily activated after the open procedure than after the laparoscopic equivalent. Neutrophil chemotaxis and superoxide elaboration were similarly studied. Similar results were noted; chemotaxis was increased and superoxide elaboration increased after open cholecystectomy [22]. Some investigators argue that these alterations in monocyte and neutrophil responsiveness might be beneficial because these patients would be better prepared to respond to an early bacterial infection. The authors, however, suggest that postoperative overproduction of these inflammatory mediators may lead to a cycle of overproduction of these mediators, which could cause dysfunction of vital organs. Therefore, the clinical relevance of these findings is not clear.

E. Interleukin 6

The cytokine interleukin 6 (IL-6) is produced by monocytes, fibroblasts, and vascular endothelial cells in response to IL-1 and TNF. IL-6 stimulates hepatocytes to synthesize fibrinogen and thus contributes to the acute-phase response. IL-6 levels are not a measure of immune function; however, they have been used as a means of assessing overall surgical stress. IL-6 levels have been shown to be elevated following major open surgery. The majority of studies comparing laparoscopic and open cholecystectomy have reported significantly lower IL-6 levels in the laparoscopic groups, which suggests that the minimally invasive approach is less stressful. Conflicting results have been noted after colectomy in humans. One study found significantly lower IL-6 levels in the laparoscopic group during the first 12 hours following laparoscopic-assisted colectomy when compared to open group levels. At 24, 48, and 72 hours after surgery no significant differences were observed [23]. Ordemann et al. noted significantly lower levels 1 day after surgery in the laparoscopic group patients. At least three other investigators, none of whom measured IL-6 levels in the first 12 hours after surgery, found no differences [24]. One study that assessed laparoscopic colectomy done via an abdominal wall lifting device found higher levels after the minimally invasive operation. To summarize, presently the impact of open and closed colectomy on IL-6 levels is not clear. There may be a short-lived difference, persisting for less than a day.

F. Peritoneal Macrophages

As mentioned earlier, although systemic cell-mediated immunity seems to be less affected by laparoscopic than open surgery, there is evidence that the carbon dioxide pneumoperitoneum may have a detrimental impact on local peritoneal immunity. Peritoneal macrophages function as the immune system's first line of defense in the abdominal cavity. A fair number of small animal studies that assessed peritoneal macrophage function after carbon dioxide pneumoperitoneum have reported diminished macrophage cytokine release and impaired ability of the macrophages to clear intraperitoneal bacterial loads [25–27]. Other animal studies, however, have reported conflicting results. There are few human data available, and the animal data remain confusing. Until further human studies are conducted, no firm conclusions can be made regarding the choice of operative technique and its impact on intraperitoneal immunity.

G. Etiology of Surgery-Related Immunosuppression

What is it about abdominal surgery that causes temporary suppression of the immune system? Probably there are a number of contributing factors. There is evidence that the overall length of the abdominal wall incision is an important factor. Others, based on the results of a murine study, believe that it is exposure of the abdominal cavity to air that is the cause of the immunosuppression after open surgery. These latter investigators believe that small amounts of lipopolysaccharide (LPS) in the air cause immunosuppression by stimulating bacteria in the intestine to elaborate LPS, which then translocates across the bowel wall, after which it is absorbed systemically [28].

H. Perioperative Immunomodulation

Is it possible to avoid surgery-related immunosuppression pharmacologically? A single small randomized study determined the impact of daily perioperative injections of granulocyte-macrophage colony-stimulating factor (GM-CSF) on immune function after open colectomy [29]. It was demonstrated that such treatment is associated with significantly better preserved postoperative DTH responses and monocyte HLA-DR expression levels than following surgery alone. It remains to be proven that this treatment will result in a lower rate of perioperative complications or improved short-term outcome. Although there are no data thus far, in theory, this type of treatment might influence oncologic outcome. Numerous animal studies, utilizing different models, have determined the impact of perioperative immunomodulation on several oncologic variables. These studies have demonstrated that such treatment decreases the rate of tumor growth and establishment as well as the rate of tumor metastasis formation [30–33]. This line of research would seem to warrant further investigation.

I. Summary

To summarize, the results of the DTH studies, the lymphocyte proliferation studies, and select lymphocyte and monocyte function studies suggest that open surgery causes more systemic immunosuppression than laparoscopic procedures. However, there are other studies, concerning a limited number of immune function indicators, that have found no significant differences in immune function between the two surgical methods. There are still other studies that have yielded results which are not easily interpreted. Although the overall interpretation of this literature is open to discussion, it is the authors' belief that there are sufficient data to support the position that minimally invasive surgery is associated with better-preserved immune function than that following traditional open surgical methods. Finally, there are some data to suggest that surgery-related immunosuppression may be avoided via perioperative immunomodulation for open surgery patients.

J. References

1. Nielsen HJ, Pedersen BK, Moesgaard F. Effect of Ranitidine on postoperative suppression of natural killer cell activity and delayed hypersensitivity. Acta Chir Scand 1989;155:377–382.
2. Christou NV, Superina R, Broadhead M, et al. Postoperative depression of host resistance: determinants and effect of peripheral protein-sparing therapy. Surgery 1982; 92:786–792.
3. Nielsen HJ, Moesgaard F, Kehlet H. Ranitidine for prevention of postoperative suppression of delayed hypersensitivity. Am J Surg 1989;157:291–294.
4. Hjortso NC, Kehlet H. Influence of surgery, age, and serum albumin on delayed hypersensitivity. Acta Chir Scand 1986;152:175–179.
5. Lennard TW, Shenton BK, Borzotta A, et al. The influence of surgical operations on components of the human immune system. Br J Surg 1985;72:771–776.
6. Lacy AM, Garcia-Valdecasas JC, Delgardo S, et al. Laparoscopically-assisted colectomy versus open colectomy for treatment of non-metastatic colon cancer: a randomised trial. Lancet 2002;359:2224–2229.
7. Trokel MJ, Bessler M, Treat MR, et al. Preservation of immune response after laparoscopy. Surg Endosc 1994;8:1385–1388.
8. Allendorf JD, Bessler M, Whelan RL, et al. Better preservation of immune function after laparoscopic-assisted versus open bowel resection in a murine model. Dis Colon Rectum 1996;39:67–72.
9. Kloosterman T, von Blomberg ME, Borgstein P, et al. Unimpaired immune functions after laparoscopic cholecystectomy. Surgery 1994;115:424–428.
10. Whelan RL, Franklin M, Donahue J, et al. Postoperative cell mediated immune response is better preserved after laparoscopic versus open colectomy in humans: a preliminary study. Surg Endosc 1998;12:551.

11. Nguyen NT, Luketich JD, Schatz S, et al. Effect of open and laparoscopic surgery on cellular immunity in a swine model. Surg Laparosc Endosc Percutan Tech 1999;9: 177–180.
12. Horgan PG, Fitzpatrick M, Couse NF, et al. Laparoscopy is less immunotraumatic than laparotomy. Minim Invasive Ther 1992;1:241–244.
13. Lee SW, Southall JC, Gleason NR, et al. Time course of differences in lymphocyte proliferation rates after laparotomy versus CO_2 insufflation. Surg Endosc 2000;14: 145–148.
14. Griffith JP, Everitt NJ, Lancaster F, et al. Influence of laparoscopic and conventional cholecystectomy upon cell-mediated immunity. Br J Surg 1995;82:677–680.
15. Perttila J, Salo M, Ovaska J, et al. Immune response after laparoscopic and conventional Nissen fundoplication. Eur J Surg 1999;165:21–28.
16. Decker D, Schöndorf M, Bidlingmaier F, et al. Surgical stress induces a shift in the type-1/type-2 T-helper cell balance, suggesting down-regulation of cell-mediated and up-regulation of antibody-mediated immunity commensurate to the trauma. Surgery 1996;119:316–325.
17. Kirman I, Cekic V, Asi Z, et al. The percentage of CD31+ T-cells decreases after open but not laparoscopic surgery in humans. Surg Endosc 2002;16(suppl 1):s192.
18. Appel SH, Wellhausen SR, Montgomery R, et al. Experimental and clinical significance of endotoxin independent HLA-DR expression on monocytes. J Surg Res 1089; 47:44–48.
19. Faist E, Mewes A, Strasser T, et al. Alteration of monocyte function following major injury. Arch Surg 1988;123:287–292.
20. Hershman MJ, Cheadle WG, Wellhausen SR, et al. Monocyte HLA-DR antigen expression characterizes clinical outcome in the trauma patient. Br J Surg 1990;77: 204–207.
21. Ordemann J, Jacobi A, Schwenk W, et al. Cellular and humoral inflammatory response after laparoscopic and conventional resections. Surg Endosc 2001;15:600–608.
22. Redmond HP, Watson WG, Houghton T, et al. Immune function in patients undergoing open vs. laparoscopic cholecystectomy. Arch Surg 1994;129:1240–1246.
23. Harmon GD, Senagore AJ, Kilbride MJ, Warzynski MJ. Interleukin-6 response to laparoscopic and open colectomy. Dis Colon Rectum 1994;37:754–759.
24. Mehigan BJ, Hartley JE, Drew PJ, et al. Changes in T cell subsets, interleukin-6, and C-reactive protein after laparoscopic and open colorectal resection for malignancy. Surg Endosc 2001;15:1289–1293.
25. Neuhaus SJ, Watson DI, Ellis T, et al. Influence of gases on intraperitoneal immunity during laparoscopy in tumor-bearing rats. World J Surg 2000;24:1227–1231.
26. Chekan EG, Nataraj C, Clary EM, et al. Intraperitoneal immunity and pneumoperitoneum. Surg Endosc 1999;13:1135–1138.
27. West MA, Hackam DJ, Baker J, et al. Mechanism of decreased in vitro murine macrophage cytokine release after exposure to carbon dioxide: relevance to laparoscopic surgery. Ann Surg 1997;226:179–190.
28. Watson RWG, Redmond HP, McCarthy J, Burke PE, Hayes DB. Exposure of the peritoneal cavity to air regulates early inflammatory responses to surgery in a murine model. Br J Surg 1995;82:1060–1065.

29. Mels AK, Statius Muller MG, van Leeuwen PAM, et al. Immune-stimulating effects of low-dose perioperative recombinant granulocyte-macrophage colony stimulating factor in patients operated on for primary colorectal carcinoma. Br J Surg 2001; 88:539–544.
30. Schuurman B, Heuff G, Beelen RHJ, et al. Enhanced killing capacity of human Kupffer cells after activation with granulocyte/macrophage-colony-stimulating factor and interferon-?. Cancer 1994;39:179–184.
31. Tanemura H, Sakata K, Kunieda T, et al. Influences of operative stress on cell-mediated immunity and on tumor metastasis and their prevention by nonspecific immunotherapy: experimental studies in rats. J Surg Oncol 1982;21:189–195.
32. Heys SD, Deehan DJ, Eremin O. Interleukin-2 treatment in colorectal cancer: current results and future prospects. Eur J Surg Oncol 1994;20:622–629.
33. Hill ADK, Redmond HP, Naama HA, et al. Granulocyte-macrophage colony-stimulating factor inhibits tumor growth during the postoperative period. Surgery 1996;119:178–185.

42. Effect of Patient Position on Cardiovascular and Pulmonary Function

Eric J. Hazebroek, M.D.
H. Jaap Bonjer, M.D., Ph.D.

The intraabdominal exposure required to perform laparoscopic surgery is most commonly provided by a carbon dioxide (CO_2) pneumoperitoneum that elevates the abdominal wall, suppresses the viscera, and creates a working space in the abdominal cavity which permits the safe introduction of trocars and instruments. The CO_2 pneumoperitoneum has a number of cardiopulmonary and physiologic effects. CO_2, which is highly soluble, is readily absorbed through the visceral and parietal peritoneum and almost always results in hypercarbia and a respiratory acidosis. In addition, the increased intraabdominal pressure (IAP) pushes the diaphragms cephalad, which makes it more difficult to ventilate the patient. To compensate for these deleterious changes the minute ventilation is increased, by increasing either the tidal volume or the respiratory rate. Elevated peak inspiratory pressures are usually required to effect these changes. The increased IAP may also have an impact on cardiovascular function.

During laparoscopic procedures, the body position of the patient is often changed to expose the organ of interest and provide the best operative field. In general, more radical body positions are used in minimally invasive surgery than in open cases because retraction of the intestine and other mobile viscera is more difficult in minimally invasive cases. Although laparotomy pads and other packs are used in conjunction with retractors to create an operative field during an open procedure, gravity is the principal means by which retraction is accomplished during a laparoscopic case. The body positioning options include Trendelenburg (head down), reverse Trendelenburg (head up), lateral "airplaning" of the table (left or right side of patient up or down), or a combination of these. Radical patient positioning, by itself, will have an impact on cardiopulmonary function. The effect, which varies depending on the position, may either exacerbate or alleviate the pneumoperitoneum effects. Although for short laparoscopic procedures the cardiopulmonary changes are not problematic, during advanced procedures and in patients with considerable cardiopulmonary disease clinically significant cardiorespiratory changes may result. In this chapter the cardiovascular and pulmonary changes associated with various patient positions during laparoscopic procedures are discussed. A brief overview of the cardiovascular and the pulmonary changes with the patient in the supine position is given, followed by discussion of the cardiopulmonary impact of the specific positions.

A. Supine Position

Cardiovascular Changes

Although not all reports agree about the impact of pneumoperitoneum on the cardiac output during laparoscopic procedures, the majority have noted increases in systemic vascular resistance (SVR) and mean arterial pressure (MAP). As mentioned, intraperitoneal insufflation with CO_2 causes hypercarbia and acidosis: hypercarbia stimulates the sympathetic nervous system, which may lead to an increase in blood pressure, heart rate, and vascular tone [1]. Increased IAP also compresses the inferior vena cava, which compromises venous return from the lower extremities. As a result cardiac preload will decrease. Afterload is increased as a result of the elevated increased SVR that is caused by compression of the abdominal vessels and increased sympathetic activity.

Reduced preload may cause a reduction of cardiac output and a compensatory increase in heart rate. Therefore, if preload is markedly reduced, it may be critical to expand the intravascular volume. The effect of increased IAP on venous return is dependent on the intravascular volume status and central venous pressure (CVP). At low or normal right atrial pressure, venous return is reduced with increased IAP by compression of the inferior vena cava (IVC). In subjects with a high right atrial pressure, the IVC remains patent despite the IAP and, in fact, venous return is augmented. Several investigators have demonstrated that femoral vein blood flow decreases with increased IAP, which implies that installation of pneumoperitoncum increases pooling of blood in the peripheral circulation [2] (Table 42.1).

Table 42.1. Effect of body position on cardiovascular and pulmonary changes during laparoscopic surgery.

	Supine	**Head-down**	**Head-up**	**Lateral**
Cardiovascular changes:				
MAP	↑	↑↑	↑↑	=/↑
SVR	↑	↑	↑	↑
Venous return	↓	↑	↓↓	=/↓[a]
Preload	↓	↑	↓↓	=/↓[a]
Afterload	↑	↑	↑↑	
Cardiac output	↓	↑	↓	
Blood pooling in legs	↑	↓	↑↑	↑
Pulmonary changes:				
Diaphragmatic cephalad shift	↑	↑↑	↓	↑
FRC	↓	↓↓	↑	↓
Chest compliance	↓	↓↓	↓	↓
Peak airway pressure	↑	↑↑	↑	↑

MAP, mean arterial pressure; SVR, system vascular resistance; FRC, functional residual capacity.
[a] Depends on right/left lateral decubitus position.

In general, the extent of the cardiovascular changes (including cardiac output) associated with creation of pneumoperitoneum depend on the IAP attained, the volume of CO_2 absorbed, the patient's intravascular volume status, the ventilation technique, surgical conditions, and the anesthetic agents employed [3].

Pulmonary Changes

Anesthesia and both open and closed abdominal surgery may cause a progressive cranial displacement of the diaphragm [4] (Figure 42.1). The sequence of events for an open procedure can be described as follows, assuming the patient is in the supine position: induction of anesthesia, causation of paralysis, and the placement of retractors and packs to provide exposure. During laparoscopic surgery, exposure is provided by the CO_2 pneumoperitoneum and fairly radical patient positioning. In both scenarios, the diaphragm is shifted in a cephalad direction, which results in a decreased functional residual capacity (FRC). With few exceptions, the alterations are significantly greater during laparoscopic surgery where the general anesthesia-related decrease in FRC is enhanced by intraperitoneal insufflation of CO_2. Decreased FRC may result in the development of intraoperative atelectasis, intrapulmonary shunting, and hypoxemia. The patient's position will influence the degree of the diaphragmatic shift and either enhance or lessen the effects of the CO_2 pneumoperitoneum.

In addition, increased IAP decreases chest compliance and thus increases peak airway pressure. As a result, the bronchial tree may expand, which increases anatomical deadspace. In patients with chronic obstructive pulmonary disease or bullous emphysema, airway pressures may be high, therefore, increased IAP during laparoscopy may pose an additional danger. Furthermore, pulmonary hypertension will increase right cardiac work. Together with the decrease of filling pressures and increased SVR, this may cause a fall in cardiac output.

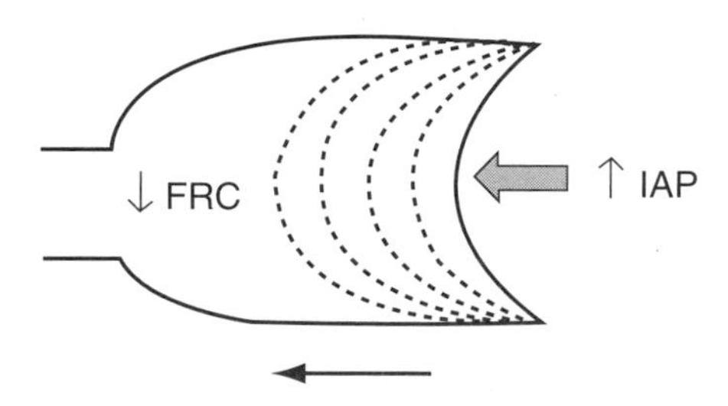

Figure 42.1. Cranial shift of the diaphragm.

B. Head-Down Position

Cardiovascular Changes

The Trendelenburg or 'head-down position' was originally described and utilized to keep the small bowel or colon out of the pelvis during gynecologic and urologic operations. It is essential to distinguish between a moderate and extreme head-down position. During creation of pneumoperitoneum, the patient is commonly placed in a 10°–20° head-down tilt to minimize complications associated with blind trocar insertion. However, some laparoscopic procedures, such as sigmoid colon or rectal resection, require a steep Trendelenburg position to provide adequate exposure.

The physiologic effects of the Trendelenburg position in normovolemic patients have been reviewed in detail by Wilcox and Vandam [5]. As generally taught: "postures with the head lowered are more favorable to the circulation." The head-down position favors venous return and, thus, improves cardiac output [6]. In addition, the Trendelenburg position decreases pooling of blood in the lower body. In a study investigating the hemodynamic effects of body position during laparoscopic surgery, peritoneal insufflation caused a significant increase in MAP, CVP, and pulmonary capillary wedge pressure (PCWP) [7]. Placement of patients in the Trendelenburg position further increased these hemodynamic changes, demonstrating an additive effect of elevated IAP and head-down positioning on hemodynamic parameters. The cardiovascular changes associated with the Trendelenburg position may be influenced by the degree of head-down tilt, the patient's age, associated cardiac disease, anesthetic drugs, and ventilation techniques.

Respiratory Changes

The Trendelenburg position reduces vital capacity because of the increased weight of the shifted abdominal viscera on the diaphragm [8]. This exacerbates the pneumoperitoneum-related cranial displacement of the diaphragm and its associated changes. Therefore, an even greater reduction of FRC is noted when pneumoperitoneum and the head-down position are applied simultaneously. Steep Trendelenburg positioning further decreases chest compliance, which may result in a decrease in the ventilation perfusion ratio and accentuated hypercarbia and hypoxemia. Studies that have assessed pulmonary function have not, in general, shown significant compromise resulting from head-down positioning itself. However, the potential for compromise exists. There may be a predilection to develop pulmonary atelectasis if deep breaths are not intermittently supplied when mechanical ventilation is employed. Increased airway pressure and the use of positive end-expiratory pressure (PEEP) may minimize this complication. The position-related changes in pulmonary function are more marked in obese, elderly, or debilitated patients and are enhanced by the placement of certain laparoscopic instruments such as liver retractors in the upper abdomen.

C. Head-Up Position

Cardiovascular changes

The reverse Trendelenburg or head-up position is commonly used in procedures such as laparoscopic cholecystectomy and Nissen fundoplication to facilitate adequate exposure of the upper abdomen and to prevent inadvertent bowel injury. Positioning in reverse Trendelenburg accentuates the CO_2 pneumoperitoneum-related decrease in venous return and may also be associated with decreased cardiac preload and cardiac index [9]. Furthermore, the head-up position may increase afterload via increases in MAP, SVR, and pulmonary vascular resistance. The decreased venous return also facilitates the pooling of blood in the lower extremities. Pneumatic compression stockings and bandages improve the venous return from the legs and thus counter the effects of both the reverse Trendelenburg position and the pneumoperitoneum. These devices should be routinely employed.

Pulmonary Changes

During laparoscopy, the change in position to reverse Trendelenburg should improve diaphragmatic function and respiratory status. Shifting the abdominal viscera away from the diaphragm toward the pelvis will improve diaphragmatic excursion, increase chest wall compliance, increase FRC, and lower the peak inspiratory pressures.

D. Lateral Position

Cardiovascular Changes

The lateral position is commonly used for laparoscopic renal and adrenal operations. In most cases, a flexed lateral decubitus position is used. Flexion enlarges the operative field by increasing the distance between the costal margin and the anterior superior iliac fossa on the exposed side and may decrease venous bleeding by decreasing venous pressure. However, this position facilitates the pooling of blood in the legs, which are dependent. During laparoscopic adrenal or renal surgery, CO_2 absorption is increased because retroperitoneal dissection often results in insufflation of the various soft tissue planes [10]. The increased $PaCO_2$ causes vasodilatation and stimulates the sympathetic nervous system, resulting in tachycardia and hypertension [11]. Few investigators have studied the hemodynamic changes associated with pneumoperitoneum and the lateral position [12]. In patients undergoing minimally invasive urologic surgery, fewer marked hemodynamic effects were noted in the left lateral position when compared to results with the patient in the right lateral position [12]. There are a few theoretical explanations for these differences. First, because of the right-sided anatomic position of the right atrium, venous return via the inferior and superior vena cava to the right atrium may be improved when the patient is in the right lateral position. Second, the heart, located in the left hemithorax, will shift to the dependent side to a different extent as a result of gravity when a patient is placed in the lateral position.

Pulmonary Changes

As in the supine position, the lateral position itself may displace the diaphragm cranially, reducing the FRC of the dependent lung and inducing a ventilation and perfusion mismatch [13]. A concomitant pneumoperitoneum is likely to further displace the diaphragm cranially and reduce FRC. Although data on pulmonary consequences following laparoscopic surgery in the lateral position are scarce, it appears that intraperitoneal insufflation of CO_2 with retroperitoneal exposure in the lateral position does not clinically affect oxygenation in healthy patients. However, ventilation is inhibited somewhat by the cephalad displacement of the dependent diaphragm and the attendant reduction in lung compliance. Furthermore, the ventilatory requirements of the patient in the lateral decubitus position are increased because of the elevated $PaCO_2$ that results from the increased absorption of CO_2.

E. Conclusion

During laparoscopic surgery, cardiopulmonary function is influenced by the CO_2 used for insufflation, elevated IAP, and body position. It is difficult to determine which of these three factors has the greatest influence on cardiovascular and respiratory function. The patient's body position can either lessen or enhance the pressure and CO_2-gas related effects. The Trendelenburg position, in general, increases venous return, cardiac output, CVP, and MAP. Pulmonary wise, the head-down position decreases chest wall compliance, inhibits ventilation, decreases the FRC, and increases $PaCO_2$. The reverse Trendelenburg position, in general, decreases venous return, cardiac preload, and cardiac index. The head-up position, however, improves pulmonary function via increased chest wall compliance and FRC in addition to lower peak inspiratory pressures.

During short laparoscopic procedures in healthy patients, alterations in body position seldom are associated with clinically significant cardiopulmonary effects beyond those noted with CO_2 insufflation in general. However, during long procedures problems may arise, most typically hypercarbia and very high peak inspiratory pressures. It is essential that the surgeon and anesthetist communicate with each other frequently during the operation in regard to insufflation pressures being used, body position, and patient respiratory status (end-tidal CO_2, $PaCO_2$, and oxygen saturation). If the end-tidal CO_2 or $PaCO_2$ becomes prohibitive, surgery should be halted, the patient placed in the neutral or reverse

Trendelenburg position, and the pneumoperitoneum released for a 5- to 10-minute period. In most cases the end-tidal CO_2 and the $PaCO_2$ will fall back into the normal range within 5 to 10 minutes, after which the pneumoperitoneum can be reestablished and the procedure resumed. The lowest acceptable peak insufflation pressure should be utilized and, if required, as little Trendelenburg as possible.

In patients with significant cardiopulmonary problems, even a relatively brief laparoscopic procedure may be poorly tolerated. An attempt should be made to use low insufflation pressures and to avoid radical positions in these patients. Further, meticulous attention must be paid to both cardiovascular and pulmonary function during the case in these patients. In patients with severe pulmonary disease, the Trendelenburg position should be avoided, whereas in those with marginal cardiac function the reverse Trendelenburg position is best avoided. In patients with the most severe cardiopulmonary disease it may not prove feasible or safe to carry out the procedure in question using a CO_2 pneumoperitoneum and minimally invasive method.

F. References

1. Joris JL, Noirot DP, Legrand MJ, Jacquet NJ, Lamy ML. Hemodynamic changes during laparoscopic cholecystectomy. Anesth Analg 1993;76:1067–1071.
2. Schwenk W, Bohm B, Fugener A, Muller JM. Intermittent pneumatic sequential compression (ISC) of the lower extremities prevents venous stasis during laparoscopic cholecystectomy. A prospective randomized study. Surg Endosc 1998;12:7–11.
3. Cunningham AJ. Anesthetic implications of laparoscopic surgery. Yale J Biol Med 1999;71:551–578.
4. Benumof JL. Anesthesia for Thoracic Surgery. Philadelphia: Saunders, 1987.
5. Wilcox S, Vandam LD. Alas, poor Trendelenburg and his position! A critique of its uses and effectiveness. Anesth Analg 1988;67:574–578.
6. Miller AH. Surgical posture with symbols for its record on the anesthetist's chart. Anesthesiology 1940;1:241–245.
7. Odeberg S, Ljungqvist O, Svenberg T, et al. Haemodynamic effects of pneumoperitoneum and the influence of posture during anaesthesia for laparoscopic surgery. Acta Anaesth Scand 1994;38:276–283.
8. Case EH, Stiles JA. The effect of various surgical positions on vital capacity. Anesthesiology 1946;7:29–31.
9. Hirvonen EA, Poikolainen EO, Paakkonen ME, Nuutinen LS. The adverse hemodynamic effects of anesthesia, head-up tilt, and carbon dioxide pneumoperitoneum during laparoscopic cholecystectomy. Surg Endosc 2000;14:272–277.
10. Mullett CE, Viale JP, Sagnard PE, et al. Pulmonary CO_2 elimination during surgical procedures using intra- or extraperitoneal CO_2 insufflation. Anesth Analg 1993;76:622–626.
11. Price HL. Effects of carbon dioxide on the cardiovascular system. Anesthesiology 1960;21:652–663.

12. Fujise K, Shingu K, Matsumoto S, Nagata A, Mikami O, Matsuda T. The effects of the lateral position on cardiopulmonary function during laparoscopic urological surgery. Anesth Analg 1998;87:925–930.
13. Rehder K, Hatch DJ, Sessler AD, Fowler WS. The function of each lung of anesthetized and paralyzed man during mechanical ventilation. Anesthesiology 1972;37:16–26.

43. Pros and Cons of Alternate Gases and Abdominal Wall Lifting Methods

Robert Talac, M.D., Ph.D.
Heidi Nelson, M.D., F.A.C.S.

Modern surgery has become complex and technically sophisticated. This is particularly true for minimally invasive surgery, in which laparoscopy replaces laparotomy as the method of exposure for abdominal surgery. Adequate exposure of the region of interest remains one of the fundamental principles of surgery, and at the same time it represents one of the limiting factors in the development of laparoscopy. Currently available data suggest that adequate exposure can be achieved using a variety of approaches. As with all surgical procedures, understanding the advantages and disadvantages of different approaches that have been used for this purpose is essential for performing laparoscopy in a safe manner, allowing for better patient care. In this chapter, the current literature is reviewed and several different techniques for exposure of the operative field in laparoscopic surgery are discussed, including pneumoperitoneum and abdominal wall lifting.

A. Pneumoperitoneum

Laparoscopy with pneumoperitoneum represents the oldest and still most common approach for establishing a working space in the peritoneal cavity.

1. Advantages
   a. **The pneumoperitoneum results in a symmetrical dome-shaped elevation of the abdominal wall that usually provides excellent exposure of the abdominal cavity and adequate working space.** In regard to intraabdominal exposure, no mechanical retraction system can compete with pneumoperitoneum. Pneumoperitoneum provides simultaneous exposure of all quadrants of the abdominal cavity, which allows the performance of more complex laparoscopic procedures. Pneumoperitoneum, therefore, is the "gold standard" against which other methods should be compared.
   b. **Establishment of pneumoperitoneum** with CO_2 is inexpensive and usually safe. Although complications can occur when the pneumoperitoneum is established, in most cases it is a safe method.

Table 43.1. Effects of increased intraabdominal pressure on cardiac functions.

Effects	Result
—↑Atrial filling pressure —↑Pressure in inferior vena cava —↓Venous return — Elevations of diaphragm —↑Intrathoracic pressure —↓Left ventricular filling	Alteration of cardiac output Stroke volume, ejection fraction

2. Disadvantages
   a. **Gas insufflation-related complications.** Complications, albeit exceedingly rare, are most likely to occur when the "blind" Veress needle insertion method is used for insufflation. The most feared complication is a gas embolus. If an "open" cut-down method is used to place the first port, through which the pneumoperitoneum is next established, then most pneumoperitoneum establishment-related complications, including gas embolism, can be avoided. However, rarely, the bowel can be injured with either the Veress or open cut-down method.
   b. **Adverse physiologic effects.** These effects limit the safety of longer, more complex laparoscopic procedures or procedures performed in high-risk patients (Tables 43.1, 43.2).
   c. **Effects of pneumoperitoneum on tumor cell implantation following laparoscopic surgery for cancer.** A number of experimental studies using animal models have demonstrated that laparoscopy with CO_2 insufflation is associated with a significant increase in the incidence of port site metastasis as well as dissemination and implantation of intraabdominal tumors. However, these findings do not correlate with results of human studies. Numerous investigators have shown that the rate of port site recurrences ranges from 0% to 2%, which is similar to incidence of wound recurrences documented after open procedures. So far, there is a paucity of information on the etiology of port site recurrences in humans. The fact that wound implants are absent in some laparoscopic series suggests that such recurrences might be related to technical details in performance of the procedure rather than to the pneumoperitoneum.

Table 43.2. Effects of increased intraabdominal pressure on renal functions.[a]

Effects	Result
—↓Cardiac output —↓Renal venous pressure — Compression of the renal parenchyma — Release of vasoconstriction Hormones (angiotensin II and vasopressin)	—↓Effective renal plasma flow —↓Glomerular filtration rate — Oliguria

[a]*Note:* Despite these effects, no long-term renal sequelae, even in patients with preexisting renal disease, have been reported after pneumoperitoneum.

d. **Technical disadvantages.** The constraints of working in a sealed environment restrict the spectrum of instruments available for laparoscopic surgery.

e. **Safety concerns.** Additional concerns related to the use of various gases and their safety in the presence of electrocautery or laser coagulation and the risk of exposure to operating room personnel must be considered.

In an effort to minimize the disadvantages of pneumoperitoneum, several insufflating agents have been explored. These include carbon dioxide, nitrous oxide, helium, and argon. Specific issues related to each agent are summarized in Table 43.3.

B. Abdominal Wall Lifting Techniques

Because of adverse physiologic effects and the technical disadvantages of the pneumoperitoneum, alternative methods of intraabdominal exposure have been designed and tested. The fundamental principle of a variety of abdominal wall lifting devices is the application of vertical upward forces to lift the anterior abdominal wall to create a space similar to that produced by pneumoperitoneum. Currently, two groups of retraction systems exist. These include (1) intraabdominal retraction systems and (2) subcutaneous lifting of the abdominal wall. Table 44.4 lists and describes the available lifting devices and methods.

1. Advantages

a. **No alteration of cardiac, pulmonary, or renal functions.** Recent studies comparing pneumoperitoneum and abdominal wall lifting in terms of hemodynamic responses demonstrated no alteration of cardiac output, stroke volume, ejection fraction, effective renal plasma flow, and glomerular filtration rate in patients operated on using the abdominal wall lifting device. These parameters do not change even in the reverse Trendelenburg position. However, no difference in stress response has been noted when patients undergoing pneumoperitoneum have been compared to those in whom an abdominal wall lifting method has been used.

b. **Combination of laparoscopic and conventional instruments.** In the absence of a pneumoperitoneum, there is the possibility of introducing conventional instruments into the abdominal cavity. The utility of conventional instruments in this setting, however, is limited due to instrument length, restrictions in opening of the jaws that result when passing such instruments through a small wound, and the narrow range of movement that the wound provides. These problems have led some to design conventional instruments for gasless laparoscopy.

c. **Regain tactile sensitivity.** The loss of tactile sensitivity of the surgeon using the minimally invasive approach to target area is a well-recognized disadvantage. The concept of laparoscopy

Table 43.3. Insufflating agents available for laparoscopy with pneumoperitoneum.

Gas	Physical characteristics	Pros	Cons	Comments
Carbon dioxide (CO_2)	— Odorless — Colorless — Stable gas	— Low risk of gas embolism — Safe with electrocautery and laser coagulation — Readily available — Inexpensive — Highly soluble	— Hypercarbia — Respiratory acidosis — Pain — Adverse effects on autonomic nerve system	Most common agent used in the US
Nitrous oxide (N_2O)	— Odorless — Colorless — Soluble in blood and body fluids	— Minimal alteration of acid-base balance — Minimal discomfort and pain	— Combustible — Safety concerns with exposure of personnel	Suitable for procedures performed under local anesthesia
Helium (He)	— Odorless — Colorless — Inert gas — Poor water solubility	— Minimal alteration of acid-base balance — Safe with electrocautery and laser coagulation — Poor solubility	— Postoperative subcutaneous emphysema — Potential risk of venous gas embolism	
Argon (Ar)	— Odorless — Colorless — Inert gas — Poor blood solubility	— Minimal alteration of acid-base balance — Safe with electrocautery and laser coagulation — Poor solubility	— Cardiac depression effect (in animal model)	Limited data available to justify feasibility of argon pneumoperitoneum

Table 43.4. Abdominal wall lifting systems.

System	Type	Lifting method	Pneumoperitoneum requirements
Abdominal Cavity Expander System	Intraabdominal retraction	Point	Permanent low-pressure pneumoperitoneum
Sling	Intraabdominal retraction	Point	Permanent low-pressure pneumoperitoneum
T-shaped endoscopic retractor	Intraabdominal retraction	Point	Permanent low-pressure pneumoperitoneum
Spreading trocars	Intraabdominal retraction	Point	Initial pneumoperitoneum
Peritoneal Cavity Augmentation	Intraabdominal retraction	Linear	Permanent low-pressure pneumoperitoneum
Winch retractor	Intraabdominal retraction	Linear	Initial pneumoperitoneum
Coathanger-shaped retractor	Intraabdominal retraction	Linear	Initial pneumoperitoneum
U-shaped retractor	Intraabdominal retraction	Linear	Initial pneumoperitoneum
Suspensor 3-X	Intraabdominal retraction	Planar	Initial pneumoperitoneum
Pelvi-Snake	Intraabdominal retraction	Planar	Initial pneumoperitoneum
Modular retraction system	Intraabdominal retraction	Planar	0
Laparolift	Intraabdominal retraction	Planar	0
Tent-shaped wiring	Subcutaneous retraction	Linear	0
Subcutaneous wiring	Subcutaneous retraction	Linear	0
Laparo Tenser	Subcutaneous retraction	Planar	0

without pneumoperitoneum allows the surgeon to combine the advantages of laparoscopic surgery (i.e., magnified visualization of target area) with well-known open surgical techniques. The ability to combine fully laparoscopic dissection of fine tissue structures with digital palpation and dissection may facilitate the performance of minimally invasive procedures.

2. Disadvantages
   a. **Suboptimal exposure of abdominal cavity** represents a major disadvantage of abdominal wall lifting devices. The distension that is provided by pneumoperitoneum is dome shaped, whereas the exposure provided by the intraabdominal retractors resembles a flat-topped pyramid and is limited to a specific quadrant of the abdomen. Quadrant-specific exposure may be adequate for certain procedures such as cholecystectomy or appendectomy. However, suboptimal exposure in more complex procedures requiring multiquadrant exposure such as laparoscopy-assisted colectomy may lead to serious complications and/or violating of sound surgical principles. It has been suggested that the "tenting" problem may be corrected by subcutaneous lifting methods.
   b. **Specific concerns.** Several abdominal wall-lifting systems require an additional permanent low-pressure pneumoperitoneum due to inadequate exposure of the target area. The advantages of this approach are minimal. Other systems require pneumoperitoneum only for the safe installation of the lifting device. This approach bears the same risk of gas insufflation-related complications such as reported for pneumoperitoneum. Because of tent-shaped suspension and suboptimal intraabdominal exposure, applications of this approach have been limited to procedures in the pelvic region. In addition, there is a possibility of ischemic injury to abdominal wall muscles with intraabdominal lifting devices. Some of these problems can be overcome using subcutaneous retraction systems. These do not require an initial pneumoperitoneum; however, to achieve adequate exposure CO_2 insufflation must be added in some situations. Moreover, setting up a system of subcutaneous wiring is more complicated.
   c. **Limited application in certain patients.** The initial experiences with abdominal wall lifting devices have shown that exposure is very poor in individuals with a muscular abdominal wall or obese patients.
   d. **The abdominal lifting device can present an obstacle** for a surgeon performing minimal-access surgery.

The concept of gasless laparoscopy is certainly valid. The technique is in its infancy, and further developments are required such that the exposure provided is comparable to that provided by pneumoperitoneum. It is conceivable that gasless laparoscopy will have value in high-risk patients, particularly those with cardiopulmonary disease.

C. Selected References

Corwin CL. Pneumoperitoneum. In: Scott-Conner CEH (ed) The SAGES Manual: Fundamentals of Laparoscopy and GI Endoscopy. New York: Springer, 1998:37–42.

Gutt CN, Daume J, Schaeff B, Paolucci V. Systems and instruments for laparoscopic surgery without pneumoperitoneum. Surg Endosc 1997;11:868–874.

Kurauchi N, Yonekawa M, Kurokawa Y, et al. Comparison between CO_2 insufflation and abdominal wall lift in laparoscopic cholecytectomy. A prospective multiinstitutional study in Japan. Surg Endosc 1999;13:705–709.

Neuhaus SJ, Ellis T, Rofe AM, Pike GK, Jamieson GG, Watson DI. Tumor implantation following laparoscopy using different insufflation gases. Surg Endosc 1998;12: 1300–1302.

Ninomiya K, Kitano S, Yoshida T, Bandoh T, Baatar D, Matsumoto T. Comparison of pneumoperitoneum and abdominal wall lifting as to hemodynamics and surgical stress response during laparoscopic cholecystectomy. Surg Endosc 1998;12:124–128.

Paolucci V, Schaeff B, Gutt CN, Litynski GS. Exposure of the operative field in laparoscopic surgery. Surg Endosc 1997;11:856–863.

Wolf JS, Stoller ML. Physiology of laparoscopy: basic principles, complications and other considerations. J Urol 1994;152:294–302.

44. Risk of Gas Embolism with CO_2 and Other Gases

David I. Watson, M.B., B.S., M.D., F.R.A.C.S.

At present, carbon dioxide (CO_2) is almost universally used to establish and maintain the pneumoperitoneum that provides exposure during laparoscopic procedures. CO_2 has properties that make it a very suitable agent; it is cheap, noncombustible, and colorless. Furthermore, it is excreted by the lungs during respiration, and it is highly soluble in water, which reduces the risk that gas which finds its way into the venous system will impair cardiac function.

More recently, debate has arisen about the metabolic and oncologic consequences of insufflating the peritoneal cavity with CO_2, and this has led to a reevaluation of the effects of CO_2 pneumoperitoneum and interest in the use of other gases for insufflation, in particular inert gases such as helium and argon [1, 2]. Although the use of these alternative gases has been predominantly in the setting of experimental studies, helium, in particular, is also being evaluated in clinical trials [3]. Among their other qualities and attributes, it is important to consider the relative risks of each type of gas in regard to venous embolism.

A. Gas Embolism

Gas embolism is one of the most serious complications of laparoscopy, and it is associated with a mortality rate of approximately 50% [4]. Fortunately, clinically significant gas embolism is rare. However, studies that utilized transesophageal echocardiography to detect gas in the cardiac chambers suggest that small asymptomatic gas embolism events are actually common during procedures such as laparoscopic cholecystectomy [5].

Pathophysiology of Gas Embolism

In the setting of laparoscopy, a gas embolism occurs when insufflated gas finds its way from the peritoneal cavity into the systemic venous circulation via an open vessel [6]. The embolus flows with the blood into the right heart, after which it is pumped into the lungs where the gas embolism is dispersed and becomes trapped as bubbles within the pulmonary capillary bed. A blocked capillary impairs both blood flow and gas exchange and results in physiologic shunting due to alterations in pulmonary vascular resistance. As the physiologic deadspace increases, these alterations are manifested by a fall in the end-tidal

PCO_2 levels. Given a large enough single embolus or a series of low-volume gas emboli, outflow obstruction develops and cardiovascular collapse follows. This is further aggravated by the trapping of gas within the right ventricle. As gas is compressible, cardiac work is wasted on compression of the gas within the ventricle rather than the expulsion of noncompressible blood. In addition to these pulmonary and cardiovascular alterations, gas embolism can also incite an inflammatory reaction via activation of Hageman factor, which, in turn, activates the complement cascade [7]. For these reasons, the end result of a sufficient volume of gas entering the systemic venous circulation is cardiovascular and circulatory collapse.

The pulmonary and hemodynamic effects of gas embolism are ultimately determined by the volume of gas entering the venous circulation, the solubility coefficient of the gas in blood, and the diffusibility of the gas in tissue. CO_2 is highly soluble in water (0.5 mL gas/mL blood); therefore, a considerable percentage of a venous embolus will be rapidly absorbed. The high solubility of CO_2 is one of the principal reasons why this gas is so widely utilized for laparoscopic procedures. What of the other gases that might be used to provide exposure during minimally invasive procedures? Helium is the best alternative presently. Helium is attractive because it is highly diffusible in tissue. It has a diffusibility constant that is three times greater than CO_2, and therefore helium which has diffused into the patient's tissues during a case is more quickly eliminated from the body after the procedure than CO_2. However, helium is poorly soluble in blood (0.008 mL gas/mL blood), and thus in the setting of a venous embolus, unlike CO_2, only a small volume is absorbed [8]. The poor solubility of helium may be a major impediment to its routine clinical use because the consequences of venous gas embolus are potentially far more serious than those relating to retention of gas in the patient's tissues.

Diagnosis

The early diagnosis of venous gas embolism can be difficult. Classical signs include cardiac dysrhythmia, elevation of pulmonary arterial pressure, elevation of central venous pressure, decrease in end-tidal CO_2 partial pressure, a fall in systemic blood pressure, and hypoxia. As the volume of CO_2 in the circulation increases, systolic blood pressure and central venous pressure initially increase, however, systemic hypotension develops later and is a preterminal event.

A number of studies have questioned the reliability of end-tidal CO_2 in the detection of venous gas embolism [6, 9, 10]. The results of a recent experimental study from Yau et al. [6] suggest that a persistently elevated central venous pressure, combined with unexplained persistent tachycardia and elevated arterial PCO_2 levels, are more reliable indicators of CO_2 gas embolism. Early signs of helium gas embolism detected using the same porcine model included a fall in systolic and diastolic blood pressure, a fall in arterial PO_2, and an elevation in central venous pressure and arterial PCO_2 [6].

Incidence and Mechanism of Gas Embolism During Laparoscopy

The clinical effect of gas embolism, or the lack thereof, depends upon the amount of gas within the circulation. Small volumes of gas are of little, if any, clinical significance; however, large-volume emboli can lead to cardiac arrest and death. Thus, it is important to distinguish small asymptomatic emboli from larger embolic events that can be fatal. In experimental and clinical studies, ultrasound has been used for the detection of small gas bubbles within the systemic circulation [5]. However, this method does not permit full characterization of the nature of the embolic material, that is, fat, thrombi, or gas. It is also not possible to determine the volume of the embolus with ultrasound. Thus, ultrasound will detect the presence of emboli but cannot determine the source of the emboli, the size of the embolus, or the clinical significance of the event.

How often does venous gas embolism occur? Mann et al. [11] have reported that transesophageal ultrasound can detect volumes of argon gas as small as 0.1 mL/kg in a pig model with a sensitivity of 100%. However, this author was unable to detect any evidence of gas embolism occurring during routine pneumoperitoneum at an insufflation pressure of 15 mmHg when using either argon or CO_2 gas. These findings are supported by another porcine study that also used transesophageal ultrasound. In this study it was demonstrated that CO_2 pneumoperitoneum at a pressure of up to 30 mmHg was not associated with gas entering the intravascular compartment during routine laparoscopy [12]. However, this study did demonstrate that a small volume of CO_2 could be detected following injury to major veins, especially after deflation of the pneumoperitoneum [12]. Similar methodology has been applied in the clinical setting: one study demonstrated that small-volume gas embolism occurred in 11 of 16 patients undergoing laparoscopic cholecystectomy [5]. These patients manifested no significant cardiorespiratory events, and thus all embolic events were minor and of no clinical significance. This study, in contrast to other reports [13], therefore, suggests that gas embolism might be common during laparoscopy. Regardless, all the studies support the position that *clinically relevant* embolism rarely occurs during laparoscopy.

Vascular injury when attempting to establish pneumoperitoneum with a Veress needle or when blindly placing the first port via a sharp trocar probably results in the majority of clinically significant gas emboli [14]. A sizable volume of gas may find its way into the bloodstream via such vascular injuries; in addition, such injuries, obviously, may also result in a major hemorrhage. Hemorrhage can lead to death from exsanguination, whereas embolism, due to direct insufflation of a large vein, can lead to cardiovascular collapse and also death. Distinguishing death from gas embolism from death due to exsanguination alone is difficult, and for this reason the mortality rate associated with gas embolism alone at the commencement of laparoscopy is uncertain. Nevertheless, published evidence suggests that the incidence of major vascular injury when using a Veress needle for the establishment of pneumoperitoneum lies somewhere between 0.8 and 7.5 injuries per 10,000 laparoscopies [14, 15], and the mortality associated with this is approximately 1 death per 10,000 procedures. It is virtually certain that the incidence of major gas embolism is less than or equal to these relatively low rates. This is supported by studies that report an incidence of clinically significant gas embolism during CO_2 pneumoperitoneum which varies between 0.001% and 0.6% [8]. Although not all these events are associated with mortality, in a recent French laparoscopy series two of seven patients who developed venous carbon dioxide embolism died [16].

It should be appreciated that major vascular injuries have not been reported following open insertion of the first laparoscopic port, and because direct intravascular insufflation is not possible during open insertion of the first port, major gas embolism is highly unlikely if the simple precaution of using an open insertion technique for the first laparoscopic trocar is followed. Clinically significant gas embolism, that is, an event that threatens life, is dependent on the balance of the volume of gas entering the circulation and the amount of gas that is removed. It is unlikely that large volumes of gas enter the circulation during routine uncomplicated laparoscopic procedures. As argued above, it is most likely that, for life-threatening gas embolism to occur, direct venous puncture with a Veress needle or the first trocar, followed by direct venous insufflation, is required. In a recent study, Welch et al. [17] investigated the pressure within the intraabdominal inferior vena cava (IVC). They demonstrated that as insufflation pressure increased, intracaval pressure also increased, and this always exceeded intraperitoneal pressure, thereby maintaining a pressure gradient from the IVC to the peritoneal cavity. A recent study (unpublished data) from the University of Adelaide Department of Surgery investigated the effect of deliberately lacerating the IVC under laparoscopic conditions. This was not followed by gas embolism. Both Jacobi et al. [18] and Dion et al. [19] conducted similar studies in which the IVC was deliberately lacerated under laparoscopic conditions, and significant venous gas embolism did not occur. A further study has found that a small volume of intravascular CO_2 gas bubbles can be detected following laparoscopic injury to major veins, especially after deflation of the pneumoperitoneum [12]. However, the volume of gas involved was again not clinically significant. These studies reinforce the view that the Veress needle insertion technique is the means by which the majority of clinically relevant gas embolism events occur.

B. The Relative Safety of Alternative Insufflation Gases

Potential oncologic and immunologic advantages demonstrated by experimental studies of inert insufflation gases have encouraged investigators to conduct experimental studies to evaluate the relative safety of these gases, in particular the consequences of iatrogenic gas embolism events. Concern has been expressed about the safety of helium insufflation if gas embolism occurs.

There is conflicting experimental evidence concerning the relative dangers of embolism when using helium insufflation compared to CO_2. Porcine studies by Rudston-Brown et al. [20], Yau et al. [6], and Wolf et al. [8] have demonstrated that helium gas embolism has a greater deleterious effect than CO_2 embolism on survival following the intravenous injection of gas. When compared to results following direct intravascular injection of CO_2, a smaller volume of helium is required to bring about cardiac arrest. This experimental model mimics the clinical situation of inadvertent insertion of a Veress needle into a vein when attempting to establish pneumoperitoneum. Jacobi et al. [18] used a different model to assess the frequency of gas embolism from a venous injury that occurs in the midst of a laparoscopic procedure, after the successful establishment of pneumoperitoneum. During these procedures the IVC was lacerated and allowed to bleed for a period of time, after which the injury was repaired. No embolic events were noted in any of the animals; these results suggested that the incidence of gas embolism during laparoscopy from accidental injury of a large vessel is likely to be low. In their dog model, Dion et al. [19] reported a similar outcome.

Helium has been used clinically for laparoscopic procedures; thus far, no complications specific to its use have been reported. Although thus far there are no reports of gas embolism, only a limited number of centers are using helium, most often in the setting of a study. As it is most likely that clinically significant and life-threatening embolism problems result from the direct injection of a large volume of gas into a large vein via a Veress needle at induction of the pneumoperitoneum, the problem of gas embolism with inert gases is potentially avoidable if care is taken to always use an open cannulation technique to commence laparoscopy.

Argon, like helium, is inert, nonflammable, and available [21]. It is also relatively insoluble in blood and, therefore, the consequences of argon gas embolism are likely to be, similar to helium, greater than for CO_2. Argon insufflation has been investigated by Mann et al. [11], also using a porcine model. During a stable pneumoperitoneum of either argon or CO_2 gas, no episodes of gas embolism were detected. However, when gas was directly injected into the venous circulation, the cardiovascular effects of gas embolism were greater with argon than for CO_2. These results mirrored those of the helium experiments mentioned above.

Nitrous oxide was used commonly for insufflation in the 1970s and 1980s [22]. Concerns about the combustibility of this gas when electrocautery is in use led to a decline in the utilization of nitrous oxide. More recently, nitrogen has been proposed for insufflation [23]. However, there is currently little evidence to support its use. The clinical implications of nitrous oxide and nitrogen gas embolism have not been investigated thus far.

C. Conclusions

Venous gas embolism is a rare, but potentially fatal, complication of laparoscopy. It is largely because of concern about this risk that CO_2, which is more rapidly eliminated from the blood than other gases, has become the standard insufflation agent for laparoscopic surgery. Life-threatening gas embolism is most likely to occur following the inadvertent introduction of a Veress needle into a large vein, followed by direct intravenous insufflation. Once the pneumoperitoneum has been established and the first port placed, clinically relevant gas embolic events are exceptionally rare. Therefore, use of an open "cut-down" cannulation technique to commence laparoscopy should drastically reduce the incidence of a major gas embolism.

The use of alternative insufflation gases, in particular the inert gas helium, is supported by experimental evidence that suggests that by utilizing an alternative gas the adverse metabolic and oncologic consequences associated with CO_2 can largely be avoided. However, because of their low solubility in blood, inert insufflation gases are inherently more dangerous than CO_2 from the point of view of embolism because cardiovascular compromise occurs following a much smaller volume of intravascular inert gas than of CO_2. However, there may be a legitimate clinical role for inert gases, provided pneumoperitoneum is not established with a Veress needle, because gas embolism is so unlikely to occur after the pneumoperitoneum has been safely established.

D. References

1. Jacobi CA, Wenger F, Sabat R, Volk T, Ordemann J, Muller JM. The impact of laparoscopy with carbon dioxide versus helium on immunologic function and tumor growth in a rat model. Dig Surg 1998;15:110–116.
2. Neuhaus SJ, Watson DI, Ellis T, et al. Wound metastasis following different insufflation gases. Surgery 1998;123:579–583.
3. Leighton TA, Liu SY, Bongard FS. Comparative cardiopulmonary effects of carbon dioxide versus helium pneumoperitoneum. Surgery 1993;113:527–531.
4. Baxter JN, O'Dwyer PJ. Pathophysiology of laparoscopy. Br J Surg 1995;82:1–2.
5. Derouin M, Couture P, Boudreault D, Girard D, Gravel D. Detection of gas embolism by transesophageal echocardiography during laparoscopic cholecystectomy. Anesth Analg 1996;82:119–124.
6. Yau P, Watson DI, Lafullarde T, Jamieson GG. An experimental study of the effect of gas embolism using different laparoscopy insufflation gases. J Laparoendosc Adv Surg Tech 2000;10:211–216.
7. Neuberger T, Andrus C, Wittgen C, Wade T, Kaminski DL. Prospective comparison of helium versus carbon dioxide pneumoperitoneum. Gastrointest Endosc 1996;43: 38–41.
8. Wolf JS, Carrier S, Stoller M. Gas embolism: helium is more lethal than carbon dioxide. J Laparoendosc Surg 1994;4:173–177.
9. Mayer K, Ho HS, Mathiesen K, Wolfe B. Cardiopulmonary responses to experimental venous carbon dioxide embolism. Surg Endosc 1998;12:1025–1030.
10. Byrick RJ, Kay JC, Mullen JB. Capnography is not as sensitive as pulmonary artery pressure monitoring in detecting marrow microembolism; studies in a canine model. Anesth Analg 1989;68:94–100.
11. Mann C, Boccara G, Grevy V, Navarro F, Fabre J, Colson P. Argon pneumoperitoneum is more dangerous than CO_2 pneumoperitoneum during venous gas embolism. Anesth Analg 1997;85:1367–1371.

12. Bazin JE, Gillart T, Rasson P, Conio N, Aigouy L, Schoeffler P. Haemodynamic conditions enhancing gas embolism after venous injury during laparoscopy: a study in pigs. Br J Anesth 1997;78:570–575.
13. Thio JM, Reichert C. Transesophageal echocardiographic assessment of venous carbon dioxide embolism during laparoscopic cholecystectomy. Anesthesiology 1994; 31:A112 [abstract].
14. Bonjer HJ, Hazebroek EJ, Kazemier G, Giuffrida MC, Meijer WS, Lange JF. Open versus closed establishment of pneumoperitoneum in laparoscopic surgery. Br J Surg 1997;84:599–602.
15. Hanney RM, Alle KM, Cregan PC. Major vascular injury and laparoscopy. Aust N Z J Surg 1995;65:533–535.
16. Cottin V, Delafosse B, Viale J. Gas embolism during laparoscopy: a report of seven cases in patients with pervious abdominal surgical history. Surg Endosc 1996;10: 166–169.
17. Welch LS, Urbach DR, Herron DM, Ludemann R, Swanstrom LL, Hansen PD. The relationship between pneumoperitoneum pressure and pressure within the intra-abdominal inferior vena cava in a pig model. Surg Endosc 2000;14:S227 [abstract].
18. Jacobi CA, Junghans T, Peter F, et al. Cardiopulmonary changes during laparoscopy and vessels injury: comparison of CO_2 and helium in an animal model. Langenbecks Arch Surg 2000;385:459–466.
19. Dion YM, Levesque C, Diollon CJ. Experimental carbon dioxide pulmonary embolisation after vena cava laceration under pneumoperitoneum. Surg Endosc 1995;9: 1065–1069.
20. Rudston-Brown B, Draper PN, Warriner B, Walley KR, Phang PT. Venous gas embolism: a comparison of carbon dioxide and helium in pigs. Can J Anaesth 1997; 44:1102–1107.
21. Eisenhauer DM, Saunders CJ, Ho HS, Wolfe BM. Hemodynamic effects of argon pneumoperitoneum. Surg Endosc 1994;8:315–320.
22. Aitola P, Airo I, Kaukinen S, Ylitalo P. Comparison of N_2O and CO_2 pneumoperitoneums during laparoscopic cholecystectomy with special reference to postoperative pain. Surg Laparosc Endosc 1998;8:140–144.
23. Aneman A, Svenson M, Stenqvist O, Dalenback J, Lonnroth H. Intestinal perfusion during pneumoperitoneum with carbon dioxide, nitrogen and nitric oxide during laparoscopic surgery. Eur J Surg 2000;166:70–76.

45. Impact of CO_2 Pneumoperitoneum on Body Temperature and the Integrity of the Peritoneal Lining

Carsten N. Gutt, M.D.
Christopher Heinbuch, M.D.
Parswa Ansari, M.D.

In addition to its well-known systemic side effects such as hypercarbia and acidosis, CO_2 pneumoperitoneum also has a number of detrimental local (i.e., intraperitoneal) effects. For example, intraabdominally, CO_2 pneumoperitonuem has been shown to reduce the blood flow to the liver [1]. Furthermore, CO_2 pneumoperitoneum may also adversely effect the peritoneal lining itself. This chapter discusses the morphological alterations of the peritoneal monolayer caused by CO_2 pneumoperitoneum. The second part of the chapter discusses the body temperature alterations associated with CO_2 pneumoperitoneum.

A. Integrity of the Peritoneal Lining

During laparoscopic procedures, a working space must be created within the closed abdomen. The most commonly employed method of exposure is CO_2 pneumoperitoneum wherein gas is insufflated until an intraabdominal pressure of 12–15 mmHg is obtained. The parietal peritoneum, which is distended and stretched by the pneumoperitoneum, is the interface between the high-pressure abdominal cavity and the abdominal wall and retroperitoneum. A sustained pneumoperitoneum initiates a variety of alterations in the mesothelial cells of the parietal peritoneum.

In a study that utilized a well-established animal model, during pneumoperitoneum, no changes from normal morphology were observed. However, 1 to 2 hours after desufflation, the surface layer of cells demonstrated drastic alterations. The mesothelial cells had partially retracted and strongly bulged so that they appeared nearly spherical. The intercellular clefts, normally difficult to identify, were enlarged and clearly visible [2]. Further, the retraction of the cells also exposed large areas of the underlying basal lamina. On the other hand, the carpet of microvilli was nearly unchanged. The normal conformation of the mesothelium is restorable. Experiments have shown that 2 hours after release of the pneumoperitoneum the process of regeneration of the monolayer tissue is initiated. After 96 hours, the intercellular gaps are shrinking. In some regions of the peritoneum, the insufflation-related alterations will have completely disappeared and the confluent layer of microvilli-covered cells is restored.

The described ultrastructural changes observed after exposure to a high-pressure CO_2 environment are the same as those found after saline injection into the peritoneal cavity [3]. Thus, one might conclude that it is the increased pressure rather than the specific agent or gas that causes the described changes. The morphologic alterations in the superficial layer of the peritoneum, induced by increased intraabdominal pressure, are related to a loss of mesothelial integrity. The exposed peritoneal basal lamina may in theory, under certain circumstances, have detrimental clinical consequences.

The parietal peritoneum functions physiologically as a barrier, with controlled pathways to remove fluids, particles, and cells from the peritoneal cavity. The abdominal secretions are drained by large lymphatics located beneath the diaphragm's mesothelial surface. This fluid is then transported to the venous system by the thoracic duct. In conditions associated with abdominal sepsis and peritonitis, the capnoperitoneum, by exposing the basal lamina, may provide intraabdominal infectious agents access to the bloodstream and the rest of the body. Such spread may result in bacteremia, endotoxemia, and, ultimately, septic shock. It should be noted that, thus far, there are no data to support this hypothesis; no studies have yet assessed bacteremia perioperatively following the instillation of bacteria into the abdominal cavity. However, several investigators have determined how well bacteria were "cleared" from the peritoneal cavity during laparoscopy.

One small animal study reported that bacterial clearance from the peritoneal cavity was decreased by CO_2 pneumoperitoneum [4]. In contrast, a second study, carried out in a porcine model, found that peritoneal bacterial clearance was increased by CO_2 pneumoperitoneum [5]. On the basis of these limited experimental data it is not possible to draw a conclusion. Can anything be gleaned from the human literature? Laparoscopic methods have been successfully used for appendectomy in the setting of perforation with complication rates similar to those noted after open surgery. Both retrospective and randomized controlled trials have failed to demonstrate a significant difference in abscess formation postoperatively [6–9]. Unfortunately, there is little literature regarding the use of laparoscopic methods for gastric or colonic perforation in humans. Clearly, further animal and human studies are needed to clarify this situation.

The uncovered basal lamina may also be a favorable environment for the attachment of viable liberated tumor cells in the abdomen. Several studies that utilized a tumor cell suspension model demonstrated that the introduction of malignant cells into the abdomen in the setting of CO_2 pneumoperitoneum leads to a higher tumor growth rate, a higher tumor load, and a lesser survival rate [10, 11]. It is important to note that other animal studies, carried out using similar tumor cell suspension models, have found that peritoneal tumors developed only at sites of peritoneal injury (trocar or laparotomy wound) and not on uninjured peritoneum [12, 13]. Thus, in these latter studies, the CO_2 pneumoperitoneum-related injury to intact parietal peritoneum was not associated with the development of peritoneal metastases in those uninjured areas. Finally, in the human arena, the recent published literature regarding laparoscopy and cancer reports no significant differences in the rate of wound or peritoneal metastases when minimally invasive (done under CO_2 pneumoperitoneum) and open surgical methods are compared.

In theory, from the standpoint of the integrity of the peritoneum, the use of CO_2 pneumoperitoneum may be problematic in the setting of peritonitis. As already noted, there are not enough human or animal data available to draw any firm conclusions. In the setting of cancer, one can raise similar concerns about CO_2 pneumoperitoneum increasing the chances of peritoneal tumor metastases. However, as per the available and ever-enlarging human literature, increased rates of wound and peritoneal tumor recurrences have not been reported. Thus, presently, it appears as though the insufflation-related peritoneal alterations are not of clinical consequence.

B. Impact of Pneumoperitoneum on Body Temperature

Perioperative hypothermia increases the morbidity of surgery. Hypothermia is associated with higher rates of postoperative wound infection [14], more adverse cardiac events [15], and greater transfusion requirements [16].

Initially, it was anticipated that laparoscopic surgery would be associated with less hypothermia than open surgery because the abdomen remains closed with the former, thus avoiding prolonged exposure of the abdominal viscera to the cool room air. However, thus far, most studies have not found a difference in the rate or extent of hypothermia when open and laparoscopic procedures are compared. Luck et al. found no statistically significant difference in the incidence of hypothermia during colorectal cases when well-matched patients undergoing open and laparoscopic surgery were compared [17]. Similarly, Nguyen et al. demonstrated a decrease in intraabdominal temperature but not core temperature when comparing laparoscopic versus open gastric bypass procedures [18].

The risk of hypothermia due to CO_2 insufflation during laparoscopic surgery was highlighted by Bessell et al. in 1995 [19]. The risk appears to be correlated with the duration of the operation and the insufflation flow rate. Modern electronic insufflator units are able to maintain the pneumoperitoneum at a constant pressure by continuous insufflation of gas to replace losses caused by leaks and the dissolution of CO_2 in the blood. This means that during a complex or advanced operation, hundreds of liters of gas may be insufflated into the abdomen.

The temperature of the gas leaving the insufflator has been shown to be about 25°C. Early after insufflation into the abdomen, the temperature of the gas is in the range of 30°–32°C. Obviously, this intraperitoneal hypothermia, relative to the core temperature, would be expected to cause a drop in the core temperature. If there is minimal leakage of CO_2 from the abdomen, then, with time, the gas will become warmer. Unfortunately, during most advanced cases there are substantial and, at times, nearly continuous leaks such that additional cold gas must be insufflated regularly to maintain the pressure and exposure. In addition, animal studies suggest that a major contributing factor to heat loss is evaporation, which can be rectified by humidifying the gas [20]. Thus, it is not surprising that laparoscopic procedures, similar to open procedures (but for different reasons), are often associated with a drop in core temperature.

There is evidence that the use of heated and humidified gas lessens the procedure-related hypothermia. In a single large animal study, the differences in core temperatures after cool and warm CO_2 insufflation were significant [19]. A recent randomized trial in humans found that patients receiving heated and humidified CO_2 demonstrated significantly higher intraabdominal temperatures; of note, no differences in core temperatures were found [21]. A second human study also reported some advantages when humidified and warmed (to body temperature) CO_2 was utilized [22]. Other studies have found that the vasodilatory effects of warmed CO_2 are not important from a thermal point of view. Therefore, some controversy exists regarding the effectiveness and impact of warmed and humidified CO_2 in regard to intraperitoneal thermoregulation. Of note, the use of warm and/or humidified CO_2 has been noted to have other effects in addition to those relating to temperature.

One study noted that warm CO_2 insufflation was associated with local vasodilatation in the kidneys; this might be beneficial to patients with borderline renal function [23]. Of uncertain significance, in another study, the use of very dry CO_2 was associated with increased peritoneal fluid viscosity [24]. The use of warm or humidified pneumoperitoneum has also been associated with decreased postoperative pain [25, 26]. Finally, Puttick et al. reported that warming and humidifying the insufflation gas led to a reduced postoperative intraperitoneal acute-phase cytokine response [27].

In summary, there are conflicting data regarding the impact of warmed and humidified CO_2 on surgery-related hypothermia; of note, postoperative pain may be reduced. There are enough encouraging reports, in the opinion of the authors, to warrant the use of gas-warming units and humidifiers, especially during lengthy cases. An effort should also be made to minimize the leakage of CO_2 from the peritoneal cavity.

C. References

1. Jakimowicz J, Stultiens G, Smulders F. Laparoscopic insufflation of the abdomen reduces portal venous flow. Surg Endosc 1998;12(2):129–132.
2. Volz J, Köster S, Spacek Z, Paweletz N. Characteristic alteration of the peritoneum after carbon dioxide pneumoperitoneum. Surg Endosc 1999;13:611–614.
3. Tsilibary EC, Wissig SL. Lymphatic absorption from the peritoneal cavity: regulation of patency of mesothelial stomata. Microvasc Res 1983;25:22–29.
4. Chekan EG, Nataraj C, Clary EM, et al. The effect of gases in the intraperitoneal space on cytokine response and bacterial translocation in a rat model. Surg Endosc 1999;13(11):1135–1138.
5. Collet D, Vitale GC, Reynolds M, Klar E, Cheadle WG. Peritoneal host defenses are less impaired by laparoscopy than by open operation. Surg Endosc 1995;9(10):1059–1064.

6. Pedersen AG, Petersen OB, Wara P, Ronning H, Qvist N, Laurberg S. Randomized clinical trial of laparoscopic versus open appendicectomy. Br J Surg 2001;88(2): 200–205.
7. Tang E, Ortega AE, Anthone GJ, Beart RW Jr. Intraabdominal abscesses following laparoscopic and open appendectomies. Surg Endosc 1996;10(3):327–328.
8. Champault GG, Barrat C, Raselli R, Elizalde A, Catheline JM. Laparoscopic versus open surgery for colorectal carcinoma: a prospective clinical trial involving 157 cases with a mean follow-up of 5 years. Surg Laparosc Endosc Percutan Tech 2002;12(2): 88–95.
9. Wullstein C, Barkhausen S, Gross E. Results of laparoscopic vs. conventional appendectomy in complicated appendicitis. Dis Colon Rectum 2001;44(11):1700–1705.
10. Volz J, Köster S, Leweling H, Melchert F. Surgical trauma and metabolic changes induced by surgical laparoscopy vs. laparotomy. Gynecol Endosc 1997;6:1–6.
11. Volz J, Köster S, Schaef B, Paolucci V. Laparoscopic surgery: the effects of insufflation gas on tumor-induced lethality in mice. Am J Obstet Gynecol 1998;174:132–140.
12. Jones DB, Guo LW, Reinhard MK, et al. Impact of pneumoperitoneum on trocar site implantation of colon cancer in hamster model. Dis Colon Rectum 1995;38:1182–1188.
13. Wu JS, Brasfield EB, Guo LW, et al. Implantation of colon cancer at trocar sites is increased by low pressure pneumoperitoneum. Surgery 1997;122(1):1–7.
14. Kurz A, Sessler DI, Lenhardt R. Perioperative normothermia to reduce the incidence of surgical-wound infection and reduce hospitalisation. N Engl J Med 1996;334: 1209–1215.
15. Jones HD, McLaren CAR. Perioperative shivering and hypoxaemia after halothane, nitrous oxide, and oxygen anaesthesia. Br J Anaesth 1965;37:35–41.
16. Schmeid H, Kurz A, Sessler DI, Kozek Z, Reiter A. Mild hypothermia increases blood loss and transfusion requirements during total hip arthroplasty. Lancet 1996;347: 289–292.
17. Luck AJ, Moyes D, Maddern GJ, Hewett PJ. Core temperature changes during open laparoscopic colorectal surgery. Surg Endosc 1999;13:480–483.
18. Nguyen NT, Fleming NW, Singh A, Lee SJ, Goldman CD, Wolfe BM. Evaluation of core temperature during laparoscopic and open gastric bypass. Obes Surg 2001;11(5): 570–575.
19. Bessell JR, Karatassas A, Patterson JR, Jamieson GG, Maddern GJ. Hypothermia induced by laparoscopic insufflation: a randomised study in a pig model. Surg Endosc 1995;9:791–796.
20. Bessell JR, Ludbrook G, Millard SH, Baxter PS, Ubhi SS, Maddern GJ. Humidified gas prevents hypothermia induced by laparoscopic insufflation: a randomized controlled study in a pig model. Surg Endosc 1999;13(2):101–105.
21. Nguyen NT, Furdui G, Fleming NW, et al. Effect of heated and humidified carbon dioxide gas on core temperature and postoperative pain: a randomized trial. Surg Endosc 2002;16(7):1050–1054.
22. Ott DE, Reich H, Love B, et al. Reduction of laparoscopic-induced hypothermia, postoperative pain and recovery room length of stay by pre-conditioning gas with the Insu-

flow device: a prospective randomized controlled multi-center study. J Soc Laparosc Surg 1998;2(4):321–329.

23. Bäcklund M, Kellokumpu I, Scheinin T, von Schmitten, Tikkanen I, Lindgren L. Effect of temperature of insufflated CO_2 during and after prolonged laparoscopic surgery. Surg Endosc 1998;12:1126–1130.
24. Ott DE. Laparoscopic and tribology: the effect of laparoscopic gas on peritoneal fluid. J Am Assoc Gynecol Laparosc 2001;8:117–123.
25. Mouton WG, Bessell JR, Millard SH, Baxter PS, Maddern GJ. A randomized controlled trial assessing the benefit of humidified insufflation gas during laparoscopic surgery. Surg Endosc 1999;13(2):106–108.
26. Mouton WG, Bessell JR, Otten KT, Maddern GJ. Pain after laparoscopy. Surg Endosc 1999;13:445–448.
27. Puttick MI, Scott-Coombes DM, Dye J, et al. Comparison of immunologic and physiologic effects of CO_2 pneumoperitoneum at room and body temperatures. Surg Endosc 1999;13:572–575.

46. Adhesion Formation

A. Brent Fruin, M.D.
Arthur F. Stucchi, Ph.D.
Ali M. Ghellai, M.D.
James M. Becker, M.D.

Intraabdominal adhesions are a significant cause of postoperative morbidity. Adhesions are the cause of approximately 75% of all cases of small bowel obstruction (SBO) [1]. Pelvic adhesions are also a significant cause of infertility in women. The incidence of adhesions after abdominal surgery ranges from 50% to 95% [2]. Adhesions are the reason for 2% of all surgical admissions and 3% of all laparotomies. In 1992, in the United Kingdom, 200,000 patients required hospitalization for SBO and at least 50,000 operations were done for the sole purpose of lysis of adhesions [3]. In a recent retrospective study [4], it was determined that bowel obstruction, adhesiolysis for obstruction, and adhesiolysis to permit performance of other abdominal procedures occurred more often after abdominal surgery than was previously suspected. Lysis of adhesions is associated with an estimated cost of $1.3 billion in direct patient care per year in the United States [5].

Of note, adhesions are the cause of significant morbidity at the time of abdominal reoperation and may increase the complication rate of the intended procedure. In one study of 270 reoperations in which lysis of adhesions was necessary, inadvertent enterotomy occurred in 19% of patients [6]. Postoperative complications such as anastomotic leak and wound infection were increased in these patients. Adhesions are also a major reason for conversion from a laparoscopic to a standard open approach.

A. Pathophysiology of Adhesion Formation

During the past two decades, there has been considerable progress in defining the pathogenesis of postsurgical adhesions [7]. Injury or insult to the peritoneum, an inevitable consequence of any abdominal surgical procedure, is the initial stimulus for adhesion formation (Figure 46.1).

Abrasion, cutting, ischemia, desiccation, and coagulation all lead to inflammation, as characterized by hyperemia, fluid exudation, an inflammatory cell infiltrate, the production of proinflammatory cytokines, and the activation of the complement and coagulation cascades.

Inflammatory exudate is rich in fibrinogen, which is converted to fibrin by thrombin. Fibrin deposition occurs and attaches adjoining damaged surfaces [7].

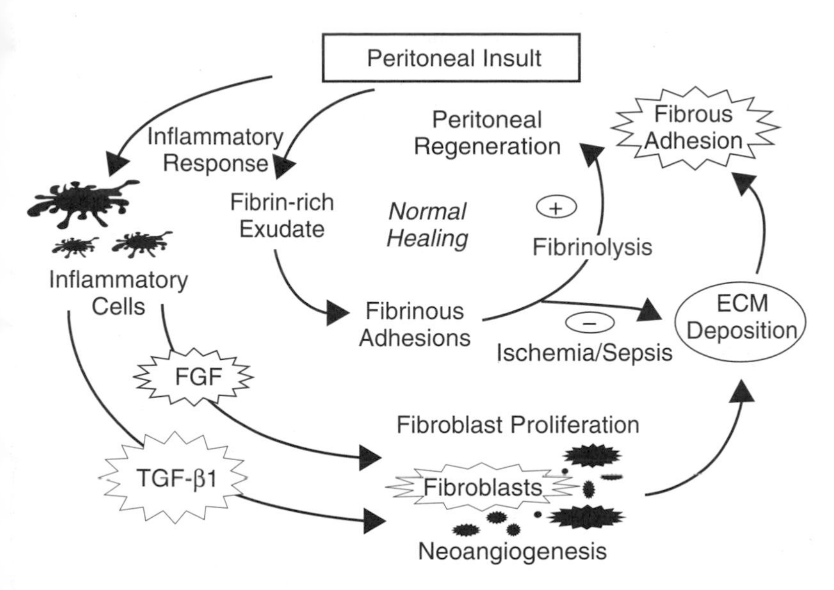

Figure 46.1. Adhesion formation begins with an insult to the peritoneum, which elicits an inflammatory cell response and results in the deposition of a fibrin-rich exudate. Newly formed fibrinous adhesions undergo fibrinolysis, facilitating normal peritoneal regeneration. However, in the presence of tissue ischemia, trauma, or infection, fibrinolytic activity is suppressed. Thereby, numerous inflammatory cells invade the persistent fibrinous adhesions and secrete potent growth and chemotactic factors such as transforming growth factor beta-1 (TGF-β1) and fibroblast growth factor (FGF). Fibroblasts attracted to the area subsequently proliferate and secrete extracellular matrix (ECM), forming fibrous adhesions.

Within days, migrating fibroblasts infiltrate the fibrin matrix in response to the production of chemoattractants secreted by inflammatory cells, and facilitate the conversion of fibrinous adhesions into fibrous adhesions by the deposition of extracellular matrix materials (ECM) such as collagen. Peritoneal tissue possesses inherent fibrinolytic activity. Injury to the peritoneum impairs this activity via an initial depletion of tissue plasminogen activator (tPA) as well as a later increase in plasminogen activator inhibitor (PAI.) This early balance between fibrin formation and degradation seems to be the major determinant of adhesion formation [8]. Transforming growth factor beta-1 (TGF-β_1), a polypeptide cytokine with potent chemoattractant and mitogenic activity, in concert with other cytokines and mitogens derived primarily from inflammatory cells, reduces peritoneal fibrinolytic activity and plays an important role in adhesion formation [9].

Recognition of the significant reduction in perioperative pain and more rapid recovery associated with laparoscopic surgical techniques has led to their wide-

Table 46.1. Potential causes of pneumoperitoneum-induced adhesions.

• Duration of insufflation
• Intraperitoneal acidosis
• Desiccation
• Excessive intraabdominal pressure
• Hypoxia
• Ischemia

spread and rapid acceptance by the surgical community and to their considerable popularity with the public at large. There was also an expectation that laparoscopic surgery would be associated with a reduction in the formation of abdominal adhesions. The ability to access the abdominal cavity with minimal peritoneal trauma should, logically, result in fewer adhesions [2]. Minimal access also prevents exposure to air, preventing the desiccation of peritoneal and serosal surfaces. In addition, some have postulated that the earlier recovery of peristalsis associated with laparoscopic surgery might facilitate the disruption of early fibrinous adhesions [10].

However, there are certain aspects unique to laparoscopic surgery that may, indeed, contribute to adhesion formation (Table 46.1). Recently, investigators have begun to examine the role of pneumoperitoneum in adhesion formation. Ordonez et al. showed that duration of pneumoperitoneum was a cofactor in adhesion formation in a rabbit model [11] and Yesildaglar et al. demonstrated similar results in a mouse model [12]. Carbon dioxide (CO_2) is generally used for pneumoperitoneum because of its high solubility in water and high exchange rates in the lungs. Carbon dioxide has been shown to cause intraperitoneal acidosis [13]. Without adequate irrigation, CO_2 pneumoperitoneum may result in the desiccation of mesothelial layers, which can exacerbate adhesion formation. Also, the increased intraabdominal pressure associated with pneumoperitoneum may result in impaired peritoneal microcirculation, leading to ischemia [14].

In a rabbit model of adhesion formation utilizing laser and bipolar coagulation, Yesildaglar and Koninckx demonstrated that adhesion formation was increased with increased insufflation pressure [15]. Molinas et al., again in a rabbit model, demonstrated a significant relationship between duration of pneumoperitoneum and adhesion formation using either CO_2 or helium pneumoperitoneum [14]. No difference was found between CO_2 and helium. The addition of 4% oxygen to either CO_2 or helium caused a decrease in adhesion formation [14]. These results suggest that the mechanism of adhesion formation caused by pneumoperitoneum is not acidosis but local hypoxemia, produced by peritoneal distension. The clinical significance of these findings is unknown. However, they do suggest that avoidance of excessively high intraabdominal pressures may reduce the risk of postoperative adhesions.

The question remains: does minimally invasive surgery result in a reduced incidence of adhesion formation when compared with conventional, open surgical methods? Various clinical trials and experimental studies using animal models have addressed this issue. The majority of studies do conclude that laparoscopic surgery is less adhesiogenic, in part due to the avoidance of risk factors associated with adhesion formation during laparotomy. For example, laparoscopy in and of itself mitigates the usage of retractors, packs, sponges, and even glove powder, all of which have been implicated in adhesion formation. The maintenance of a closed abdomen significantly reduces peritoneal desiccation. Other factors potentially contributing to reduced adhesion formation during laparoscopic procedures include the decreased need for blind dissection of adhesions during abdominal exploration and less visceral tissue damage from excess handling. However, the degree to which minimally invasive surgery reduces adhesions has not been determined and it has become clear, similar to the situation following open surgery, that adhesion formation varies considerably among patients. Furthermore, the clinical significance of the purported reduced adhesion formation rate following laparoscopic surgery is not known yet.

In a study of cecal resection in a canine model, Schippers et al. found a marked reduction in adhesion formation in a laparoscopic group when compared to a laparotomy group [16]. There was no difference in adhesions between the two groups at the intraabdominal operative site, but there were fewer adhesions to abdominal wall incision sites and fewer enteroenteric adhesions in the laparoscopic group. In a study of open versus laparoscopic Nissen fundoplication in the rat, Krahenbuhl et al. found a significantly greater number of adhesions to the abdominal wall in the laparoscopic group than in the open group [17]. Luciano et al. found lower adhesion formation after laser injury to the uterus and peritoneum during laparoscopy in the rabbit [18]. However, Jorgenson et al. found no difference in adhesion formation between laparoscopic and laparotomy groups in a model of cecal abrasion in the rabbit [19]. Similar studies with pigs have also shown a reduction of adhesion formation after laparoscopic procedures [20]. The variable results of these studies is undoubtedly a result of the different methods used to produce adhesions, the different species used, as well as the subjective nature of most standardized methods of grading adhesions. The majority of animal studies do show at least some degree of reduction in adhesion formation when minimally invasive techniques are used.

Inherent ethical and practical limitations preclude most potential attempts to evaluate adhesion formation in the human population. Hence, there is little evidence in the literature to support a lower incidence of adhesion formation following laparoscopic surgery rather than laparotomy. The largest studies have been performed in the gynecologic population. The Operative Laparoscopic Study Group evaluated 68 women who had undergone laparoscopic adhesiolysis and then underwent a "second-look" laparoscopy within 90 days of the initial procedure. Of the 68 women studied, 66 showed recurrence of adhesions in areas where adhesions had been lysed [21]. This result was similar to, or greater than, the results of similar open surgery studies that also assessed the results of adhesiolysis. However, it should be noted that only 8 of the 68 women formed de novo adhesions, which was less than the 50% incidence of de novo adhesions noted in prior studies evaluating laparotomy and lysis of adhesions [22]. Lundorff et al. conducted a trial in which 105 women presenting with a tubal pregnancy were randomly assigned to either laparoscopic or open surgery. Seventy-three of these women underwent a "second-look" laparoscopy to assess adhesion formation. Women who had undergone an initial laparoscopic procedure had a significant decrease in adhesions at the operative site [23].

Polymeneas et al. conducted a study of 28 patients, 18 status post laparoscopic cholecystectomy and 8 status post open cholecystectomy, who underwent later laparoscopy for various indications. Patients who had undergone laparoscopic cholecystectomy had fewer adhesions at the operative site, as well as at the incision sites, than did patients who had undergone the open procedure [24]. De Wilde reported a prospective randomized trial examining postoperative adhesion formation after laparoscopic or conventional appendectomy as assessed by "second-look" laparoscopy. The incidence of adhesions was 10% (2/20) in the laparoscopic group versus 80% (16/20) in the conventional group [25].

Only one study has attempted to evaluate the prevalence of small bowel obstruction after laparoscopic abdominal surgery. In a multicenter retrospective study, Duron et al. identified 24 patients who underwent surgery for small bowel obstruction and whose only prior abdominal surgical history was a single laparoscopic procedure [26]. Either cholecystectomy, appendectomy, or transperitoneal hernia repair was the procedure in 19 of 24 cases. Fifty percent of the cases were found to be caused by adhesions, and 50% of cases were found to be caused by incarceration of small intestine in a port site. Twenty-six percent of all cases were severe enough to require a small bowel resection. All cases occurred less than 2 years after the laparoscopic procedure. The prevalence of early SBO requiring surgery in the context of the total population of patients who had undergone laparoscopic surgery was similar to that reported by Stewart et al. in 1987, looking at the occurrence of early SBO after common abdominal surgical procedures [27].

B. Adhesion Prevention During Laparoscopic Surgery

Laparoscopic surgery generally results in reduced adhesiogenesis; however, there are several general principles germane to good surgical technique that can further minimize adhesion formation during laparoscopic procedures (Table 46.2).

Parameters unique to laparoscopy that appear to be associated with adhesion formation such as extended insufflation times as well as excessive intraabdominal pressures are easily controllable. However, strict adherence to those surgical principles used to avoid adhesions during laparotomy also applies to

Table 46.2. Techniques to avoid pneumoperitoneum- and laparoscopic-induced adhesions.

- Minimize length of insufflation
- Minimize intraabdominal pressure
- Use adequate irrigation to avoid desiccation
- Gentle tissue manipulation
- Meticulous hemostasis
- Use of adhesion prevention adjuvant when appropriate

laparoscopic procedures. These include meticulous attention to minimizing tissue damage, desiccation, and hemostasis. In addition, adhesion prevention adjuvants should be used when appropriate.

Although numerous adjuvants and physical barriers are currently utilized to prevent adhesions during laparotomy [7], laparoscopic application of the more clinically efficacious products are limited [28]. For example, physical barriers such as sodium hyaluronate-based bioresorbable membrane or Sepafilm, which has been shown to significantly reduce adhesion formation [29], cannot be readily applied via a laparoscope. However, other barriers such as modified oxidized regenerated cellulose or Interceed have been successfully applied through the laparoscope with proven efficacy [30, 31], but only in the absence of blood. For obvious reasons, adhesion prevention adjuvants that can be applied as aqueous solutions or low-viscosity gels, such as polyethylene glycol hydrogel [32], SprayGel [33], or ACP gel [34], will most likely be the focus of emerging technologies in laparoscopic adhesion prevention [35].

In summary, adhesion formation after abdominal and pelvic surgery is a significant cause of morbidity. Pneumoperitoneum causes peritoneal hypoxemia, which may be a risk factor for adhesion formation that is unique to laparoscopic surgery. Minimizing the duration and insufflation pressure of pneumoperitoneum may reduce this risk. Laparoscopic techniques result in less direct peritoneal trauma: the primary stimulus for adhesiogenesis. This difference results in a reduction in adhesion formation when compared to open techniques, albeit to a variable degree in different settings. However, the clinical significance of reduced adhesion formation following minimally invasive surgery has yet to be demonstrated.

C. References

1. Menzies D. Postoperative adhesions: their treatment and relevance in clinical practice. Ann R Coll Surg Engl 1993;75:147–153.
2. Schafter M, Krahenbhl L, Buchler MW. Comparison of adhesion formation in open and laparoscopic surgery. Dig Surg 1998;15:148–152.
3. Ellis H. The clinical significance of adhesions: focus on intestinal obstruction. Eur J Surg Suppl 1997;21:5–9.
4. Beck DE, Opelka FG, Bailey HR, Rauh SM, Pashos CL. Incidence of small-bowel obstruction and adhesiolysis after open colorectal and general surgery. Dis Colon Rectum 1999;42:241–248.
5. Ray NF, Denton WG, Thamer M, Henderson SC, Perry S. Abdominal adhesiolysis: inpatient care and expenditures in the United States in 1994. J Am Coll Surg 1998; 186:1–9.
6. Van Der Krabben AA, Dijkstra FR, Nieuwenhuijzen M, Reijnen MM, Schaapveld M, Van Goor H. Morbidity and mortality of inadvertent enterotomy during adhesiotomy. Br J Surg 2000;87:467–471.
7. Dijkstra FR, Nieuwenhuijzen M, Reijnen MM, van Goor H. Recent clinical developments in pathophysiology, epidemiology, diagnosis and treatment of intra-abdominal adhesions. Scand J Gastroenterol Suppl 2000;232:52–59.

8. Thompson J. Pathogenesis and prevention of adhesion formation. Dig Surg 1998; 15:153–157.
9. Ghellai AM, Stucchi AF, Chegini N, et al. Role of transforming growth factor beta-1 in peritonitis-induced adhesions. J Gastrointest Surg 2000;4:316–323.
10. Menzies D, Ellis H. The role of plasminogen activator in adhesion prevention. Surg Gynecol Obstet 1991;172:362–366.
11. Ordonez JL, Dominguez J, Evrard V, Koninckx PR. The effect of training and duration of surgery on adhesion formation in the rabbit model. Hum Reprod 1997;12: 2654–2657.
12. Yesildaglar N, Ordonez JL, Laermans I, Koninckx PR. The mouse as a model to study adhesion formation following endoscopic surgery: a preliminary report. Hum Reprod 1999;14:55–59.
13. Volz J, Koster S, Weiss M, et al. Pathophysiologic features of a pneumoperitoneum at laparoscopy: a swine model. Am J Obstet Gynecol 1996;174:132–140.
14. Molinas CR, Koninckx PR. Hypoxaemia induced by CO_2 or helium pneumoperitoneum is a co-factor in adhesion formation in rabbits. Hum Reprod 2000;15: 1758–1763.
15. Yesildaglar N, Koninckx PR. Adhesion formation in intubated rabbits increases with high insufflation pressure during endoscopic surgery. Hum Reprod 2000;15:687–691.
16. Schippers E, Tittel A, Ottinger A, Schumpelick V. Laparoscopy versus laparotomy: comparison of adhesion-formation after bowel resection in a canine model. Dig Surg 1998;15:145–147.
17. Krahenbuhl L, Schafer M, Kuzinkovas V, Renzulli P, Baer HU, Buchler MW. Experimental study of adhesion formation in open and laparoscopic fundoplication. Br J Surg 1998;85:826–830.
18. Luciano AA, Frishman GN, Maier DB. A comparative analysis of adhesion reduction, tissue effects, and incising characteristics of electrosurgery, CO_2 laser, and Nd:YAG laser at operative laparoscopy: an animal study. J Laparoendosc Surg 1992;2:287–292.
19. Jorgensen JO, Lalak NJ, Hunt DR. Is laparoscopy associated with a lower rate of postoperative adhesions than laparotomy? A comparative study in the rabbit. Aust N Z J Surg 1995;65:342–344.
20. Garrard CL, Clements RH, Nanney L, Davidson JM, Richards WO. Adhesion formation is reduced after laparoscopic surgery. Surg Endosc 1999;13:10–13.
21. Diamond MP. Postoperative adhesion development after operative laparoscopy: evaluation at early second-look procedures. Operative Laparoscopy Study Group. Fertil Steril 1991;55:700–704.
22. Diamond MP, Daniell JF, Feste J, et al. Adhesion reformation and de novo adhesion formation after reproductive pelvic surgery. Fertil Steril 1987;47:846–866.
23. Lundorff P, Hahlin M, Kallfelt B, Thorburn J, Lindblom B. Adhesion formation after laparoscopic surgery in tubal pregnancy: a randomized trial versus laparotomy. Fertil Steril 1991;55:911–915.
24. Polymeneas G, Theodosopoulos T, Stamatiadis A, Kourias E. A comparative study of postoperative adhesion formation after laparoscopic vs open cholecystectomy. Surg Endosc 2001;15:41–43.

25. De Wilde RL. Goodbye to late bowel obstruction after appendicectomy. Lancet 1991; 338:1012.
26. Duron JJ, Hay JM, Msika S, et al. Prevalence and mechanisms of small intestinal obstruction following laparoscopic abdominal surgery: a retrospective multicenter study. French Association for Surgical Research. Arch Surg 2000;135:208–212.
27. Stwart RM, Page CP, Brender J, Schwesinger W, Eisenhut D. The incidence and risk of early postoperative small bowel obstruction. A cohort study. Am J Surg 1987; 154:643–647.
28. Tulandi T. How can we avoid adhesions after laparoscopic surgery? Curr Opin Obstet Gynecol 1997;9:239–243.
29. Becker JM, Dayton MT, Fazio VW, et al. Prevention of postoperative abdominal adhesions by a sodium hyaluronate-based bioresorbable membrane: a prospective, randomized, double-blind multicenter study [see comments]. J Am Coll Surg 1996; 183:297–306.
30. Mais V, Ajossa S, Piras B, Guerriero S, Marongiu D, Melis GB. Prevention of de-novo adhesion formation after laparoscopic myomectomy: a randomized trial to evaluate the effectiveness of an oxidized regenerated cellulose absorbable barrier. Hum Reprod 1995;10:3133–3135.
31. Keckstein J, Ulrich U, Sasse V, Roth A, Tuttlies F, Karageorgieva E. Reduction of postoperative adhesion formation after laparoscopic ovarian cystectomy. Hum Reprod 1996;11:579–582.
32. West JL, Chowdhury SM, Sawhney AS, Pathak CP, Dunn RC, Hubbell JA. Efficacy of adhesion barriers. Resorbable hydrogel, oxidized regenerated cellulose and hyaluronic acid. J Reprod Med 1996;41:149–154.
33. Dunn R, Lyman MD, Edelman PG, Campbell PK. Evaluation of the SprayGel adhesion barrier in the rat cecum abrasion and rabbit uterine horn adhesion models. Fertil Steril 2001;75:411–416.
34. De Iaco PA, Stefanetti M, Pressato D, et al. A novel hyaluronan-based gel in laparoscopic adhesion prevention: preclinical evaluation in an animal model. Fertil Steril 1998;69:318–323.
35. Wiseman DM. Adhesion prevention: past the future. In: diZerega GS (ed) Peritoneal Surgery. New York: Springer, 2000:401–417.

47. Impact of Minimally Invasive Methods on Postoperative Pain and Pulmonary Function

Alessandro Fichera, M.D.
Jeffrey W. Milsom, M.D.

During the past two decades, minimally invasive surgery (MIS) has changed the way we treat many disease entities. The management of biliary disease, gastroesophageal reflux, and morbid obesity, to mention just a few conditions, has radically changed since the introduction of laparoscopy. The reported short-term advantages of MIS over conventional surgery are faster recovery, shorter length of stay, early return of gastrointestinal function, decreased pain, early return to work, and decreased morbidity. In this chapter we address the effect of laparoscopy on postoperative pain and pulmonary function.

Pain perception and the characteristics of pain after any surgical procedure are influenced by several complex factors. Multiple objective and subjective components complicate the clinical evaluation of pain. Another confounding factor is that under the broad heading of MIS are grouped a variety of procedures that vary in regard to the extent of abdominal wall and intraabdominal tissue damage incurred as well as the duration of the procedure. Although many investigators have reported that operations carried out using laparoscopic methods are associated with less pain than procedures done using open techniques, it is clear that minimally invasive patients are not exempt from postoperative pain; up to 80% of patients require opiod analgesics after surgery. One of the benefits of the MIS "revolution" is that it has led to a reevaluation of surgeons' assumptions, attitudes, and practices regarding postoperative care. As a result of this introspection, it has become clear that by altering our behavior and practices and by using a multimodality approach we can improve the outcome of patients undergoing either minimally invasive or traditional surgery.

A. Postoperative Pain

In regards to pain, the most thoroughly studied procedure is cholecystectomy. In contrast, only a few high-quality studies have been carried out concerning colorectal, morbid obesity, and gynecologic surgery.

Most trials utilized a visual analogue scale (VAS) or a verbal rating scale to assess pain. Similar results, for the most part, were noted regardless of which method was employed; however, the VAS method appears to be more sensitive in detecting small differences in pain levels.

Most studies comparing laparoscopic and open cholecystectomy have noted that the former group of patients experience less pain and/or require less pain medication than patients in the latter group. Presently, there is little or no controversy regarding this well-documented benefit of minimally invasive cholecystectomy [1, 2, 4, 13].

A significant reduction in postoperative pain after laparoscopic colorectal surgery has been demonstrated in several studies [10, 12]. A well-designed prospective randomized study from Germany demonstrated significantly decreased postoperative pain, as assessed by VAS at rest and while coughing. This finding was associated with a reduced analgesic requirement, less fatigue, shorter hospital stay, and improved postoperative quality of life [10].

The results of several studies suggest that morbidly obese patients undergoing laparoscopic gastric bypass also benefit from the minimally invasive approach in regards to decreased postoperative pain and narcotic usage [5, 9]. These patients often present with right-sided heart failure secondary to pulmonary hypertension. Opioid narcotic drug-related respiratory depression worsens these patients' borderline respiratory function, and in some cases made necessitate long-term ventilatory support with all the sequelae associated with it.

Laparoscopic hysterectomy versus the open equivalent was similarly associated with less pain in one randomized gynecologic study [3]. Several other prospective, randomized trials have demonstrated a reduction in the narcotic requirement after laparoscopic procedures when compared to the equivalent open procedure. A reduction in postoperative narcotic requirements may be associated with earlier return of bowel function, earlier discharge, and improved pulmonary function.

B. Nature of Pain

Of the several classifications available in the literature, the authors believe the one proposed by Joris et al. [5] is the most comprehensive. According to this concept, pain following laparoscopy falls into one of three categories: visceral, abdominal wall, or shoulder tip pain (Table 47.1). Visceral pain, which is related to the intraperitoneal dissection and the specific procedure performed, in theory should be similar after equivalent open and closed operations. Abdominal wall pain is secondary to the incision(s) made to gain access to the abdominal cavity; laparoscopic patients should have less of this type of pain when compared to open surgery patients who have lengthier and more traumatic incisions. Shoulder tip pain, which has been reported to occur in 20%–40% of patients after laparoscopic cholecystectomy (LC), can also occur, albeit less frequently, after open surgery. In a study that compared LC with cholecystectomy carried out via a minilaparotomy, the incidence of shoulder tip pain was 23% after LC and 13% following open surgery. Several mechanisms have been proposed to explain this type of pain after laparoscopy, including irritation of somatic nerve fibers by overdistension of the diaphragm and the CO_2 pneumoperitoneum-related acidic intraperitoneal milieu.

It can be difficult to break down postoperative pain as to the relative contribution from each component. Among the laparoscopic operations, LC best lends

Table 47.1. Nature of pain.

Visceral pain
Abdominal wall pain
Shoulder tip pain

itself to this type of analysis because the procedure is limited to a single quadrant, the target organ is removed via limited dissection, and the procedure is performed via a limited number of ports. During the first 24 hours after LC, when the pain is most severe, the visceral component is predominant. A second pain peak is noted later; port wound-related abdominal pain and shoulder tip pain are thought to account for most of the pain during this period. Such a detailed evaluation is almost impossible after more complex procedures that require suturing, a bowel anastomosis, working in multiple quadrants, or, possibly, a small incision for extraction of the specimen.

C. Mechanisms of Pain

It is important to identify and clarify the pathophysiologic mechanisms behind laparoscopic procedure-related pain so that more effective treatment strategies can be devised.

Parietal peritoneal irritation is likely to account for some of the visceral and shoulder tip pain that is experienced after minimally invasive surgery. The CO_2 pneumoperitoneum, in a variety of ways, may have an impact on the peritoneum. Numerous studies have been carried out to assess the effect that the pneumoperitoneum has on the peritoneal surfaces (Table 47.2).

The total volume of gas insufflated, the rate of insufflation, the intraperitoneal pressure, the humidity, the intraabdominal temperature, the type of gas used, and the volume of residual gas all may influence the condition of the peritoneum, which, in turn, may contribute to the pain the patient experiences. It has been documented, via peritoneal biopsies, that pneumoperitoneum is associated with peritoneal inflammation, capillary and neuronal rupture, and granulocyte infiltration.

Table 47.2. Mechanisms of pain.

Direct traumatic effect of pneumoperitoneum
Localized acidosis
Peritoneal ischemia
Distension neuropraxia
Wound size and location
Port size and location
Drain
Anesthetic regimen
Individual sociocultural factors

The intraperitoneal carbonic acid that forms from the insufflated CO_2 gas may also irritate the peritoneum. Localized peritoneal acidosis has been demonstrated in a porcine model following CO_2 but not air pneumoperitoneum, and the degree of acidosis has been related to the duration of pneumoperitoneum and the intraabdominal pressure. In a human study similar findings were noted, but interestingly, peritoneal acidosis was also found in a small number of patients who underwent an argon pneumoperitoneum. This latter finding suggests that the increased intraabdominal pressure, independent of the type of gas used, may impede the peritoneal circulation, cause localized ischemia, and lead to acidosis. One of the benefits of saline lavage at the end of the procedure may be the dilution and, it is hoped, removal of the pneumoperitoneum-related carbonic acid.

What is the etiology of shoulder tip pain? One theory purports that the pneumoperitoneum stretches the diaphragm and the phrenic nerve, resulting in a neuropraxic injury that is the source of the shoulder pain. Other possible causes of this neuropathic pain include chemical irritation, nerve ischemia, and nerve compression. Aspiration of residual gas at the end of the case and the injection of local anesthetic into the diaphragm have been only moderately successful. In contrast, phrenic nerve block after the induction of anesthesia has been shown to significantly reduce the incidence of shoulder tip pain after LC.

The number, size, and location of the incision(s), obviously, play a large role in determining the amount of abdominal wall pain experienced by patients. The use of drains, the particular anesthetic regimen utilized, and individual sociocultural factors also influence the degree of postoperative pain.

Clearly the origin of pain after laparoscopy is multifactorial, with pain arising from the incision sites, the peritoneal surface, the phrenic nerve, and the intraabdominal operative site. In managing postoperative pain, an analgesic regimen that addresses the varied causes and mechanisms of pain is likely to be the most effective.

D. Methods of Reducing Postoperative Pain

It is not surprising that many different anesthetic regimens have been proposed and evaluated for the management of pain after MIS when one considers the multifactorial nature of pain and our limited understanding of the problem (Table 47.3). There is an abundant literature on this topic.

In brief, the infiltration of abdominal wall incision sites with local anesthetics provides short-lived benefits. The best results are obtained if the anesthetic is injected down to the level of the peritoneum and the injections are given at the end of the procedure.

The use of intraperitoneal local anesthetic, either lidocaine or bupivacaine, has been validated by several trials that have, for the most part, shown a short-lived benefit in terms of pain reduction. No benefit was shown with respect to earlier discharge or return to normal activity. No clinical toxicity has been reported as a consequence of peritoneal absorption. The intraperitoneal instillation of saline at the end of a procedure is a simple and safe approach, associated with a reduction in postoperative pain. It seems to work better when mixed with local anesthetics.

Table 47.3. Methods of reducing postoperative pain.

Methods of reducing postoperative pain
Local anesthesia preoperative vs. postoperative
Intraperitoneal local anesthetic
Intraperitoneal saline solution
NSAID preoperative vs. postoperative
Epidural analgesia
Removal of insufflation gas
Alternative gases
Increase temperature/humidity
Decrease pressure/volume

Nonsteroidal antiinflammatory agents (NSAIDs) seem to improve some aspects of postoperative pain, but only for the first 24 hours after the operation. The benefit of preemptive administration of NSAIDs has not been demonstrated. The principal role of NSAIDS, presently, are as opiate-sparing agents. Epidural analgesia has been shown to reduce postoperative pain and to be associated with reduced postoperative stress, as reflected by lower serum cortisol and catecholamine levels after surgery [14]. Epidural analgesia is also associated with improved postoperative pulmonary function. In the open surgery setting, epidural analgesia has been associated with a reduction in postoperative morbidity, specifically cardiac and respiratory complications, a reduced postoperative infection rate, and lower overall hospital cost.

The gynecologic literature suggests that removal of residual gas after surgery by mean of a gas drain reduces shoulder tip pain. After other major laparoscopic procedures, the reduction of shoulder tip pain by this method was very short lived and this method had minimal impact on the overall pain experienced. Adding a drain for active aspiration of residual pneumoperitoneum is not routinely recommended at this point.

Alternate insufflation gases have been assessed in an attempt to minimize or avoid the deleterious effects associated with CO_2. In regard to postoperative pain, neither nitrous oxide, argon, nor helium has been found to be superior to CO_2. Furthermore, there has been concern about the possibility of combustion with the use of cautery during nitrous oxide pneumoperitoneum. For these reasons, carbon dioxide remains the gas of choice at this time for all laparoscopic procedures.

Eliminating the pneumoperitoneum altogether by using a mechanical lifting device, surprisingly, has not been shown to decrease postoperative pain. Rather, lifting methods have been reported to increase the difficulty of carrying out the operation, owing to the inferior exposure provided, and are also associated with prolonged operative times.

The use of humidified and heated gas has been suggested as a means of minimizing peritoneal inflammation and injury. A reduction of peritoneal trauma may diminish pain postoperatively. There are currently several insufflators commercially available that are capable of warming and humidifying CO_2 before insufflation. Although some preliminary results are promising, the clinical impact of this approach has yet to be determined. It remains to be proven that the use of warmed and humidified gas translates into shortened length of stay, improved quality of life, or more rapid return to work.

A very inexpensive way to decrease postoperative pain is to decrease the maximum insufflation pressure to 12 mmHg or less and to limit gas leakage from around and through the ports. These maneuvers should decrease the extent of pneumoperitoneum-related diaphragmatic stretching and limit the overall volume of insufflated gas required for the case. The total volume of gas and the maximal insufflation pressure have been shown to correlate with the degree of postoperative pain.

In conclusion, because pain after laparoscopy is multifactorial, it is likely that a multimodality analgesia regimen will best reduce postoperative pain. Local anesthetic injections into the peritoneal and abdominal wall wounds, saline irrigation, and NSAIDs may reduce pain after laparoscopy. However, this benefit is short lived and does not translate into an improved functional outcome. Heated and humidified gas and the use of lower insufflation pressures and lower total gas volumes are also promising measures that should be considered.

E. Postoperative Pulmonary Function

The postoperative deterioration of respiratory function is a well-known sequela of abdominal surgery and is most marked for operations carried out via upper abdominal incisions. Numerous pulmonary function parameters, including functional residual capacity (FRC), forced vital capacity (FVC), and forced expiratory volume in 1 second (FEV_1) are reduced by as much as 60% after major abdominal surgery. These alterations have been attributed to temporary diaphragmatic dysfunction, which has been directly and proportionately correlated to postoperative pain. Regardless of anesthesia technique and aggressive postoperative pulmonary toilet, in the majority of cases pulmonary function does not return to preoperative values for up to a week to 10 days after conventional surgery. As a result of the reduced FRC, small airways collapse and atelectasis often develops. In the elderly and debilitated as well as in those patients with underlying pulmonary conditions, if atelectasis is not treated and corrected early, pneumonia may develop. Postoperative pneumonia, which occurs in about 5% of patients after major abdominal surgery, is one of the most commonly noted general complications.

It has been well established that LC is associated with significantly less marked pulmonary function changes and more rapid postoperative recovery of pulmonary function when compared with open cholecystectomy [4] (Table 47.4).

Morbidly obese patients who undergo laparoscopic gastric bypass not uncommonly present with right-sided heart failure and pulmonary hypertension. In this population, the ramifications of diminished pulmonary function after surgery are

Table 47.4. Pulmonary function and laparoscopy.

Less impairment of pulmonary function
Faster postoperative recovery of pulmonary function
Decreased postoperative complications

more serious than in the general population. So feared are major respiratory problems that it is the practice of some surgeons to perform prophylactic tracheostomy at the time of surgery in selected extremely obese patients [body mass index (BMI) $\geq 50\,kg/m^2$) with severe pulmonary hypertension. In this high-risk population, laparoscopic methods have been shown to be associated with less impairment of pulmonary function [5, 9]. Furthermore, in the great majority, respiratory function parameters return to preoperative levels by the first week postoperatively. Clinically these findings translate into a lower incidence of postoperative hypoxemia and segmental atelectasis.

In laparoscopic colorectal surgery, three prospective randomized trials have assessed postoperative pulmonary function; these studies not only determined the functional changes associated with each surgical method but also sought to clarify the mechanisms by which these alterations came about [6, 7, 11]. The respiratory parameters that were followed perioperatively included forced vital capacity (FVC), forced expiratory volume in 1 second (FEV_1), peak expiratory flow (PEF), midexpiratory phase of forced expiratory flow ($FEF_{25\%-75\%}$), and oxygen saturation of arterial blood preoperatively and daily postoperatively until discharge. These trials included patients with a variety of colorectal pathologies, including inflammatory bowel disease and cancer; all three studies reached the same conclusions.

First of all, the laparoscopic approach was associated with less impairment of pulmonary function on the first postoperative day than noted after open surgery. The FVC and the FEV_1 were more profoundly suppressed in patients having conventional resection than in those undergoing laparoscopic surgery. Similar results were found for PEF and $FEF_{25\%-75\%}$. The oxygen saturation of arterial blood, measured while the patients were breathing room air, also was noted to be lower after conventional surgery than after laparoscopic bowel resection. Furthermore, after laparoscopic colorectal resection there was a more rapid recovery of the FVC and FEV_1 to 80% of the preoperative value than following open resection. Intuitively, less postoperative pulmonary compromise should translate into a lower rate of respiratory complications; however, the available clinical data have not yet demonstrated such differences.

F. Conclusions

The reduction of postoperative pain, the better preservation of pulmonary function, and the reduction of pulmonary complications after surgery are goals that all surgeons strive to achieve. It has been demonstrated, in the majority of studies that assessed these parameters, that laparoscopic patients experience less pain and manifest less profound decreases in pulmonary function. Despite these benefits, dramatic differences in pain have not been demonstrated, and no one has yet shown that there are significantly fewer pulmonary complications after minimally invasive procedures. Regardless, the dialogue regarding MIS methods has heightened surgeons' awareness of the needs of our patients and has stimulated surgeons to renew the search for new methods to improve outcomes after both open and closed surgery.

G. References

1. Bisgaard T, Klarskov B, Trap R, Kehlet H, Rosenberg J. Pain after microlaparoscopic cholecystectomy. a randomized double-blind controlled study. Surg Endosc 2000; 14(4):340–344.
2. Blanc-Louvry I, Coquerel A, Koning E, Maillot C, Ducrotte P. Operative stress response is reduced after laparoscopic compared to open cholecystectomy: the relationship with postoperative pain and ileus. Dig Dis Sci 2000;45(9):1703–1713.
3. Ellstrom M, Olsen MF, Olsson JH, Nordberg G, Bengtsson A, Hahlin M. Pain and pulmonary function following laparoscopic and abdominal hysterectomy: a randomized study. Acta Obstet Gynecol Scand 1998;77(9):923–928.
4. Hendolin HI, Paakonen ME, Alhava EM, Tarvainen R, Kemppinen T, Lahtinen P. Laparoscopic or open cholecystectomy: a prospective randomized trial to compare postoperative pain, pulmonary function, and stress response. Eur J Surg 2000; 166(5):394–399.
5. Joris JL, Hinque VL, Laurent PE, Desaive CJ, Lamy ML. Pulmonary function and pain after gastroplasty performed via laparotomy or laparoscopy in morbidly obese patients. Br J Anaesth 1998;80(3):283–288.
6. Milsom JW, Hammerhofer KA, Bohm B, Marcello PW, Elson P, Fazio VW. Prospective randomized trial comparing laparoscopic vs. conventional surgery for refractory ileocolic Crohn's disease. Dis Colon Rectum 2001;44(1):1–9.
7. Milsom JW, Bohm B, Hammerhofer KA, Fazio V, Steiger E, Elson PA. Prospective, randomized trial comparing laparoscopic versus conventional techniques in colorectal cancer surgery: a preliminary report. J Am Coll Surg 1998;187(1):46–54.
8. Mouton WG, Bessell JR, Otten KT, Maddern GJ. Pain after laparoscopy. Surg Endosc 1999;13(5):445–448.
9. Nguyen NT, Lee SL, Goldman C, et al. Comparison of pulmonary function and postoperative pain after laparoscopic versus open gastric bypass: a randomized trial. J Am Coll Surg 2001;192(4):469–476.
10. Schwenk W, Bohm B, Muller JM. Postoperative pain and fatigue after laparoscopic or conventional colorectal resections. A prospective randomized trial. Surg Endosc 1998;12(9):1131–1136.
11. Schwenk W, Bohm B, Witt C, et al. Pulmonary function following laparoscopic or conventional colorectal resection: a randomized controlled evaluation. Arch Surg 1999; 134(1):6–12.
12. Schwenk W, Neudecker J, Mall J, Bohm B, Muller JM. Prospective randomized blinded trial of pulmonary function, pain, and cosmetic results after laparoscopic vs. microlaparoscopic cholecystectomy. Surg Endosc 2000;14(4):345–348.
13. Wills VL, Hunt DR. Pain after laparoscopic cholecystectomy. Br J Surg 2000; 87(3):273–284.
14. Yeager MP, Glass DD, Neff RK, Brinck-Johnsen T. Epidural anesthesia and analgesia in high-risk surgical patients. Anesthesiology 1987;66(6):729–736.

48. Ergonomics in Laparoscopic Surgery

Ramon Berguer, M.D.

As surgeons, we use tools to carry out our trade. How well—or awkwardly—we work with these tools has a sizable impact on the length of the procedure and the overall morbidity. The "relationship" between the surgeon and their tools also determines how much effort is expended by the surgeon. Ergonomics (often called human factors in the United States) is the study of the psychologic and physical interaction between the user (e.g., surgeons, assistants, or nurse) and their tools [12]. Because the costs of surgical errors and delays are substantial in both economic and human terms, ergonomic principles should be applied in the operating room (OR) to make the best possible use of our surgical tools.

A. Ergonomics and Laparoscopic Surgery

In open surgery, we look at and touch the patient's tissues directly using our hands or relatively simple instruments. In this situation, our senses of vision, touch, and position are working under normal conditions and with a large performance reserve so that standard surgical instruments, although not perfect, serve us well. During laparoscopic surgery, the situation is very different [11]. The surgeon indirectly views the operative field and can only touch the intraabdominal tissues with long instruments via ports that are in fixed positions. Our senses are now working much harder to achieve the same goals. The proper design of the instruments and the layout of the operating room now become critical to avoid fatigue and human errors. In other words, because simple tasks are more stressful and fatiguing during laparoscopic surgery, we have less physical and mental reserve to compensate for the poor design of instruments or the poor layout of the OR environment [1] (Figure 48.1). This is why ergonomics is important.

B. Critical Ergonomic Adjustments for Laparoscopic Surgery

The goal of proper posture is comfort, efficiency of movement, and minimization of the risk of musculoskeletal injuries to the operator. The surgeon's neck and back should be maintained in a comfortable and upright position facing

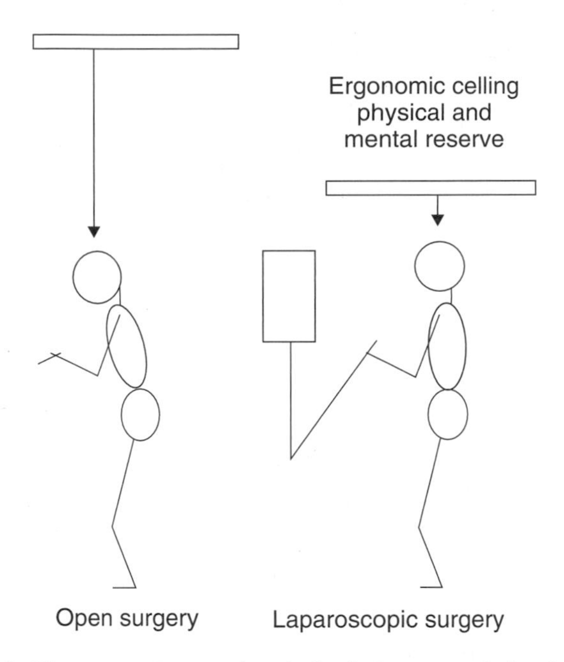

Figure 48.1. The surgeon's mental and physical reserve during laparoscopic surgery is significantly reduced compared to open surgery.

forward. During laparoscopic surgery, the ability to achieve this ideal posture is determined by:

1. The height of the operating room table
2. The position of the visual display (e.g., monitor)
3. Foot pedal locations
4. The selection of hand instruments

Although back posture tends to be straighter in laparoscopic surgery (because the surgeon no longer has to bend and twist to look directly inside the patient), more than 15% of surgeons still report frequent back pain and stiffness following laparoscopic operations [2]. These symptoms are likely due to the adoption of a more static posture (standing stiffly without moving) [3], which is the result of increased concentration and the frequent need to look in one direction at the monitor while manipulating instruments or foot pedals in another direction.

Although individual adjustment in the layout of the OR (patient and monitor position) can decrease this problem, it is always beneficial to periodically relax your mind and body, move around, look away from the monitor, and let go of the instruments. We unconsciously take these "minibreaks" during open surgery but often forget them during laparoscopic operations, which are more "intense."

C. Operating Table Height

The proper adjustment of the operating table height is very important in laparoscopic surgery. Ergonomically, the angle between the lower and upper arm should be between 90° and 120° when performing manual work [4, 15]. The operating table should be elevated or lowered such that the surgeon will be able to work within this ideal "window."

1. Specifically, in regard to setting the table position for laparoscopic operations, the table's height should be adjusted so that laparoscopic instrument handles (after the instruments have been inserted into the ports) are roughly at, or slightly below, the level of the surgeon's elbows.
2. Because laparoscopic instruments are much longer than their open counterparts, this requires lowering the table substantially. This may be difficult in some cases, and you many need to stand on one or more lifts to achieve the proper table height.

D. Foot Pedals

Foot pedals are commonly used during laparoscopic surgery to activate instruments such as the cautery, ultrasonic shears, bipolar device, or other tissue welding/dividing instruments. Foot pedals, which are often poorly positioned, demand awkward and unnatural postures and should be avoided in favor of hand controls when possible.

1. Pedals should be placed near the foot and aligned in the same direction as the instruments, toward the target quadrant and the principal laparoscopic monitor. Such positioning will permit the surgeon to activate the pedal without twisting their body or leg. If the surgeon is standing on a lifting platform, the pedal must be placed at the same level off the ground.
2. A pedal with a built-in foot rest is preferable so the surgeon does not have to hold their foot in the air or move it back and forth on the floor. If there are two pedals (for different devices), the surgeon must be careful not to confuse them in the darkness.

E. Vertical Positioning of Video Monitor

Because the surgeon views the surgical field through a visual display (e.g., video monitor) for lengthy periods during laparoscopic surgery, the position of the video monitor will affect neck and back posture.

1. The display should be placed directly in front of the surgeon, 15°–40°C below eye level for maximum comfort [9, 14].
2. Although standard video monitors still provide the best picture quality, the quality of the image of flat panel screens, displays suspended from

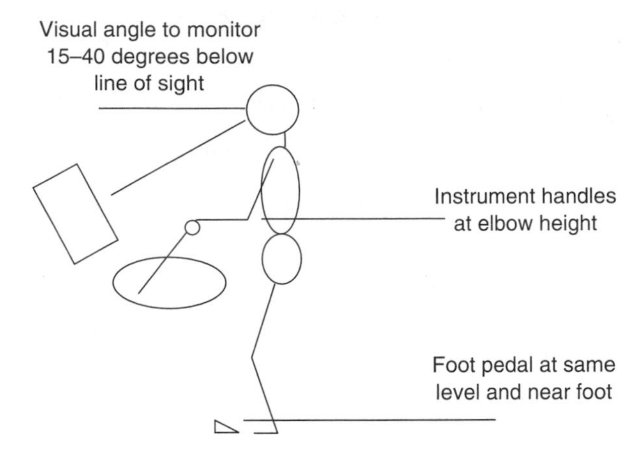

Figure 48.2. Key elements of the ergonomic laparoscopic surgeon.

booms, and head-mounted displays is improving. These alternative display devices are now acceptable alternatives to the standard video monitor.

3. Video display devices that are mounted on flexible booms allow the surgeon to alter the vertical position of the monitor to obtain the ideal angle between eye level and the monitor, as described above (Figure 48.2).

F. Choosing Laparoscopic Instruments

1. Laparoscopic instruments are lengthy because they must reach inside the inflated but closed abdomen. Unlike open surgery, the surgeon works a considerable distance from the target organ. The instruments are passed through narrow ports that are in fixed positions. Given these restrictions, it is not surprising that these instruments are more awkward and difficult to use than open instruments. Various attributes of the laparoscopic instruments account for their handling characteristics, including decreased mechanical efficiency, increased length, movement about a fulcrum on the body wall (the port), and the design of the handle. In general terms, the surgeon needs to squeeze harder, bend the wrists more, and hold their arms higher when using laparoscopic instruments compared to open instruments. These factors, together, can produce substantial hand and shoulder fatigue and discomfort during laparoscopic surgery [2].

No single laparoscopic instrument design is substantially superior to others, so each surgeon needs to choose the design(s) that best achieves the following goals:

a. Enables the surgeon to keep both wrists in a neutral (unbent) position
b. Permits the surgeon to keep both arms at the sides of their body
c. Avoids pressure points on the hands
d. Allows the surgeon to apply force with a power grip (hammer or gun-style) hand position
e. Allows fine manipulation with a precision grip (pencil or forceps-style) hand position

When it is necessary to apply continuous grasping force to tissues, seek an instrument that incorporates a locking or ratchet mechanism that will maintain the force. "Palming" an instrument (removing the thumb from the ring and placing the palm against the handle) can reduce the amount of wrist flexion and increase the surgeon's power when grasping tissues for a long period of time or when an especially forceful grip is required. When even larger forces must be applied to tissue, such as during stapling, seek instruments that provide a power-grip handle with large smooth contact surfaces.

Most laparoscopic instruments are designed with either a pistol grip-type handle or an axial (in-line) handle. The pistol grip allows the hand to remain at an angle to the instrument shaft and can lessen the ulnar deviation needed to use the axial handles. However, the axial handles permit the use of a fine grasp and rotation of the instrument in the hand that can be useful in fine manipulation and suturing. The most important features to look for in laparoscopic instruments are these:

a. Instrument handles that are smooth and broad surfaced to avoid pressure points and finger entrapment
b. An internal mechanism that is smooth, precise, and allows good tactile feedback from the tip of the instrument to the handle
c. Easy and intuitive access for the fingers to any additional controls that govern shaft rotation, jaw-locking, or electrocautery or suction activation
d. Sturdy insulation of the instrument shaft all the way to the base of the jaws to avoid stray electrocautery injury during use
e. An electrocautery connector pin that keeps the electrocautery cable out of the way of the surgeon's hand during use of the instrument
f. Instruments that require substantial force to use (staplers, clip appliers, heavy graspers) should have a broad and smooth pistol-type hand that permits the surgeon to use a power-grasp hand position

G. Laparoscopic Surgical Technique

Performing laparoscopic surgery requires the proper placement of the access ports and the efficient and safe use of the instruments to accomplish tissue dissection, division, sealing, and reapproximation. The location of the access ports is critical because they determine the reach and the working angle of the instruments passed through them. A manipulation angle range of 45°–75° (in the horizontal plane, the acceptable range of angles between the instruments inserted through the different ports) with equal azimuth angles (the elevation angle range in the vertical plane) is recommended [8]. Ideally, the surgeon maintains similar elevation angles for each of the instruments that they hold.

Instruments should be inserted such that at least half of the instrument is inside the patient. If the instrument is utilized while inserted less than half of its length, excessive motion at the shoulder will be required, which is likely to fatigue the surgeon [7]. There are no data to strongly support the use of one type of laparoscopic instrument handle design over another. Laparoscopic suturing is generally best performed with axial (in-line) instruments because they allow the surgeon to finely grasp the needle holder and facilitate rotation of the instrument with simple wrist motions. Laparoscopic needle drivers and forceps should incorporate a locking mechanism to hold the needle, thus obviating the need for the constant application of force by the surgeon. Several excellent reviews of suturing technique have been published [6, 13]. In addition to the choice of instruments and port locations, the ergonomic principles stated in the previous sections should always be followed.

H. Team Performance in Laparoscopic Surgery

A well-trained team always outperforms a less cohesive group. This dictum is also true in surgery, and particularly during laparoscopic surgery where more complex technology is being used [10]. The anesthesiologist must be aware of the potential complications of both pneumoperitoneum and the specific laparoscopic procedure to be performed and must communicate well with the surgical team throughout the procedure, especially during critical parts of the operation. Likewise, when problems arise, frequent and thorough communication between the surgeons and anesthetists must be maintained. The operating room nurses must be trained in the setup and use of the equipment and instruments. Often a medical technician or biomedical engineer is employed to set up and maintain the equipment. It is invaluable to have a trained and knowledgeable team to troubleshoot the not-infrequent equipment and instrument problems that arise during laparoscopic operations.

Ideally, each hospital or ambulatory center should create a dedicated laparoscopic surgery team. The members of this team would train together and develop a common understanding of the instrumentation and equipment needed for each procedure. The other nurses of the OR staff, who usually do nonlaparoscopic cases, should all undergo a basic equipment, instrument, and procedure orientation so that they will be able to staff laparoscopic procedures at night or when emergency cases arise.

I. Errors and Complications in Laparoscopic Surgery

1. Since the publication of the Institute of Medicine report *To Err Is Human* in 1999 [5], the prevention of human error in medicine has become a priority in the U.S. health care system. Human error and adverse patient events (complications) in laparoscopic surgery can be minimized by proper training and supervision along with attention to

key ergonomic and human factors issues in the operating room. Nevertheless, experience has shown that even experts are subject to human error. Thus, it is important that we create a system of patient care that minimizes the possibility of errors, promptly detects errors when they occur, responds appropriately to errors to minimize the adverse effect, and allows us to learn from our mistakes. Errors and complications should be seen as an opportunity to learn and to make positive changes, and not used to blame or criticize those involved.

Errors can be categorized as follows:

a. **Mistakes:** The surgeon makes a mistake because of an incorrect interpretation of the anatomy or situation [e.g., mistaking the common bile duct (CBD) for the cystic duct and dividing it]. Similarly, the overzealous application of a "rule" that may be inappropriate in certain situations may lead to an error (e.g., CBD filling defects found on cystic duct cholangiogram should result in CBD exploration).
b. **Slips:** The surgeon makes the right decision but carries out the wrong action (e.g., presses the "cut" pedal instead of the "coagulation" pedal on the electrocautery).
c. **Lapses:** The Surgeon forgets to perform a procedure or a specific step in a procedure (e.g., forgets to check the integrity of a colonic anastomosis using air insufflation before closing).

2. Slips are much more easy to detect and correct ("oops, I stepped on the wrong pedal!") than mistakes. Slips can best be prevented by better design and layout of the workplace, instruments, and controls following the guidelines in this chapter. Mistakes are harder to detect and are best prevented through better feedback (visual, auditory, manual) to the surgeon and improved training.

We can avoid common slips and mistakes in laparoscopic surgery by:

a. Ensuring that all OR personnel obtain adequate training and proctoring for all procedures
b. Striving to be in good physical and mental condition before surgery
c. Positioning all the equipment and instruments in a comfortable, efficient, and ergonomic manner
d. Maintaining a clear view of the operative field and instruments at all times
e. Converting to open surgery if the exposure is poor or the potential for complications seems higher than usual

When slips or mistakes occur, the surgeon should view them as a learning experience and try to make changes in the above areas to lessen the likelihood that they will occur again.

J. Operating Room Setup

1. The overall OR layout is important because it affects setup and turn-around times and the efficiency of surgery, as well as patient and staff safety. The modern OR is a temperature-controlled and, it is hoped, aseptic environment that must accommodate the presence and movement of multiple people as well as numerous small and large equipment items.
2. The OR for laparoscopic cases should be larger (at least 400 square feet in area) than a typical room used for open surgery to accommodate the additional equipment. The traditional laparoscopic setup makes use of large multilevel wheeled carts to house the equipment. This system has several disadvantages. It requires multiple power cables from the wall to the cart as well as numerous cables and tubes coursing from the cart to the surgical field and from cart to cart. Equipment carts are large and heavy and cannot be ergonomically positioned in the OR; carts also do not permit each piece of equipment to be individually placed in its optimal position. Finally, carts are cumbersome to move in, out, and about the OR. A better solution is to place the large equipment items on movable ceiling-mounted booms or wall-mounted storage areas and to route all cables and tubes through single conduits that are off the floor (e.g., ceiling-mounted booms) to the surgical field.
3. Unfortunately, because of cost issues, it is not always possible to work in a room with ceiling-mounted booms; when working in a room where the equipment is on carts it is important to develop a strategy to deal with the myriad of associated cables, wires, and tubes coursing through the OR. The latter, unless carefully arranged and secured, are hazards and obstacles that impede the movement of both surgeons and OR staff and can result in the inadvertent disconnection of equipment, falls, or electrical injury. When setting up for a laparoscopic operation, pay particular attention to the location of large pieces of equipment that may be needed later during the case such as a fluoroscopy unit or ultrasound machine. Position these before surgery such that they can easily be moved toward the surgical field to a place where the device can be readily utilized and their displays easily seen by the surgeons. A well-thought-out plan is needed for the routing of cables and tubes from the equipment and devices to the surgical field and to the control pedals so that the cables are as out of the way as possible and the foot pedals comfortably placed. Where feasible, cables and tubes that run to the operative field should be grouped and run off the field together (either off the head or the foot of the table) such that movement of the surgeons is not impeded. Floor-based tubes and cables can be taped to the floor to decrease the chances that someone will trip and fall. Ideally, the numerous cables, wires, and tubes should not pose a contamination hazard and their position should not interfere with the operation.
4. The surgical lights can interfere with laparoscopic equipment, fluoroscopy units, or ceiling-mounted booms holding equipment or visual

displays. The lights should be positioned in the desired location (often in the midline of the patient and to each side of the surgeon's head) before prepping the patient.

K. Summary

1. Adjust the operating table height so that the instrument handles, once inserted into the abdomen, are at your elbow height.
2. Place the visual display (monitor) directly in front of you and 15°–40° below the line of sight.
3. Choose laparoscopic instruments that minimize wrist flexion and rotation and ulnar deviation.
4. Choose instruments with comfortable and efficient handles that are matched to the task you are performing (e.g., power grip for grasping chores or fine grip for suturing).
5. If foot pedals must be used, place them close to your foot and use a foot rest.
6. Where possible, use large ORs with integrated and moveable storage systems that decrease clutter and turnaround times.
7. When using floor-based equipment carts, carefully position all equipment so that movement in the room is not impeded and so that devices required for only one portion of the case can be easily moved to the field when needed.
8. Similarly, the cables and tubes associated with laparoscopic cases must be intelligently grouped and secured, both in the operative field and on the floor, so as to minimize the hazard they represent and to permit the flow of OR personnel and the surgeons.
9. Emphasize team training for the laparoscopic OR crew.
10. Learn to minimize the risk of slips and mistakes and learn from them when they occur.

L. Conclusion

Ergonomics describes the interaction between the user and their work environment. Laparoscopic surgery requires more physical and mental effort on the part of the surgeon and therefore mandates that very close attention be paid to the proper arrangement of the OR workspace, the choice and proper use of surgical instruments, the training of the OR staff, and ensuring that all staff communicate well with each other.

M. References

1. Berguer R. Surgery and ergonomics. Arch Surg 1999;134:1011–1016.
2. Berguer R, Forkey D, Smith W. Ergonomic problems associated with laparoscopic surgery. Surg Endosc 1999;13:466–468.
3. Berguer R, Rab GT, Abu-Ghaida H, Alarcon A, Chung J. A comparison of surgeons' posture during laparoscopic and open surgical procedures. Surg Endosc 1997;11: 139–142.
4. Berguer R, Smith W, Davis S. An Ergonomic Study of the Optimum Operating Table Height for Laparoscopic Surgery. Maastrich, Netherlands: European Association of Endoscopic Surgery, 2001.
5. Corrigan J, Kohn LT, Donaldson MS. To Err Is Human: Building a Safer Health System. Washington, DC: National Academy Press, 2000:xxi, 287.
6. Cuschieri A, Szabo Z. Tissue approximation in endoscopic surgery: suturing and knotting techniques. Oxford: Isis Medical Media, 1995.
7. Emam TA, Hanna GB, Kimber C, Dunkley P, Cuschieri A. Effect of intracorporeal-extracorporeal instrument length ratio on endoscopic task performance and surgeon movements. Arch Surg 2000;135:62–65; discussion 66.
8. Hanna GB, Shimi S, Cuschieri A. Optimal port locations for endoscopic intracorporeal knotting. Surg Endosc 1997;11:397–401.
9. Hanna GB, Shimi SM, Cuschieri A. Task performance in endoscopic surgery is influenced by location of the image display. Ann Surg 1998;227:481–484.
10. Kenyon TA, Lenker MP, Bax TW, Swanstrom LL. Cost and benefit of the trained laparoscopic team. A comparative study of a designated nursing team vs a nontrained team. Surg Endosc 1997;11:812–814.
11. Patkin M, Isabel L. Ergonomics, engineering and surgery of endosurgical dissection. J Rl Coll Surg Edinb 1995;40:120–132.
12. Salvendy G. Handbook of Human Factors and Ergonomics. New York: Wiley, 1997: xxii, 2137.
13. Szabo Z, Hunter J, Berci G, Sackier J, Cuschieri A. Analysis of surgical movements during suturing in laparoscopy. Endosc Surg Allied Technol 1994;2:55–61.
14. van Veelan M, Jakimowicz JJ, Goosens R, Meijer DW, Bussman H. Evaluation of the Usability of Two Types of Image Display Systems During Laparoscopy. Maastrich, Netherlands: European Association of Endoscopic Surgery, 2001.
15. van Veelen M, Kazemier G, Koopman J, Goosens R, Meijer DW. Assessment of the Ergonomically Optimal Operating Surface Height for Laparoscopic Surgery. Maastrich, Netherlands: European Association of Endoscopic Surgery, 2001.

Appendix
Operative Management and Evaluation: Bowel Preparation

Peter Marcello, M.D.

A. Introduction

The major risk of sepsis following colorectal resection relates to the high bacterial concentration within the colon. Therefore, appropriate preoperative preparation to "clean" the colon and rectum has become the standard of practice within the United States.

To reduce the septic complications following elective colon and rectal resection, a combination of dietary restriction (clear liquids), mechanical cleansing of the colon and both oral and parenteral antibiotics are commonly utilized (Table A.1).

B. Mechanical Bowel Preparation

Historically the preparation of the large bowel prior to elective resection was extended over 3–5 days which resulted in severe metabolic disturbances secondary to prolonged fasting, catharsis, and enema usage.

Irrigation of the colon with large volume electrolyte solutions (10–12 L) began in the 1970s and offered the advantages of reducing the preparation time to 24 hours and avoided the need for enemas. However, the use of these electrolyte solutions resulted in fluid and sodium retention and were contraindicated in elderly patients with cardiac or renal insufficiency and patients often did not tolerate the large volume of solution required to cleanse the colon.

Mannitol, an oligosaccharide which is neither absorbed nor digested was introduced in 1979. Mannitol has a rapid transit through the small intestine which causes an osmotic catharsis, but may be associated with dehydration and hyponatremia. Mannitol also allows for methane production by bacterial fermentation and has been reported to cause potentially fatal explosions when used with electrocautery.

In 1980, polyethylene glycol, an inert nonabsorbable nonfermentable compound which acts as an osmotic agent was introduced. Combined with an electrolyte solution containing sodium sulfate instead of sodium chloride, this osmotically balanced solution minimizes fluid and electrolyte disturbances during colon lavage. However, three to four liters of the solution must be ingested over a four-hour period in order to achieve optimal colon cleansing. This large

Table A.1. Elective Bowel Preparation Regimens.

Polyethylene Glycol Prep	Sodium Phosphate Prep*
Diet	
Clear liquids beginning the day before surgery	same
Mechanical preparation	
Polyethylene glycol lavage 4 L over 4 hours starting at 8 AM, the day before surgery	Sodium Phosphate prep 45 mL at 8 AM and 1 PM, the day before surgery 8 glasses of clear liquids between 1st and 2nd dose
Oral antibiotic preparation	
Neomycin 1–2 gm and Metronidazole 1–2 gm, or Erythromycin 1–2 gm orally at 7 PM and 11 PM, the day before surgery	same
Parenteral antibiotic preparation	
Appropriate aerobic and anaerobic antimicrobial coverage, single dose given within 30 minutes of incision (example—cefoxitin 1 gm IV, cefotetan 2 gm IV)	same

* Contraindicated inpatients with renal and cardiac insufficiency.

volume over a relatively short period often results in nausea, vomiting, and fullness, with roughly 5–15 percent of patients unable to complete the full preparation. Prolonged consumption of the preparation may cause absorption of excess fluid and salts leading to more dramatic fluid shifts. Despite this, polyethylene glycol solutions remain one of the leading preparations for elective bowel surgery and colonoscopy.

Sodium phosphate is a low volume electrolyte solution which may be better tolerated than polyethylene glycol solutions. Two 45 mL doses are given several hours apart, but require the ingestion of a large volume of clear liquids in-between to effectively prepare the colon. In a number of prospective randomized trials, polyethylene glycol and sodium phosphate preparations were equally effective in cleansing the colon. The lower volume sodium phosphate preparation however, is contraindicated in patients with renal and cardiac insufficiency due to intravascular volume shifts and phosphate absorption. In a recent survey of 520 colorectal and general surgeons, 46% routinely use sodium phosphate for bowel preparation, 32% routinely use polyethylene glycol, and 15% selectively alternate between the two methods.

In the past decade there have been at least four published randomized trials outside the United States which have compared elective bowel preparation to no mechanical preparation. These studies have not demonstrated a significantly higher rate of wound infection or anastomotic leakage in the unprepared patients and the converse was true in several of the studies. Despite the lack of clear evidence in favor of mechanical bowel preparation, it remains the standard of care for elective colorectal surgery throughout the world. In addition to reducing the risk of infection, mechanical bowel preparation of the colon allows for direct colon palpation during conventional surgery. During laparoscopic colon resection, mechanical preparation could potentially reduce the risk of inadvertent bowel injury by laparoscopic instruments during manipulation of a heavy stool laden colon.

C. Oral Antibiotic Prophylaxis

Preoperative antibiotic prophylaxis is aimed to provide both adequate tissue levels of antimicrobial agents and reducing the bacterial load of the colon. There are more published controlled studies comparing oral and intravenous antimicrobial agents than there are comparing mechanical preparations, however, the results are inconsistent. This may in part be due to the small number of patients enrolled in the published trials which have never achieved appropriate statistical power.

Preoperative oral antibiotic preparations have been shown to produce a high level of antimicrobial within the colon with limited systemic toxicity. The most common preparation uses a combination of neomycin (1 gm) with either erythromycin (1 gm) or metronidazole (1 gm) in two doses following mechanical bowel preparation the evening before surgery. Despite the lack of strong scientific evidence, 70% of surgeons utilize oral antibiotic prophylaxis in elective colorectal surgery. While nausea and vomiting may occur, these medications are generally well tolerated.

D. Parenteral Antibiotic Prophylaxis

While conflicting, a large number of prospective studies have demonstrated that broad-spectrum intravenous antibiotics, given just prior to the surgical incision, significantly reduces the septic complications following elective colorectal resection. In studies comparing intravenous antibiotics to placebo, most have shown a reduction in postoperative wound infection. When compared to oral antibiotic prophylaxis, parenteral prophylaxis is equally effective. If used alone, parenteral antibiotic agents must provide adequate coverage of both anaerobic and aerobic colonic bacteria. The intravenous agent should be given within 30 minutes of incision time and should be repeated intraoperatively in cases that last more than 2–4 hours. While single-agent or combination therapy are both recommended, no single regimen has consistently been demonstrated superior to others. Long-acting second-generation cephalosporin, penicillin based combination agent, and other broad-spectrum regimens are all effective options.

E. Conclusions

Most surgeons commonly practice elective preparation of the large intestine prior to colorectal resection. A combination of preoperative bowel cleansing and antibiotic prophylaxis (both oral and parneteral agents) is recommended. The choice of bowel cleansing and antibiotic agents should be individualized to the patient's history and the surgeon's practice.

F. Selected References

Holmes JWC, Nichols RL. Bowel Preparation in colorectal surgery. In Mazier WP, Levien DH, Lutchtefeld MA, Senagore AJ, eds. Surgery of the colon, rectum, and Anus. WB Sauders, Philadelphia, Pennsylvania, 1995; pp 200–204.

Solla JA, Rothenberger DA. Preoperative bowel preparation: a survey of colon and rectal surgeons. Dis Colon Rectum 1990;33:154–159.

Zmora O, Pikarsky AJ, Wexner SD. Bowel preparation for colorectal surgery. Dis Colon Rectum 2001;44:1537–1549.

Index

W

X